Atlas of Ulcers in Systemic Sclerosis

Marco Matucci-Cerinic • Christopher P. Denton
Editors

Atlas of Ulcers in Systemic Sclerosis

Diagnosis and Management

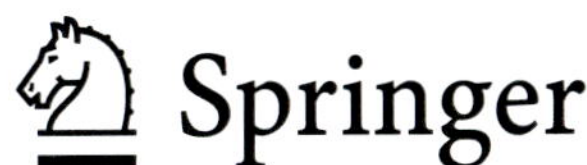 Springer

Editors
Marco Matucci-Cerinic
Department of Experimental and Clinical
Medicine
University of Florence
Florence
Italy

Department of Geriatric Medicine
Division of Rheumatology
AOUC
Florence
Italy

Christopher P. Denton
Division of Medicine
University College London
Centre for Rheumatology
Royal Free Hospital
London
England

ISBN 978-3-319-98475-9   ISBN 978-3-319-98477-3   (eBook)
https://doi.org/10.1007/978-3-319-98477-3

Library of Congress Control Number: 2018959558

This Springer imprint is published by the registered company Springer Nature Switzerland AG
The registered company address is: Gewerbestrasse 11, 6330 Cham, Switzerland

Preface

Systemic sclerosis (SSc), also called scleroderma, is an intransigent disease with many manifestations and has high mortality due to involvement of the vital organs such as the heart, lungs, gut and kidneys. However, it also has an enormous burden of non-lethal complications, and it is these features of the disease that challenge patients and health-care professionals daily. Of the non-life-threatening aspects of the disease, digital ulceration provides perhaps the most striking external manifestation of vasculopathy. Although they are not life-threatening, digital ulcers cause enormous pain, impact function and quality of life and can lead to serious local complications such as gangrene, osteomyelitis and permanent tissue loss. This atlas has been compiled to provide practical advice and information about management of digital ulcers and to address the diversity of the ulcers that can occur. The wide range in appearance and features of ulcers reflects their complex and multifaceted pathogenesis but also underlies some of the well-recognised difficulty of undertaking clinical trials to underpin evidence-based management of ulcers.

The first topic considered in this book is definition of ulcers. Definition is linked to pathology but also requires attention to the practical aspects of diagnosis and classification. Definition necessitates consideration of pathology therefore of the pathobiology that underlies SSc, vasculopathy, ulceration and repair. It is ironic that SSc, which in its worst forms is associated with severe "scar-like" thickening of the skin, also leads to ulceration and slow repair of skin lesions at sites of poor blood supply or minor physical trauma. This is perhaps a reminder that SSc is perhaps best regarded as a disease of "dysregulated connective tissue repair" where scar tissue forms in sites and to an extent that is not needed but cannot be developed at areas that need to heal appropriately. This dilemma may underlie the complex challenges of treatment and prevention of ulcers and explain the paradox that some drugs, such as bosentan, may reduce the formation of new ulcers but not necessarily speed up healing of lesions that are already present.

Consideration of definition and pathogenesis provides the foundation for the later sections of the book covering key topics in a series of chapters written by experts in the field. The relationship of digital ulcers to other aspects of scleroderma such as Raynaud's phenomenon is considered together with the best methods of predicting patients at risk. Comorbidity is also relevant in determining the complications of ulcers. The important complications of ulcers are outlined in specific chapters in a practical way that provided advice about investigation and management.

Treatment and prevention of ulcers is now a key focus of management of SSc. Availability of guidelines and recommendations to support current therapy and regulatory approval of drugs for digital ulcer disease in some countries are testament to the ability for medical therapy to improve and treat this problem. There is an emerging evidence base to support current practice but also a need to critically evaluate available evidence and to balance the needs of prevention of ulcers with the most effective treatment of established lesions. Local and systemic aspects of management are carefully outlined and discussed.

The final section of this book provides a pictorial descriptive guide to the types and appearance of ulcers and other related lesions in SSc. Current management and future research and clinical trials in the area of ulcerations will depend on rigorous and consistent definitions and classification. In addition, it is important that terminology and descriptors are harmonised and standardised where possible. This will benefit patients through better communication and provide a platform for improved education and learning for patients and health-care professionals. Eventually patients will be better able to manage their disease, and it is a realistic hope that the large number of ongoing clinical trials to treat aspects of SSc including the skin and other organ-based diseases will together have true disease-modifying potential. Thus, ulcers may become less frequent, management may be more consistent and effective, and clinical trials specifically addressing ulcers can be targeted to areas of greatest unmet medical need.

This volume represents substantial and sustained effort fuelled by the desire to improve outcomes for our patients and shed light on a common but previously neglected aspect of SSc. It is our hope that by sharing experience and expertise in this way, the outlook for patients with SSc and ulcers will be less bleak.

London, UK
Florence, Italy

Christopher P. Denton
Marco Matucci-Cerinic

Contents

Contributors

Yannick Allanore, MD, PhD Service de Rheumatologie A, Hôpital Cochin, Paris, France

Marina E. Anderson, FRCP, PhD Institute of Ageing and Chronic Disease, University of Liverpool and Aintree University Hospital NHS Foundation Trust, Liverpool, UK

Francesca Bartoli, MD Rheumatology Department, Azienda Ospedaliero – Universitaria Careggi, Florence, Italy

Silvia Bellando-Randone Department of Experimental and Clinical Medicine, University of Florence, Florence, Italy
Department of Geriatric Medicine, Division of Rheumatology, AOUC, Florence, Italy

Laura Benelli Nurse Independent Contractor, Florence, Italy

Jelena Blagojevic, MD Department of Experimental and Clinical Medicine, Division of Rheumatology, University of Florence, Florence, Italy

Francesca Braschi, MSN, RN Department of Experimental and Clinical Medicine, University of Florence, Florence, Italy
Department of Geriatric Medicine, Division of Rheumatology, AOUC, Florence, Italy
Health Professional Department, AOUC, Florence, Italy

Cosimo Bruni, MD Department of Experimental and Clinical Medicine, Division of Rheumatology, University of Florence, Florence, Italy

Benjamin Chaigne, MD National Referral Center for Rare Systemic Autoimmune Diseases, Department of Internal Medicine, Hôpital Cochin, Assistance Publique-Hôpitaux de Paris (APHP), Université Paris Descartes, Paris, France

Kuntal Chakravarty, FRCP(Lond., Ireland, Glasgow) Rheumatology, Royal Free Hospital NHS Foundation Trust, London, UK

Laura Cometi, MD Rheumatology Department, Azienda Ospedaliero – Universitaria Careggi, Florence, Italy

Maurizio Cutolo, MD Research Laboratory and Academic Division of Clinical Rheumatology, Department of Internal Medicine, University of Genova, Genoa, Italy

Nicoletta Del Papa, MD Department of Rheumatology, ASST Gaetano Pini, Milan, Italy

Christopher P. Denton, PhD, FRCP Division of Medicine, University College London, Centre for Rheumatology, Royal Free Hospital, London, UK

Gabriele Di Luca, MD Department of Rheumatology, ASST Gaetano Pini, Milan, Italy

Oliver Distler, MD Department of Rheumatology, University Hospital Zurich, Zurich, Switzerland

Sabine A. Eming, MD Dermatology, University of Cologne, Cologne, Germany

Claudia Fantauzzo Department of Experimental and Clinical Medicine, University of Florence, Florence, Italy

Department of Geriatric Medicine, Division of Rheumatology, AOUC, Florence, Italy

Health Professional Department, AOUC, Florence, Italy

Daniel E. Furst, MD Department of Medicine, University of California Los Angeles, Los Angeles, CA, USA

University of Washington, Seattle, WA, USA

Department of Experimental and Clinical Medicine, University of Florence, Florence, Italy

Carina Gaertner, MD Department of Dermatology, University of Cologne, Cologne, Germany

Felice Galluccio, MD Division of Rheumatology, Department of Clinical and Experimental Medicine, University of Firenze – Aou Careggi, Firenze, Italy

Nabil George, BSc, MSc, MBBS Medicine/Surgery, North Middlesex University Hospital, London, UK

Loïc Guillevin, MD National Referral Center for Rare Systemic Autoimmune Diseases, Department of Internal Medicine, Hôpital Cochin, Assistance Publique-Hôpitaux de Paris (APHP), Université Paris Descartes, Paris, France

Ariane L. Herrick, MD, FRCP NIHR Manchester Musculoskeletal Biomedical Research Unit, Central Manchester NHS Foundation Trust, Manchester Academic Health Science Centre, Manchester, UK

Michael Hughes, BSc(Hons), MSc, MBBS, MCRP(UK), PhD Centre for Musculoskeletal Research, The University of Manchester, Salford Royal NHS Foundation Trust, Manchester Academic Health Science Centre, Manchester, UK

Nicolas Hunzelmann, MD Department of Dermatology, University of Cologne, Cologne, Germany

Todd Kanzara, MBBS, LLB(Hons) Otolaryngology, Southend Hospital, Southend, Essex, UK

Paul Legendre, MD Internal Medicine Department, Reference Center for Rare Systemic Autoimmune Diseases of Ile de France, Hospital Cochin, Paris, France

Gemma Lepri Department of Clinical and Experimental Medicine, University of Florence, Florence, Italy

Department of Geriatric Medicine, Division of Rheumatology AOUC, Florence, Italy

Wanda Maglione, MD Department of Rheumatology, ASST Gaetano Pini, Milan, Italy

Marco Matucci-Cerinic, MD, PhD Department of Experimental and Clinical Medicine, University of Florence, Florence, Italy

Department of Geriatric Medicine, Division of Rheumatology, AOUC, Florence, Italy

Britta Maurer, MD Department of Rheumatology, University Hospital Zurich, Zurich, Switzerland

Luc Mouthon, MD, PhD Internal Medicine Department, Reference Center for Rare Systemic Autoimmune Diseases of Ile de France, Hospital Cochin, Paris, France

Lindsay Muir, MB, MChOrth, FRCS(Orth) Manchester Hand Centre, Salford Royal NHS Foundation Trust, Salford, Lancashire, UK

Voon H. Ong, PhD, FRCP Centre for Rheumatology and Connective Tissue Diseases, UCL Medical School Royal Free Campus, London, UK

Lucia Paganelli Department of Experimental and Clinical Medicine, University of Florence, Florence, Italy

Department of Geriatric Medicine, Division of Rheumatology, AOUC, Florence, Italy

Health Professional Department, AOUC, Florence, Italy

Oana-Diana Persa, MD Department of Dermatology, University of Cologne, Cologne, Germany

Guya Piemonte, RN, PhD Candidate Department of Health Science, University of Florence, Florence, Italy

Tiziana Pucci, Digital Ulcer Speciality Nurse Department of Experimental and Clinical Medicine, University of Florence, Florence, Italy

Department of Geriatric Medicine, Division of Rheumatology, AOUC, Florence, Italy

Health Professional Department, AOUC, Florence, Italy

Jasmin Raja, MBBS, MMED Division of Rheumatology, Department of Medicine, University of Malaya, Kuala Lumpur, Malaysia

Laura Rasero, Professor of Nursing Department of Health Sciences, University of Florence – Careggi of Hospital, Florence, Tuscany, Italy

Janine Schniering, MSc Department of Rheumatology, University Hospital Zurich, Zurich, Switzerland

Vanessa Smith, MD, PhD Department of Internal Medicine, Ghent University, Ghent, Belgium

Department of Rheumatology, Ghent University Hospital, Ghent, Belgium

Yossra Atef Suliman, MD, PhD Rheumatology and Rehabilitation Department, Assiut University Hospital, Assiut, Egypt

Alberto Sulli, MD Research Laboratory and Academic Division of Clinical Rheumatology, Department of Internal Medicine, University of Genova, Genoa, Italy

Eleonora Zaccara, MD Department of Rheumatology, ASST Gaetano Pini, Milan, Italy

Part I

Definition and Classification

Defining Digital Ulcers in Systemic Sclerosis: The State of the Art

Daniel E. Furst, Yossra Atef Suliman, Christopher P. Denton, and Marco Matucci-Cerinic

Significance

1. A definition of digital ulcer in scleroderma is needed to enhance the ability to test therapies and compare results across treatments.
2. A uniform clinical definition of ulcers has been partially validated which can help physicians do credible research.
3. A definition of DU based on ultrasound is being developed, another step toward a more objective definition.

Skin ulcers are a major problem in systemic sclerosis (SSc). Pathogenesis is complex and likely reflects poor microvascular function in the skin, susceptibility to trauma and local injury due to contractures and intrinsic defects in skin wound healing related to altered angiogenesis and dermal and epidermal repair [1]. Skin ulcers are common and occur in up to 58% of SSc patients. They may appear nearly anywhere, although they most often occur at sites of skin trauma [2]. They may occur on the tips of fingers or toes, over the extensor surfaces and bony prominences (such as the elbow) secondary to trauma or caused by underlying calcinosis.

Most ulcers are very painful and often result in considerable impairment of hand function [3]. Digital ulcers (DUs) tend to recur, with up to 66% of patients having more than one episode, despite routine use of vasodilators [4]. There is a risk for multiple complications including osteomyelitis, gangrene, and amputation, with 5–20% of SSc patients experiencing gangrene or amputation [5–9]. The risk of gangrene and amputation is 5–10% and rises to 20% in patients with DUs, while the incidence of amputation ranges from 1% to 2% of patients/year [4–9]. Not surprisingly, patients with active DU have significant pain, impaired hand function and decreased quality of life (QOL) as well as an increased financial burden from more hospitalizations and decreased ability to work [5, 10, 11].

Ulcer endpoints have been used in clinical trials, but these trials have often failed, perhaps because there has not been a uniform, validated definition of DUs in SSc [11]. There are a variety of indicators for assessing the severity: ulcer size, number, location, loss of function, pain, and tissue loss. A larger ulcer may be associated with longer healing time, tissue loss, increased risk of infection, and increased pain [12]. Ulcer site may be important if the ulcer prevents the patient from working, and loss of function is important since it hinders normal daily activities [4].

Given the impact of SSc skin ulcers and the obvious need, efforts have been made to develop a valid definition of skin ulcers in SSc. Thus, for example, Baron et al. developed a definition of DU, although it was not validated [13]. Their consensus definition was: "A digital ulcer is a lesion with visually discernable depth and a loss of continuity of epithelial coverage, which could be denuded or covered by a scab or necrotic tissue."

Recent efforts have focused on developing a more robust and pragmatic definition of DU. Initially, a systematic litera-

D. E. Furst
Department of Medicine, University of California Los Angeles, Los Angeles, CA, USA

University of Washington, Seattle, WA, USA

Department of Experimental and Clinical Medicine, University of Florence, Florence, Italy

Y. A. Suliman
Rheumatology and Rehabilitation Department, Assiut University Hospital, Assiut, Egypt

C. P. Denton
Division of Medicine, University College London, Centre for Rheumatology, Royal Free Hospital, London, England

M. Matucci-Cerinic (✉)
Department of Experimental and Clinical Medicine, University of Florence, Florence, Italy

Department of Geriatric Medicine, Division of Rheumatology, AOUC, Florence, Italy
e-mail: marco.matuccicerinic@unifi.it

© Springer Nature Switzerland AG 2019
M. Matucci-Cerinic, C. P. Denton (eds.), *Atlas of Ulcers in Systemic Sclerosis*, https://doi.org/10.1007/978-3-319-98477-3_1

ture review was done with the goal of defining digital ulcers for the purposes of a clinical trial. From 3475 references, 74 definitions were ultimately found [11]. The most frequent definitions included "loss of epidermis with or without dermis, with depth", "denuded," and most often the definition was unclear (e.g., 27 of the 74 definitions). Examples of particularly unclear definitions were such terms as "open wound," "skin break," "necrotic ulcer." A number of mitigating or clarifying factors were found such as referring to site (DU, PIP, malleolus), size (0.2–30 cm^2), calcinosis, gangrene, fissures, pitting scars, and traumatic ulcers. From this systematic literature review, it was clear no consensus definition other than that by Baron et al. had been developed and that there was a clear need for such a definition for SSc.

Initial efforts to develop a valid DU definition were undertaken. In a face-to-face meeting, 11 expert rheumatologists and 1 dermatologist voted on definition domains and mitigating factors for inclusion. The final definition was developed by consensus (i.e., greater than 70% agreement for each

> "Loss of epidermal covering with a break in the basement membrane (which separates dermis from epidermis).
>
> It appears clinically as visible blood vessels, fibrin, granulation tissue and/or underlying deeper structures (e.g. muscle, ligament, fat) or as it would appear on debridement" [12].

domain and factor) and was as follows:

Validation of the definition was then begun. Initially there was a face-to-face meeting among 11 rheumatologists expert in SSc +1 dermatologist. Face validity and feasibility were tested by examining the photos of 11 SSc skin lesions in the context of the new definition. Face validity and feasibility were agreed unanimously. During a second face-to-face meeting among rheumatologists, further discussion resulted in polishing of exclusionary states that might hinder a patient with a skin ulcer from being included in a clinical trial (remembering that this definition was for clinical trials and not for clinical practice). For example, the presence of clinical counsel gnosis, it was agreed by consensus (greater than 70% agreement among the experts), would exclude a patient from a clinical trial. Reliability and reproducibility were tested by having each expert examine each of seven actual patients with skin ulcers twice, with approximately 1 hour between examinations and after patients had been reallocated to different seats. Fleiss' kappa coefficient for interrater agreement during the first round was 0.511 and during round two was 0.488. The intraclass correlation (ICC) using a logistic regression model with a random slope is 0.868. The mean intra-rater Cohen's kappa is 0.901. This indicated that in clinical trials of DU, as for other measures such as joint counts, it is important that the same investigator examine the ulcers throughout. Further evaluations for visual clinical validation of this definition continue. Concurrent with the above efforts, the use of an 18 MHz ultrasound (US) probe to examine DU was initiated in 21 skin ulcers from 10 SSc patients. Using a simple dichotomous definition (US either breaking the basement membrane or not doing so), pain (100 mm visual analog scale) and function (HAQ disability index), ulcers were examined clinically and by US. By US, 8 lesions were defined as ulcers and 13 as nonulcers. Incidentally three ulcers had high-power Doppler signals suggesting infection; after treatment with antibiotic, the power Doppler signal and pain VAS's decreased concomitantly. Five lesions showed subclinical calcinosis. There was only a 48% concordance between clinical and US estimations of the presence of ulcers.

In conclusion, there is a clear need to develop and uniform valid definition of digital ulcers for clinical trials. Validation of a visual definition is underway, and validation of ultrasound-defined ulcers is also advancing [14, 15].

References

1. Suliman YA, Distler O. Novel aspects in the pathophysiology of peripheral vasculopathy in systemic sclerosis. Curr Rheumatol Rev. 2013;9:237–44.
2. Mouthon L, Carpentier PH, Lok C, Clerson P, Gressin V, Hachulla E, et al. Ischemic digital ulcers affect hand disability and pain in systemic sclerosis. J Rheumatol. 2014;41:1317–23.
3. Sunderkötter C, Herrgott I, Brückner C, Moinzadeh P, Pfeiffer C, Gerss J, et al. Comparison of patients with and without digital ulcers in systemic sclerosis: detection of possible risk factors. Br J Dermatol. 2009;160(4):835–43.
4. Hachulla E, Clerson P, Launay D, Lambert M, Morell-Dubois S, Queyrel V, Hatron PY. Natural history of ischemic digital ulcers in systemic sclerosis: single-center retrospective longitudinal study. J Rheumatol. 2007;34:2423–30.
5. Steen V, Denton CP, Pope JE, Matucci-Cerinic M. Digital ulcers: overt vascular disease in systemic sclerosis. Rheumatology (Oxford). 2009;48(Suppl 3):19–24.
6. Poormoghim H, Moghadam AS, Moradi-Lakeh M, Jafarzadeh M, Asadifar B, Ghelman M, Andalib E. Systemic sclerosis: demographic, clinical and serological features in 100 Iranian patients. Rheumatol Int. 2013;33(8):1943–50.
7. Muangchan C, Baron M, Pope J. The 15% rule in scleroderma: the frequency of severe organ complications in systemic sclerosis. A systematic review. J Rheumatol. 2013;40(9):1545–56.
8. Denton CP, Krieg T, Guillevin L, Schwierin B, Rosenberg D, Silkey M, Zultak M, Matucci-Cerinic M, DUO Registry Investigators. Demographic, clinical and antibody characteristics of patients with digital ulcers in systemic sclerosis: data from the DUO Registry. Ann Rheum Dis. 2012;71(5):718–21.
9. Allanore Y, Denton CP, Krieg T, Cornelisse P, Rosenberg D, Schwierin B, Matucci-Cerinic M. Clinical characteristics of systemic sclerosis patients with digital ulcer disease who

developed gangrene: data from DUO registry. Ann Rheum Dis. 2015;74(Suppl2):818.

10. Bérezné A, Seror R, Morell-Dubois S, de Menthon M, Fois E, Dzeing-Ella A, et al. Impact of systemic sclerosis on occupational and professional activity with attention to patients with digital ulcers. Arthritis Care Res (Hoboken). 2011;63(2):277–85.

11. Suliman YA, Bruni C, Johnson SR, Praino E, Alemam M, Borazan N, et al. Defining skin ulcers in systemic sclerosis: systematic literature review and proposed World Scleroderma Foundation (WSF) definition. J Scleroderma Rel Dis. 2017;2:115–20.

12. Amanzi L, Braschi F, Fiori G, Galluccio F, Miniati I, Guiducci S, et al. Digital ulcers in scleroderma: staging, characteristics and sub-

setting through observation of 1614 digital lesions. Rheumatology (Oxford). 2010;49:1374–82.

13. Baron M, Chung L, Gyger G, Hummers L, Khanna D, Mayes MM, et al. Consensus Opinion of a North American Working Group regarding the classification of digital ulcers in systemic sclerosis. Clin Rheum. 2014;33:207–14.

14. Hughes M, Moore T, Manning J, Dinsdale G, Herrick AL, Murray A. A pilot study using high-frequency ultrasound to measure digital ulcers: a possible outcome measure in systemic sclerosis clinical trials? Clin Exp Rheumatol. 2017;35:218. [Epub ahead of print].

15. Suliman Y, Kafaja S, Fitzgerald J, Wortsman X, Matucci-Cerinic M, Ranganath VG, Furst DE. Ultrasound characterization of cutaneous ulcers in systemic sclerosis. Clin Rheumatol. 2018;37:1555.

Digital Ulcerations and Classification of SSc Subsets and Overlap Syndromes

Carina Gaertner, Oana-Diana Persa, and Nicolas Hunzelmann

Digital ulcerations (DUs) belong to the most characteristic visible clinical signs of SSc. However, only very recently DU became a defined component of a classification system, i.e., the 2013 ACR/EUSTAR classification. The appreciation of the clinical symptom DU reflects the breadth of data generated in large registry studies in recent years that delineated the characteristics of SSc patients suffering from DU and underlines the importance of this major clinical symptom [1].

The prevalence rates of DU reported in cross-sectional studies ranged from 8% to 41% of patients with SSc [2–6]. This relatively large range has been attributed to many factors, e.g., the definition of DU, the geographic area surveyed, the population investigated containing different ethnic backgrounds, the composition of disease subsets, as well as differences in study methods and design.

The differences of DU frequency observed between different geographic areas could reflect genetic influences from different backgrounds. For example, DUs are more frequent in the western part of Europe compared to Eastern Europe [7]. Also, it was shown that black patients with SSc are more likely to develop DU [8] and white females appear more likely to develop digital infarcts compared to black females [9].

Differences observed between cohorts in the prevalence of DU could be due to the heterogeneous distribution of patients in different stages of the disease in these cohorts. A number of studies indicate that in approximately 75% of patients with SSc, the initial DU develops within 5 years from the beginning of their first non-Raynaud symptom [6–11].

When data obtained in different countries are compared, the differential access to the health-care system and specialist care including the large variation of reimbursement policies for diagnostic procedures and treatment should also be considered.

The clinical importance of DU is only partially reflected in the earliest classification of SSc, which was developed in 1980 by the American College of Rheumatology (ACR) [12]. The ACR criteria included one major criterion, proximal sclerodermatous skin changes, and three minor criteria: (1) sclerodactyly, (2) digital pitting scars of fingertips or loss of substance of the distal finger pads, and (3) bibasilar pulmonary fibrosis (Table 2.1). A patient could be classified as having systemic sclerosis either if he fulfilled the major criterion or if he fulfilled two of the three minor criteria. In this context it is important to note that digital pitting scars but not DU themselves were included as one of the three minor criteria of the earliest so-called preliminary classification of systemic sclerosis of the American College of Rheumatology (ACR) [12]. In the literature the percentages of patients fulfilling the minor criterion for SSc of digital pitting scars range from 8% to 31% [2–6].

It is important to keep in mind that this earliest classification published in 1980 was developed in patients with established disease showing a 97% sensitivity and 98% specificity for SSc [12]. Therefore it is not surprising that subsequently it became clear that in daily clinical practice, this classification was of limited usefulness as some of the criteria are not present during earlier disease phases (e.g., sclerodactyly, loss of substance of the distal finger pads). The aim of the ACR criteria was to enable physicians to distinguish between scleroderma patients and patients with a different connective tissue disease. However, the ACR criteria did not take into account to a sufficient degree the heterogeneity of patients and the wide range of symptoms and prognosis of patients with SSc.

A better description of patient subsets with different organ involvement and prognosis was the aim of a new classification of systemic sclerosis, which was proposed by LeRoy et al. in 1988. This classification distinguished between two types of systemic sclerosis (Table 2.2): diffuse cutaneous SSc (dcSSc) and limited cutaneous SSc (lcSSc). Among additional clinical symptoms, the LeRoy classification for the first

C. Gaertner · O.-D. Persa · N. Hunzelmann (✉)
Department of Dermatology, University of Cologne, Cologne, Germany
e-mail: nico.hunzelmann@uni-koeln.de

© Springer Nature Switzerland AG 2019
M. Matucci-Cerinic, C. P. Denton (eds.), *Atlas of Ulcers in Systemic Sclerosis*, https://doi.org/10.1007/978-3-319-98477-3_2

Table 2.1 ACR classification criteria for systemic sclerosis [12]

Major criterion	Proximal sclerodermatous skin changes (proximal to the metacarpophalangeal joints)
Minor criteria	1. Sclerodactyly
	2. Digital pitting scars of fingertips or loss of substance of the distal finger pads
	3. Bibasilar pulmonary fibrosis

The patient should fulfill the major criterion or two of the three minor criteria

ACR American College of Rheumatology

Table 2.2 LeRoy classification of systemic sclerosis in limited and diffuse cutaneous scleroderma [13]

	Limited form	Diffuse form
Skin fibrosis	Skin thickening limited to sites distal to elbows and knees, face and neck also involved but no truncal involvement	Skin thickening present in the trunk in addition to the face and extremities
Internal organ involvement	Late onset: Pulmonary arterial hypertension (especially in older age at onset and long-standing disease). Telangiectasia Esophageal dysmotility	Early onset: Lung fibrosis Gastrointestinal, heart and renal involvement
Raynaud's phenomenon	Often Raynaud's phenomenon occurs years prior to the skin fibrosis	Raynaud's phenomenon may onset around the same time that the skin changes start
Antibodies	Often anti-centromere antibodies	Often anti-topoisomerase I antibodies (Scl-70)

time introduced autoantibodies into a classification of SSc. Two SSc-specific autoantibodies, i.e., anti-centromere autoantibodies (ACA) and anti-topoisomerase 1-autoantibodies (topo-1), were included. ACA were described as being part of the lcSSc subset; topo-1 belonged to the dcSSc subset [13]. Subsequently, this classification received widespread recognition and became the basis for many clinical studies and registries. In this classification, DU or digital pits are not mentioned. However, many studies performed in the years following the publication of this classification addressed the issue of DU in these subsets. It is of interest to mention that in the publication of LeRoy et al., the existence of SSc-overlap syndromes was addressed and recognized, however not yet included in their classification. The subset of SSc-overlap syndromes has increasingly been acknowledged in recent years and will be part of this chapter (see below).

Limited Cutaneous SSc (lcSSc)

The limited form of SSc is characterized by skin fibrosis limited to the acral body parts. Patients affected by the limited subset develop Raynaud phenomenon often years before the first non-Raynaud symptoms occur. Regarding the occurrence of DU, it has been found that patients with limited disease run a lower risk to develop DU [4–10, 13, 14] than patients with dcSSc (Table 2.3). The association of DU with lcSSc and with anti-centromere antibodies observed by Brand et al. was most probably related to the relative higher number of these patients in general [15]. DUs in lcSSc are reportedly more often accompanied by inflammation of perilesional skin and edema. In addition DUs in limited disease develop more often on the basis of calcinosis and are more often localized at the dorsal side of the fingers [16–19]. It has been noted that due to their development on the basis of calcinosis, these ulcers are more likely to come along with inflammation. Other than DU deriving from digital pitting scars, DUs deriving from calcinosis are stated to be mostly deep, seldom intermediate and usually never superficial [16]. Digital amputation secondary to occlusion of digital arteries has been reported to occur in a subset of patients (11%), usually with limited skin disease and the presence of ACA [20]. DUs seen in patients with lcSSc, especially those deriving from calcinosis, are less often associated with visceral involvement [21].

Table 2.3 Frequency of digital ulcers in systemic sclerosis subsets

Subset of systemic sclerosis						
	N	Diffuse systemic sclerosis	Limited systemic sclerosis	Overlap syndrome	Systemic sclerosis sine scleroderma	Undifferentiated connective tissue disease
Poormoghim et al. [24]	555	n.d.	59%	n.d.	33%	n.d.
Ferri et al. [2]	1012	51%	43%	n.d.	n.d.	n.d.
Ostojic et al. [19].	91	67.3%	46.2%	n.d.	n.d.	n.d.
Tiso et al. [47]	333	46.8%	37.8%	n.d.	n.d.	n.d.
Walker et al. [10]	3656	42.7%	32.9%	22.3%	n.d.	n.d.
Hunzelmann et al. [30]	1483	34.4%	23.8%	21.2%	9.9%	n.d.
Sunderkötter et al. [14]	1881	33.9%	21.8%	20%	25%	11.9%
Amanzi et al. [16]	100	61.5%	44.43%	n.d.	n.d.	n.d.
Mouthon et al. [6]	213	27.9%	27%	n.d.	25%	n.d.
Khimdas et al. [4]	938	54.6%	38.4%	n.d.	n.d.	n.d.
Simeon-Aznar et al. [48]	916	63.8%	39%	n.d.	14.5%	n.d.
Marangoni et al. [49]	947	n.d.	n.d.	n.d.	24.1%	n.d.
Diab et al. [25]	1417	58.4%	48.1%	n.d.	18.5%	n.d.
Minier et al. [41]	466	n.d.	n.d.	n.d.	n.d.	6.9%
Moinzadeh et al. [28]	3240	33.3%	23.3%	18.2%	n.d.	n.d.
Tolosa-Vilella et al. [50]	1326	62.8%	38.7%	n.d.	16%	20%
Range	91–3656	27.9–67.3%	21.8–59%	18.2–22.3%	14.5–33%	6.9–20%

n.d. not determined

SSc Sine Scleroderma

SSc sine scleroderma is a subset of patients that presents with virtually no scleroderma, but has Raynaud phenomenon (RP), pulmonary hypertension or other scleroderma features as well as ACA (in the majority) or other scleroderma-associated autoantibodies [22, 23]. This subset is nowadays generally considered to belong to the limited subset. In one of the largest patient series, Poormoghim et al. described a significantly lower frequency of digital pitting scars (27%) and digital tip ulcers (33%) than in the limited subset of their cohort (62% and 59%, respectively) [24]. Similar data were reported by Diab et al. In their study, a frequency of digital pits in 11% and digital ulcers in 18.5% was found in the SSc sine scleroderma subset being markedly lower than the frequency (43.6% and 48.1%, respectively) found in the lcSSc subset of the same cohort [25].

Diffuse Cutaneous SSc (dcSSc)

Patients with dcSSc often progress rapidly and develop internal organ involvement significantly earlier when compared to patients with limited disease. In this subset, DUs are most frequent with frequencies reported between 28% and 67% (Table 2.3) [4–10, 13, 14, 26]. Early occurrence of DU in the disease course (i.e., within 5 years after disease onset) is especially seen in this subset. In the DUO registry, Denton et al. observed that topo-1-positive patients suffered from DU approximately 6 years earlier than ACA-positive patients [16, 19, 21]. DUs occurring in the dcSSc subset are more often associated with gangrene. They lead the ranking in severity. Amanzi et al. stated that these DUs are always presenting as deep ulcers partly with bone or tendon exposure and always associated with severe spontaneous pain [16]. Not surprisingly, DUs seen in patients with dcSSc are more often associated with visceral involvement [21]. However, recent data indicate that even in this subset, a substantial proportion of patients will probably never develop DU [11, 27].

SSc-Overlap Syndrome

In addition to patients with limited and diffuse disease, patients with SSc-overlap syndrome have emerged as a different subgroup of patients with systemic sclerosis [28, 29]. Patients with SSc-overlap syndrome do not only display the typical symptoms of systemic sclerosis but also develop symptoms specific for other autoimmune diseases such as lupus erythematosus, rheumatoid arthritis, Sjögren syndrome, and dermatomyositis. Approximately 10–20% of the patients with SSc can be classified as having an overlap syndrome [30, 31]. This particular subset of patients with systemic sclerosis

is often positive for U1-RNP and Pm-Scl antibodies, which are present in 33% and 16.7% of patients with an SSc-overlap syndrome [22, 28, 31–35]. Recently, it was shown that patients with an SSc-overlap syndrome have a distinct disease progression compared to patients with limited and diffuse disease [28]. DUs occur in this subset of patients, however, less frequently than in patients with lcSSc and dcSSc [28]. Data indicate that approximately 20% of the patients suffering from an overlap syndrome develop DU in the course of disease (Table 2.3) [14, 30]. A recent study by Balbir-Gurman indicates that the frequency of DU may differ between different SSc-overlap syndromes as they report a frequency of DU in the myositis group of 42.1% versus 11.8% in the Sjögren syndrome group [36]. Reiseter et al. (2015) reported a DU frequency of 32% in mixed connective tissue disease (MCTD) patients of the Norwegian cohort [37].

Very Early SSc, Early SSc, and Undifferentiated Form of SSc

The clinical usefulness of the preliminary ACR criteria from 1980 and the LeRoy classification of systemic sclerosis in daily clinical practice have been limited by the fact that these criteria do not take into consideration patients in an early stage of systemic sclerosis. Due to improved health care, activity of patients' associations, and the rise of the Internet in recent years, many patients present early or very early in the course of the disease. Therefore, presenting symptoms of a patient are often suggestive of but not conclusive for a diagnosis of definite systemic sclerosis, e.g., RP, capillaroscopic findings, scleroderma-specific antinuclear antibodies (ANA) or puffy hands.

Currently there is a controversy in the field whether patients with a set of laboratory parameters (i.e., autoantibodies) or symptoms (i.e., RP, puffy fingers) compatible with SSc, however not fulfilling criteria for the diagnosis of SSc, should be classified as undifferentiated connective tissue disease (UCTD), very early SSc, or early SSc [38–40].

In a preliminary analysis of the very early diagnosis of SSc (VEDOSS) EUSTAR multicentre study, it was found that among patients presenting with RP, DUs were present in 6.0% of ANA positive and 8.7% of ANA-negative patients [41]. Bruni et al. investigated 110 patients with the diagnosis of very early systemic sclerosis for the presence of digital lesions and the potential association with internal organ involvement. In order to be classified as very early diagnosis of systemic sclerosis, the presence of preliminary criteria, i.e., RP, puffy fingers, ANA, capillaroscopic abnormalities, and/or disease-specific antibodies, was required. Subjects were then screened for internal organ involvement, and according to the involvement pattern, derived into four groups as follows: (1) patients without internal involvement, (2) patients with pulmonary involvement only, (3) patients with gastrointestinal involvement only, and (4) patients with gastrointestinal and pulmonary involvement. DUs were not seen in the group without internal involvement, whereas they were present in the other groups. Patients with gastrointestinal involvement had the highest frequency with 43.3%, patients with pulmonary and gastrointestinal involvement had DU in 26.6%, and patients only showing pulmonary involvement had DU in 14.8%. These data suggest that DU is a marker of early organ involvement and indicates a transition from very early SSc to early SSc, potentially as a clinical sign of a more generalized vascular pathology [11, 42, 43].

2013 ACR/EULAR Criteria

In 2013 the ACR/EULAR criteria for classification of systemic sclerosis were developed to reflect the considerable advancement in the knowledge of the disease with the goal to overcome the weaknesses of previous classifications. Symptoms and findings often present in very early disease stages as nailfold capillaroscopic changes, antibodies specific for systemic sclerosis including RNA polymerase 3 antibodies, as well as puffy hands were included in this set of eight items (Table 2.4) [44]. After adding the scores for each item, a patient can be classified as having systemic sclerosis if the patient reaches a score of at least 9 points. Both DU and fingertip pitting scars were included in this new classification. DUs were defined as ulcers distal to or at the proximal interphalangeal joint not thought to be due to trauma. The implementation of these criteria has already led to new data on the prevalence of digital ulcers in patients with systemic sclerosis. For instance, a recent study has shown that patients who met the 2013 ACR/EULAR criteria but not the 1980 ACR criteria had a lower frequency of digital ulcers (i.e., 11.8%) in comparison to patients that were already

Table 2.4 The ACR-EULAR criteria for classification of systemic sclerosis [44]

Criteria	Sub-item	Score
Skin fibrosis[a]	Skin thickening of the fingers of both hands extending proximal to the metacarpophalangeal joints	9
	Puffy fingers	2
	Sclerodactyly of the fingers (distal to the metacarpophalangeal joints but proximal to the proximal interphalangeal joints)	4
Fingertip lesions[a]	Digital tip ulcers	2
	Fingertip pitting scars	3
Telangiectasia		2
Abnormal nailfold capillaries		2
Lung involvement	Pulmonary arterial hypertension and/or interstitial lung disease	2
Raynaud phenomenon		3
Scleroderma-related autoantibodies	Any of centromere-, topoisomerase I- and RNA polymerase III-specific antibodies	3

These criteria are applicable to any patient considered for inclusion in a systemic sclerosis study. The criteria are not applicable to patients with skin thickening sparing the fingers or to patients who have a scleroderma-like disorder that better explains their manifestations such as nephrogenic sclerosing fibrosis, generalized morphea, eosinophilic fasciitis, scleredema diabeticorum, scleromyxedema, erythromelalgia, porphyria, lichen sclerosus, graft-versus-host disease and diabetic cheiroarthropathy. The score for each category is added. A summary score of 9 is sufficient to fulfill the criteria
ACR American College of Rheumatology, EULAR European League Against Rheumatism
[a]Only the highest score is counted

classified as having systemic sclerosis according to the 1980 ACR criteria (33.3%) [45]. This finding probably reflects the inclusion of patients in earlier disease stages.

Hoffmann-Vold et al. assessed the 1980 ACR and the 2013 EULAR classification criteria on defined subgroups of patients suffering from SSc or MCTD. It was shown that out of the SSc subgroup, the ACR/EULAR criteria were met by 96%, whereas the ACR classification criteria were only met by 75%. In addition, the SSc patients initially presented quite often with the novel items of the EULAR criteria suggesting that the EULAR criteria are more sensitive than the ACR criteria. Interestingly, in the MCTD subgroup, 8% of patients had DU or pitting scars in contrast to 40% in the SSc group [46].

Conclusion

The highest frequency of DU is observed in dcSSc followed by the lcSSc and the overlap subset. In the dcSSc subset, DUs occur earlier in the disease course and are a marker of disease severity and internal organ involvement. As a substantial share of patients in all subsets will never develop DU, it will be a major aim to identify biomarkers to differentiate prospectively these two populations.

References

1. Guillevin L, Hunsche E, Denton CP, Krieg T, Schwierin B, Rosenberg D, et al. Functional impairment of systemic scleroderma patients with digital ulcerations: results from the duo registry. Clin Exp Rheumatol. 2013;31(Suppl 76):71–80.
2. Ferri C, Valentini G, Cozzi F, Sebastiani M, Michelassi C, La Montagna G, et al. Systemic sclerosis: demographic, clinical, and serologic features and survival in 1,012 Italian patients. Medicine (Baltimore). 2002;81:139–53.
3. Tiev KP, Diot E, Clerson P, Dupuis-Siméon F, Hachulla E, Hatron PY, et al. Clinical features of scleroderma patients with or without prior or current ischemic digital ulcers: post-hoc analysis of a nationwide multicenter cohort (Itinérair-Sclérodermie). J Rheumatol. 2009;36:1470–6.
4. Khimdas S, Harding S, Bonner A, Zummer B, Baron M, Pope J, C.S.R. Group. Associations with digital ulcers in a large cohort of systemic sclerosis: results from the Canadian Scleroderma Research Group Registry. Arthritis Care Res (Hoboken). 2011;63:142–9.
5. Hachulla E, Clerson P, Launay D, Lambert M, Morell-Dubois S, Queyrel V, et al. Natural history of ischemic digital ulcers in systemic sclerosis: single-center retrospective longitudinal study. J Rheumatol. 2007;34:2423–30.
6. Mouthon L, Mestre-Stanislas C, Bérezné A, Rannou F, Guilpain P, Revel M, et al. Impact of digital ulcers on disability and health-related quality of life in systemic sclerosis. Ann Rheum Dis. 2010;69:214–7.
7. Walker UA, Tyndall A, Czirják L, Denton CP, Farge-Bancel D, Kowal-Bielecka O, et al. Geographical variation of disease manifestations in systemic sclerosis: a report from the Eular Scleroderma Trials and Research (Eustar) group database. Ann Rheum Dis. 2009;68:856–62.
8. Nietert PJ, Mitchell HC, Bolster MB, Shaftman SR, Tilley BC, Silver RM. Racial variation in clinical and immunological manifestations of systemic sclerosis. J Rheumatol. 2006;33:263–8.
9. Laing TJ, Gillespie BW, Toth MB, Mayes MD, Gallavan RH, Burns CJ, et al. Racial Differences in Scleroderma among Women in Michigan. Arthritis Rheum. 1997;40:734–42.
10. Walker UA, Tyndall A, Czirják L, Denton C, Farge-Bancel D, Kowal-Bielecka O, et al. Clinical Risk Assessment of Organ Manifestations in Systemic Sclerosis: A Report from the Eular Scleroderma Trials and Research Group Database. Ann Rheum Dis. 2007;66:754–63.
11. Mihai C, Landewé R, van der Heijde D, Walker UA, Constantin PI, Gherghe AM, et al. Digital Ulcers Predict a Worse Disease Course in Patients with Systemic Sclerosis. Ann Rheum Dis. 2016;75:681–6.
12. Preliminary Criteria for the Classification of Systemic Sclerosis (Scleroderma). Subcommittee for Scleroderma Criteria of the American Rheumatism Association Diagnostic and Therapeutic Criteria Committee. Arthritis Rheum. 1980;23:581–90.
13. LeRoy EC, Black C, Fleischmajer R, Jablonska S, Krieg T, Medsger TA, Rowell N, et al. Scleroderma (Systemic Sclerosis): Classification. Subsets and Pathogenesis. J Rheumatol. 1988;15:202–5.
14. Sunderkötter C, Herrgott I, Brückner C, Moinzadeh P, Pfeiffer C, Gerss J, et al. Comparison of Patients with and without Digital Ulcers in Systemic Sclerosis: Detection of Possible Risk Factors. Br J Dermatol. 2009;160:835–43.
15. Brand M, Hollaender R, Rosenberg D, Scott M, Hunsche E, Tyndall A, et al. An observational cohort study of patients with newly diagnosed digital ulcer disease secondary to systemic sclerosis registered in the EUSTAR database. Clin Exp Rheumatol. 2015;33:47–54.
16. Amanzi L, Braschi F, Fiori G, Galluccio F, Miniati I, Guiducci S, et al. Digital Ulcers in Scleroderma: Staging, Characteristics and Sub-Setting through Observation of 1614 Digital Lesions. Rheumatology (Oxford). 2010;49:1374–82.
17. Ennis H, Vail A, Wragg E, Taylor A, Moore T, Murray A, et al. A Prospective Study of Systemic Sclerosis-Related Digital Ulcers: Prevalence, Location, and Functional Impact. Scand J Rheumatol. 2013;42:483–6.
18. Baron M, Chung L, Gyger G, Hummers L, Khanna D, Mayes MD, et al. Consensus Opinion of a North American Working Group Regarding the Classification of Digital Ulcers in Systemic Sclerosis. Clin Rheumatol. 2014;33:207–14.
19. Ostojić P, Damjanov N, Pavlov-Dolijanovic S, Radunović G. Peripheral Vasculopathy in Patients with Systemic Sclerosis: Difference in Limited and Diffuse Subset of Disease. Clin Hemorheol Microcirc. 2004;31:281–5.
20. Wigley FM, Wise RA, Miller R, Needleman BW, Spence RJ. Anticentromere Antibody as a Predictor of Digital Ischemic Loss in Patients with Systemic Sclerosis. Arthritis Rheum. 1992;35:688–93.
21. Denton CP, Krieg T, Guillevin L, Schwierin B, Rosenberg D, Silkey M, et al. Demographic, Clinical and Antibody Characteristics of Patients with Digital Ulcers in Systemic Sclerosis: Data from the Duo Registry. Ann Rheum Dis. 2012;71:718–21.
22. Steen VD. Autoantibodies in Systemic Sclerosis. Semin Arthritis Rheum. 2005;35:35–42.
23. Nihtyanova SI, Denton CP. Autoantibodies as Predictive Tools in Systemic Sclerosis. Nat Rev Rheumatol. 2010;6:112–6.
24. Poormoghim H, Lucas M, Fertig N, Medsger TA Jr. Systemic sclerosis sine scleroderma: demographic, clinical, and serologic features and survival in forty-eight patients. Arthritis Rheum. 2000;43:444–51.
25. Diab S, Dostrovsky N, Hudson M, Tatibouet S, Fritzler MJ, Baron M, et al. Systemic sclerosis sine scleroderma: a multicenter study of 1417 subjects. J Rheumatol. 2014;41:2179–85.

26. Wirz EG, Jaeger VK, Allanore Y, Riemekasten G, Hachulla E, Distler O, et al. Incidence and predictors of cutaneous manifestations during the early course of systemic sclerosis: a 10-year longitudinal study from the EUSTAR database. Ann Rheum Dis. 2016;75:1285–92.
27. Hunzelmann N, Riemekasten G, Becker M, Moinzadeh P, Kreuter A, Melchers I, et al. The Predict Study: Low Risk for Digital Ulcer Development in Systemic Sclerosis Patients with Increasing Disease Duration and Lack of Topoisomerase-1 Antibodies. Br J Dermatol. 2016;174:1384–7.
28. Moinzadeh P, Aberer E, Ahmadi-Simab K, Blank N, Distler JH, Fierlbeck G, et al. Disease Progression in Systemic Sclerosis-Overlap Syndrome Is Significantly Different from Limited and Diffuse Cutaneous Systemic Sclerosis. Ann Rheum Dis. 2015;74:730–7.
29. Varga J, Hinchcliff M. Connective tissue diseases: systemic sclerosis: beyond limited and diffuse subsets? Nat Rev Rheumatol. 2014;10:200–2.
30. Hunzelmann N, Genth E, Krieg T, Lehmacher W, Melchers I, Meurer M, et al. The Registry of the German Network for Systemic Scleroderma: Frequency of Disease Subsets and Patterns of Organ Involvement. Rheumatology (Oxford). 2008;47:1185–92.
31. Pakozdi A, Nihtyanova S, Moinzadeh P, Ong VH, Black CM, Denton CP. Clinical and Serological Hallmarks of Systemic Sclerosis Overlap Syndromes. J Rheumatol. 2011;38:2406–9.
32. Steen VD, Medsger TA. Severe Organ Involvement in Systemic Sclerosis with Diffuse Scleroderma. Arthritis Rheum. 2000;43:2437–44.
33. Cepeda EJ, Reveille JD. Autoantibodies in Systemic Sclerosis and Fibrosing Syndromes: Clinical Indications and Relevance. Curr Opin Rheumatol. 2004;16:723–32.
34. Oddis CV, Okano Y, Rudert WA, Trucco M, Duquesnoy RJ, Medsger TA. Serum Autoantibody to the Nucleolar Antigen Pm-Scl. Clinical and Immunogenetic Associations. Arthritis Rheum. 1992;35:1211–7.
35. Mierau R, Moinzadeh P, Riemekasten G, Melchers I, Meurer M, Reichenberger F, et al. Frequency of Disease-Associated and Other Nuclear Autoantibodies in Patients of the German Network for Systemic Scleroderma: Correlation with Characteristic Clinical Features. Arthritis Res Ther. 2011;13:R172.
36. Balbir-Gurman A, Braun-Moscovici Y. Scleroderma overlap syndrome. Isr Med Assoc J. 2011;13:14–20.
37. Reiseter S, Molberg Ø, Gunnarsson R, Lund MB, Aalokken TM, Aukrust P, et al. Associations between circulating endostatin levels and vascular organ damage in systemic sclerosis and mixed connective tissue disease: an observational study. Arthritis Res Ther. 2015;28:17–231.
38. Valentini G, Marcoccia A, Cuomo G, Vettori S, Iudici M, Bondanini F, et al. Early systemic sclerosis: analysis of the disease course in patients with marker autoantibody and/or capillaroscopic positivity. Arthritis Care Res (Hoboken). 2014;66:1520–7.
39. Valentini G, Marcoccia A, Cuomo G, Iudici M, Vettori S. The concept of early systemic sclerosis following 2013 ACR\EULAR criteria for the classification of systemic sclerosis. Curr Rheumatol Rev. 2014;10:38–44.
40. Valentini G. Undifferentiated Connective Tissue Disease at risk for systemic sclerosis (SSc) (so far referred to as very early/early SSc or pre-SSc). Autoimmun Rev. 2015;14:210–3.
41. Minier T, Guiducci S, Bellando-Randone S, Bruni C, Lepri G, Czirják L, et al. Preliminary analysis of the very early diagnosis of systemic sclerosis (VEDOSS) EUSTAR multicentre study: evidence for puffy fingers as a pivotal sign for suspicion of systemic sclerosis. Ann Rheum Dis. 2014;73:2087–93.
42. Matucci-Cerinic M, Bellando-Randone S, Lepri G, Bruni C, Guiducci S. Very early versus early disease: the evolving definition of the 'many faces' of systemic sclerosis. Ann Rheum Dis. 2013;72:319–21.
43. Bruni C, Guiducci S, Bellando-Randone S, Lepri G, Braschi F, Fiori G, et al. Digital ulcers as a sentinel sign for early internal organ involvement in very early systemic sclerosis. Rheumatology (Oxford). 2015;54:72–6.
44. van den Hoogen F, Khanna D, Fransen J, Johnson SR, Baron M, Tyndall A, et al. 2013 Classification Criteria for Systemic Sclerosis: An American College of Rheumatology/European League against Rheumatism Collaborative Initiative. Arthritis Rheum. 2013;65:2737–47.
45. Park JS, Park MC, Song JJ, Park YB, Lee SK, Lee SW. Application of the 2013 ACR/Eular Classification Criteria for Systemic Sclerosis to Patients with Raynaud's Phenomenon. Arthritis Res Ther. 2015;17:77.
46. Hoffmann-Vold AM, Gunnarsson R, Garen T, Midtvedt Ø, Molberg Ø. Performance of the 2013 American College of Rheumatology/European League Against Rheumatism Classification Criteria for Systemic Sclerosis (SSc) in large, well-defined cohorts of SSc and mixed connective tissue disease. J Rheumatol. 2015;42:60–3.
47. Tiso F, Favaro M, Ciprian L, Cardarelli S, Rizzo M, Tonello M, et al. Digital Ulcers in a Cohort of 333 Scleroderma Patients. Reumatismo. 2007;59:215–20.
48. Simeón-Aznar CP, Fonollosa-Plá V, Tolosa-Vilella C, Espinosa-Garriga G, Ramos-Casals M, Campillo-Grau M, et al. Registry of the Spanish network for systemic sclerosis: clinical pattern according to cutaneous subsets and immunological status. Semin Arthritis Rheum. 2012;41:789–800.
49. Marangoni RG, Rocha LF, Del Rio AP, Yoshinari NH, Marques-Neto JF, Sampaio-Barros PD. Systemic Sclerosis Sine Scleroderma: Distinct Features in a Large Brazilian Cohort. Rheumatology (Oxford). 2013;52:1520–4.
50. Tolosa-Vilella C, Morera-Morales ML, Simeón-Aznar CP, Marí-Alfonso B, Colunga-Arguelles D. Callejas_Rubio JL. Digital ulcers and cutaneous subsets of systemic sclerosis: Clinical immunological, nailfold capillaroscopy, and survival differences in the Spanish RESCLE Registry. Semin Arthritis Rheum. 2016;46:200–8.

Jelena Blagojevic

Classification of DU in SSc

Over the past decades, rheumatologists have been using the classification of pressure ulcers to classify cutaneous lesions in SSc [1]. This classification has been created in order to determine the severity of pressure ulcers, and it defines different ulcer stages according to different degrees of tissue damage. The deeper the ulcers are and more extensive the tissue damage is, the higher the ulcer stage is. Though very diffuse and useful for other types of ulcers, this classification is not adequate for digital lesions seen in SSc, because of their multifactorial aetiology that may differ depending on ulcer localization.

In addition to SSc-related vasculopathy, other pathogenic factors as repetitive microtrauma at sites of joint contractures, calcinosis and dry skin may contribute to ulcer formation [2].

DUs located on the fingertips are usually related to chronic ischaemic tissue damage secondary to microvascular (*Raynaud's phenomenon, intimal proliferation and intravascular thrombosis*) [3] and sometimes also macrovascular involvement [4]. DUs on the dorsal aspect of the fingers are in the largest part of cases related to epidermal thinning and cutaneous retraction leading to cracks on the atrophic skin overlying the joints that are subject to microtrauma; poor vascularization may contribute to the impaired healing of these lesions [3].

DU may also develop as a consequence of pre-existing calcinosis. If the calcinosis is very superficial or extends superficially, it can reach the epithelial layer, causing skin rupture and a loss of tissue and thus leading to DU [5].

Furthermore, there are DUs that develop under digital pitting scars (DPS) and that can be discovered only after their removal. DPS are defined as small-sized digital concave depressions with hyperkeratosis. They can be commonly observed on the fingertips of scleroderma patients, but may often have other locations, as subungual area, radial border of the index and middle finger, the ulnar side of the thumb and dorsal surface of the proximal interphalangeal joints [6]. Dry skin and recurrent trauma in addition to chronic ischaemia may play a role in their formation. Sometimes an ulcer can be hidden below the hyperkeratotic layers of DPS. It can be suspected when there is an inflammation and oedema of the skin that surrounds DPS and when DPS are spontaneously painful. It is possible that DPS may foster development of DU by pressing soft tissues underneath, thus causing their inflammation and maceration.

Therefore, fundamentally four potential types of DUs may be identified in SSc:

1. DUs secondary to DPS.
2. DUs secondary to calcinosis.
3. Pure DUs (DUs not occurring as a consequence of DPS or calcinosis). These DUs may have pure ischaemic origin (usually located on the fingertips) or can be secondary to skin retraction and joint contractures, in addition to SSc-related vasculopathy.

In the most severe cases, gangrene may occur in SSc patients. It consists in necrosis of soft tissues, occurring when the arterial blood supply falls below minimal metabolic requirements. Gangrene can be classified as dry or wet gangrene. Dry gangrene is a more common type of gangrene in SSc, and it is related to chronic ischaemia leading slowly to tissue death, dehydration and eventually mummification of tissues that become dark brown and then black, dry, horny and shrunken. Wet gangrene is not frequent in SSc and it is usually a result of an infection of dry gangrene. If dry gangrene is not treated surgically, a layer of granulation tissue will form between the dead and living tissue, allowing gradual separation of two parts. Ulceration follows and finally gangrenous part will fall off; this process is called autoamputation. The ulcer that has been created between living and gangrenous tissue is now on the top of the part that was previously covered by gangrene. This type of ulcer can be defined as ulcer secondary to or derived from gangrene.

J. Blagojevic
Department of Experimental and Clinical Medicine, Division of
Rheumatology, University of Florence, Florence, Italy

© Springer Nature Switzerland AG 2019
M. Matucci-Cerinic, C. P. Denton (eds.), *Atlas of Ulcers in Systemic Sclerosis*, https://doi.org/10.1007/978-3-319-98477-3_3

Our study group on SSc proposed a comprehensive classification of DU, based on observations extrapolated from every day "real-life" clinical practice [5]. Morphological and clinical characteristics, natural course and time to healing of 1614 digital lesions in a cohort of 100 SSc patients (70 with limited and 30 with cutaneous subset), followed for 4 years, were analysed.

Cutaneous finger lesions were classified as follows:

1. *Digital pitting scars (DPS)*: They were defined as small-sized hyperkeratotic lesions and were most frequently observed on fingertips and dorsal area of fingers (Fig. 3.1). When exfoliated or debrided, they usually harbour an intact epithelium below. However, they may also hide small DU underneath hyperkeratotic layers.
2. *DU:* It was defined as a loss of epithelialization and tissues involving, to a different degree, the epidermis and underlying tissues (Fig. 3.2).

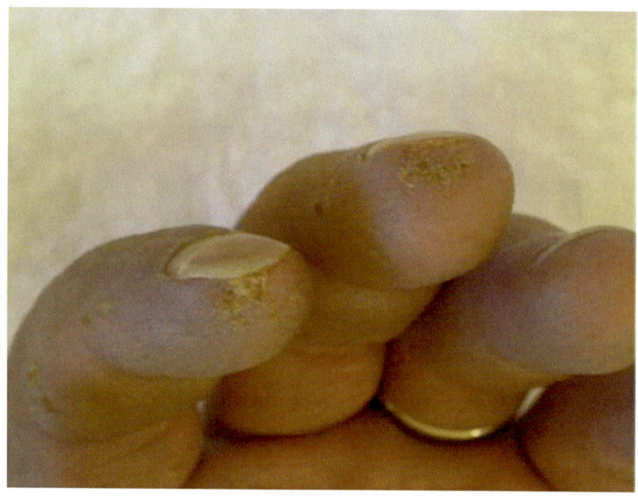

Fig. 3.1 Digital pitting scars

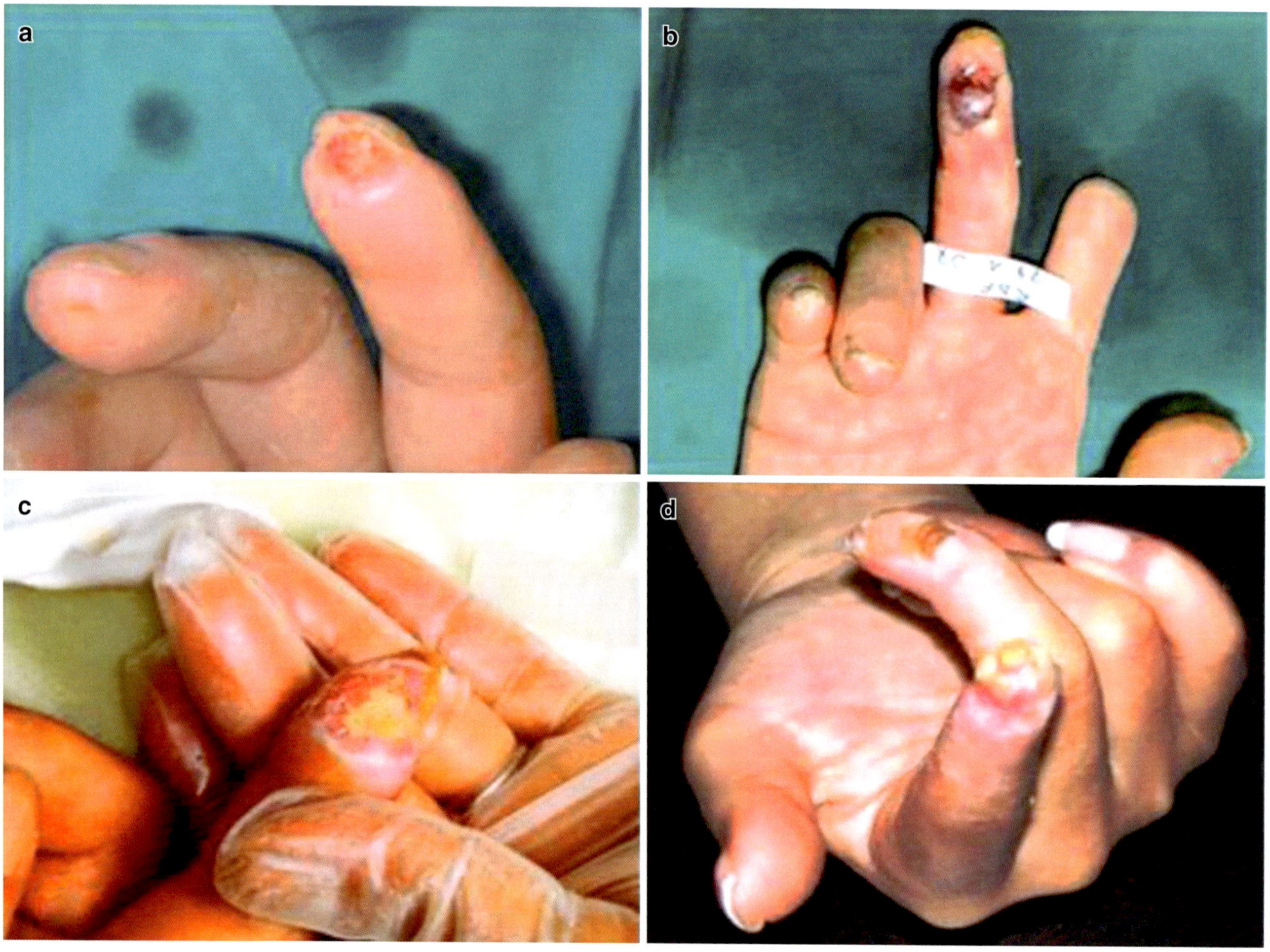

Fig. 3.2 Digital ulcers. (**a**) DU with granulation tissue. (**b**) Third finger DU with necrosis on the bottom of the lesion. DPS on the fourth and fifth finger. Amputation of the second finger. (**c**) DU with irregular borders, fibrin and granulation tissue. (**d**) Bone and tendon exposure resulting from the initial gangrene on the second finger. (From Amanzi et al. [5]. Reprinted with permission from Oxford University Press)

3. *Calcinosis*: It was defined as soft tissue deposits of calcium phosphate, visible to the naked eye (Fig. 3.3) and/or confirmed by X-ray. Visible calcinosis on fingers usually present as white-yellow creamy material ("mousse" calcinosis) or as white material of hard consistency ("stone" calcinosis). The authors observed that calcinosis was mainly located on the fingertips.

4. *Gangrene*: It was defined as the death of tissues caused by a total lack of blood supply. Gangrene can be dry or wet. In dry gangrene, the affected part is dry, shrivelled and dark black (Fig. 3.4a). The area affected by wet gangrene is moist, oedematous and macerated containing dark-coloured fluids and emanates a characteristic odour (Fig. 3.4b).

Amanzi et al. subsequently divided DUs into subsets according to their origin and main features (location, dimensions, bed and borders of the lesion, perilesional skin, presence of exudate, bone and tendon exposure and autoamputation) [5].

In addition, every DU was staged, according to the stages used for the pressure ulcers and modified by authors, in:

(a) Superficial: Defined as partial skin loss involving epidermis and presenting as an abrasion, blister or tiny crater.

(b) Intermediate: Defined as full-thickness skin loss involving subcutaneous tissues, but not underlying fascia. The ulcer presents as a deep crater with or without undermining of the adjacent tissue.

(c) Deep: Defined as full-thickness skin loss over the fascia with extensive damage to muscles, tendon and eventually joint capsule and bone.

The authors proposed the following classification of DU:

1. *DU derived from DPS*: These ulcers were hidden below the hyperkeratotic layers of DPS, were very small and superficial and were most frequently located on fingertips and dorsal aspect of fingers, as DPS. They can be usually easily identified, as they are characterized by inflammation and oedema of perilesional skin (Fig. 3.5). Spontaneous pain was also one of the indicators of their occurrence. Amanzi et al. observed hidden DU in 8.8% of DPS [5]. It is very important to distinguish these lesions from simple DPS, as they are more difficult to heal. Moreover, as it is possible that DPS may foster the ulcer development, surgical debridement of every DPS is recommended in order to prevent ulcer formation. However, these superficial DUs tend to have a benign course, as suggested by Amanzi et al. [5]. In fact, infection, gangrene and/or autoamputation never complicated DU derived from DPS within the study duration, and their mean time to healing was inferior to 1 month (26 ± 15 days).

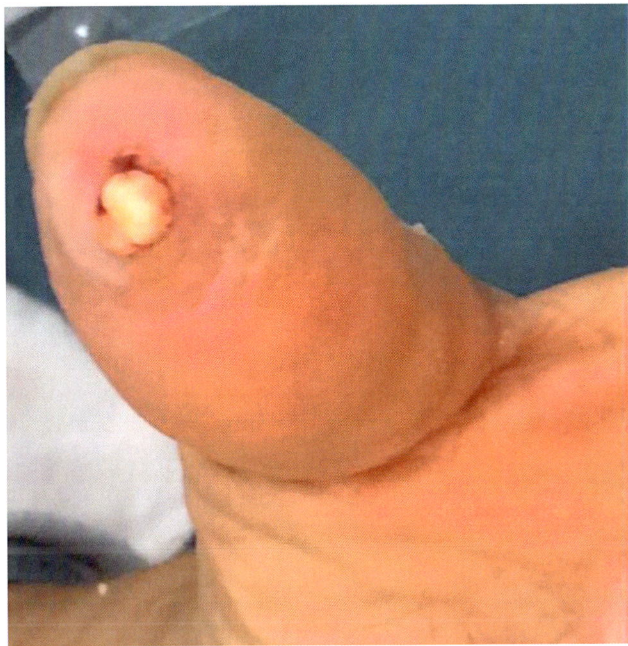

Fig. 3.3 Calcinosis and DU derived from calcinosis (fingertip)

Fig. 3.4 Gangrene. (**a**) Dry gangrene. (**b**) Wet gangrene

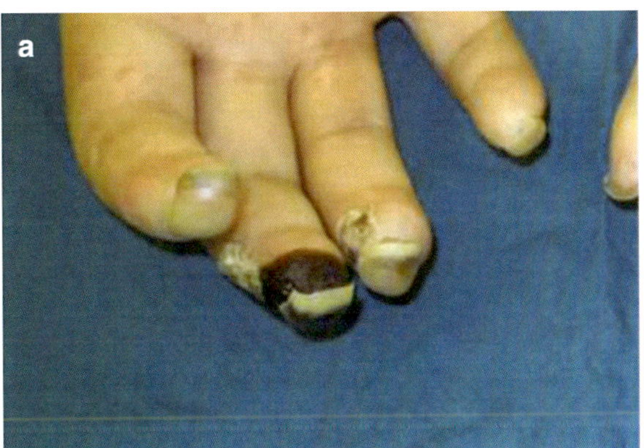

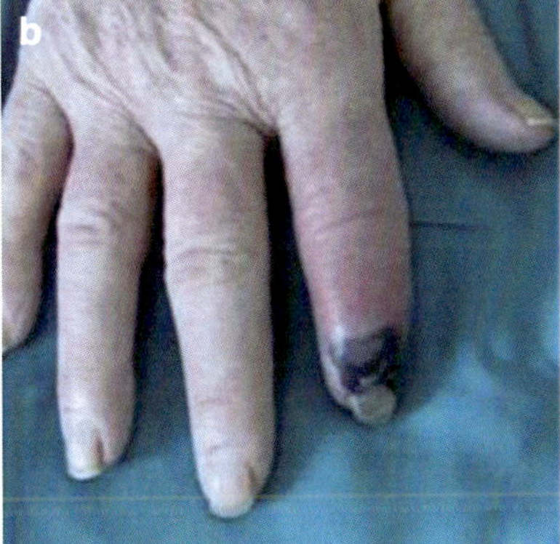

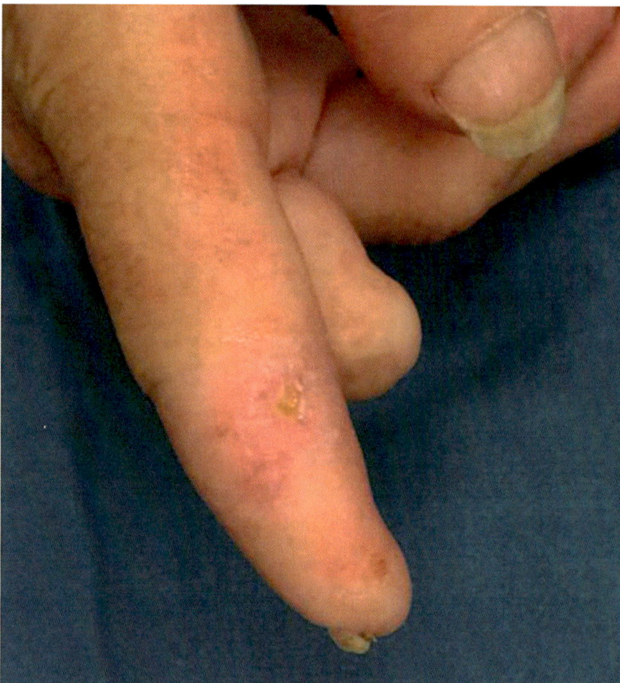

Fig. 3.5 DU secondary to DPS

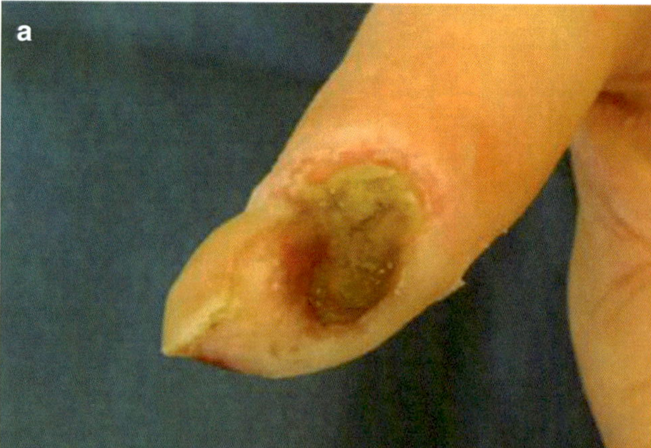

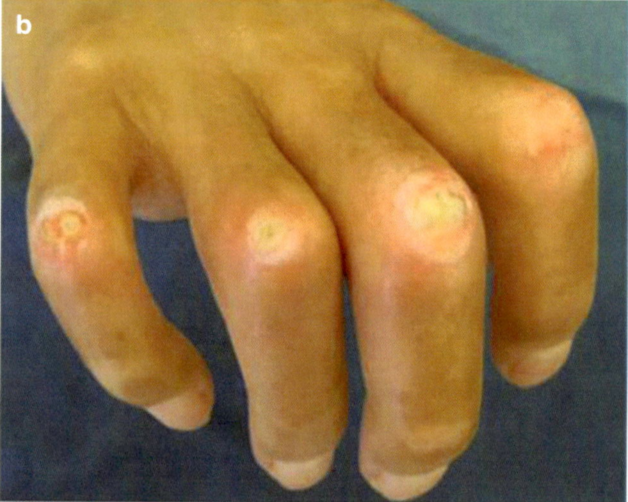

Fig. 3.6 Pure DUs. (**a**) Pure DU on the fingertip. (**b**) Pure DUs on the bony prominences

2. *DU derived from calcinosis*: These DUs develop as a consequence of calcinotic deposits in the skin and soft tissues and present as a visible stone or mousse calcinosis that emerges from the inflamed skin (Fig. 3.3). They were located most frequently on the fingertips, had irregular borders and perilesional oedema and were frequently associated with severe spontaneous pain. Amanzi observed that DU derived from calcinosis had almost always deep and had rarely intermediate stage [5]. Their mean time to healing was around 3 months (93 ± 59 days). They had higher infection rate than other subsets of DU, and the infection was associated with the presence of pus exudate ("mousse pus").

3. *Pure DU*: These DU ulcers do not occur in association with DPS or in association with calcinosis. Pure DUs have been defined as a loss of epithelialization and tissues involving, in different degrees, the epidermis, dermis and subcutaneous tissue. They can be situated anywhere in the fingers but were most frequently observed on the fingertips and on the dorsal surface of the proximal interphalangeal joints (Fig. 3.6). Pure DUs had frequently irregular borders and inflamed perilesional skin. These ulcers may have different dimensions; the bed of the lesions may consist of granulation tissue, fibrin and wet or dry necrosis (Fig. 3.2a–c). The stage was usually intermediate or deep. The majority of pure DUs did not have exudate, but when present, it was always associated with infection. Severe spontaneous pain was associated with the presence of infection too.

Gangrene and bone and tendon exposure were fortunately rare; they complicated 1.7% of pure DU; autoamputation occurred in 0.5% of cases. The mean time to healing of pure DUs was 76 ± 64 days.

The authors did not make a distinction between pure DU of pure ischaemic origin and pure DUs that occur as a consequence of skin retraction and joint contractures, in addition to SSc-related vasculopathy. If pure DUs are located on the fingertips, they are likely caused by the ischaemia. When they are located over the bony prominences, other factors may be also involved in their pathogenesis, as skin retraction and joint contractures and microtrauma. However, all these lesions are characterized by a loss of tissue and epithelialization, occurring in the absence of DPS or calcinosis.

4. *DU derived from gangrene*: These DUs form at the level of the demarcation line separating gangrene and viable tissue. DUs derived from gangrene were always deep and characterized by irregular borders, inflammation and oedema of perilesional skin. Spontaneous severe pain was

always present as well. The mean time to healing was around 9 months (281 ± 263 days). Bone and tendon exposure was frequent (around 40%) and autoamputation occurred in 14.2% of cases.

This classification is easy to apply both in clinical practice and in clinical trials, and its performance requires a minimal training. However, its inter- and intra-observer variability has not been tested.

There is ongoing European multicentre observational study named DeSScipher (acronym for "to decipher the optimal management of systemic sclerosis") that involves more than 10 000 patients (www.desscipher.eu). Its sub-study on DU called OT1 has adopted this classification in order to validate it.

Classification of Lower Limb Ulcers

Lower limb ulcers are traditionally classified in arterial, venous and ulcers of another pathogenesis (vasculitic ulcers, microangiopathic ulcers, pressure ulcers, etc.) [7]. They are usually long-lasting and represent a real clinical challenge.

Although lower limb ulcers have been recognized as one of the clinical features of SSc [8–11], they have not been described accurately and no classification of them has been proposed up to now.

The prevalence of lower limb cutaneous lesions has not been explicitly investigated in SSc, but it seems to be lower than the prevalence of finger DU [12, 13]. The pathogenesis of these lesions is more complex than the pathogenesis of DU in the upper limbs. In SSc, disease-related microangiopathy may be the primary cause of lower limb ulcers, but concomitant macrovascular arterial and/or venous disease may also overlap. Moreover, lymphatic system pathology, mechanical factors (as altered foot posture, loss of the fat pad, articular deformities and repetitive trauma) and calcinosis may all contribute to the ulcer formation.

We have recently performed a retrospective study on 554 cutaneous lower limb lesions detected in 60 patients during the 5-year observational period, with aim to assess pathogenesis of lower limb ulcers and to propose their classification [12]. Data have been extrapolated from everyday "real-life" clinical practice, as previously done for DU in the upper limbs [5].

We observed four types of lower limb lesions in SSc patients: hyperkeratoses, ulcers, calcinosis and gangrene. Some of the hyperkeratoses hid ulcers underneath hyperkeratotic skin layers, similarly as DPS harboured ulcers secondary to DPS in the upper limbs. There were ulcers that developed as a consequence of calcinosis erupting through the skin. We also observed ulcers that were not secondary to calcinosis nor associated with hyperkeratosis (pure ulcers).

The classification that we have proposed was the following [12]:

1. *Hyperkeratoses:* They were defined as hypertrophy of the stratum corneum of the skin and were mainly represented by callus and corns. These lesions were located mostly in areas submitted to increased friction or pressure (Fig. 3.7). Foot deformities and loss of the fat pad, as well as altered posture and microtrauma, represent risk factor for the occurrence of hyperkeratosis in SSc patients.
2. *Ulcers*: They were defined as a loss of epithelialization that may involve to a different extent the underneath tissues (Fig. 3.8).
3. *Calcinosis:* It was defined in the same was as in the upper limbs.
4. *Gangrene*: It was defined as necrosis of soft tissues caused by a total lack of blood supply (Fig. 3.9).

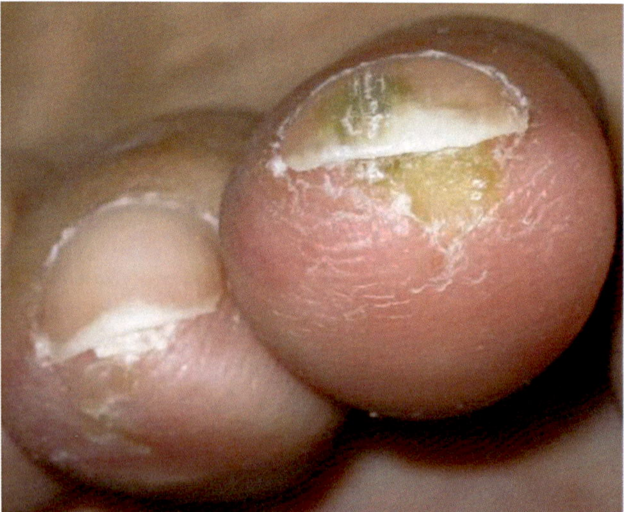

Fig. 3.7 Hyperkeratosis in the lower limbs (toes)

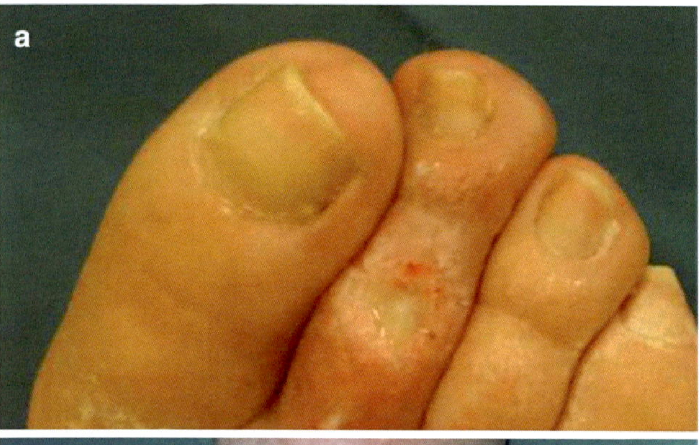

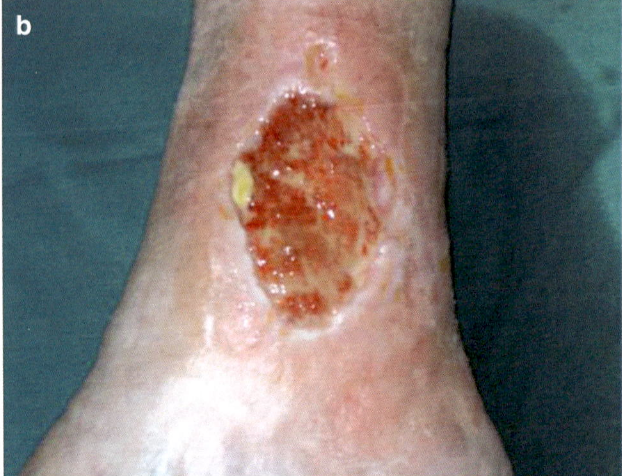

Fig. 3.8 Pure ulcers in the lower limb. (**a**) Pure toe ulcer. (**b**) Pure ulcer in the perimalleolar medial region

Every ulcer was staged using the same system applied for DU; stages were defined as superficial, intermediate and deep.

Lower limb ulcers were then classified into subsets according to their origin and main features into [12]:

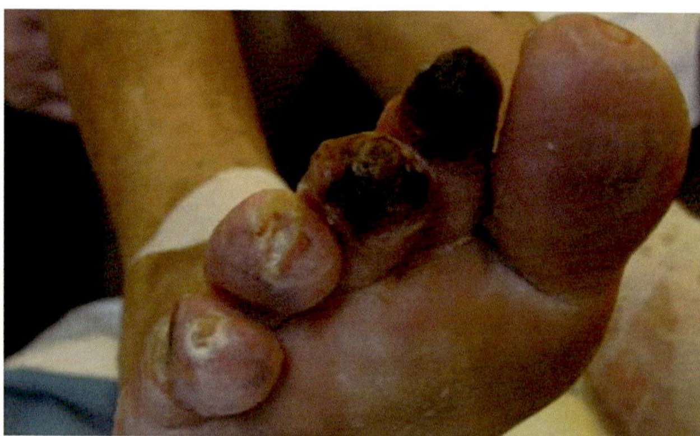

Fig. 3.9 Lower limb gangrene

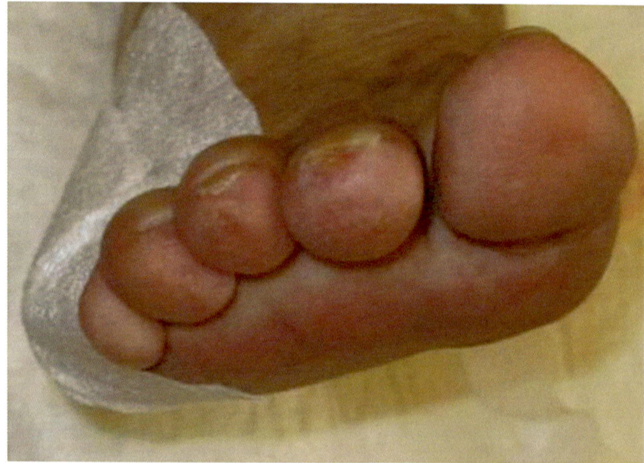

Fig. 3.10 Ulcer associated with hyperkeratosis in the lower limbs (toe)

(a) *Ulcers associated with hyperkeratosis*: If not promptly debrided, hyperkeratosis may evolve to a secondary ulcer. Hyperkeratosis may foster ulcer development by pressing underneath tissues and causing their maceration, haematoma and autolysis, as occur in diabetic foot [14]; thus the debridement of hyperkeratosis is mandatory. In our study hyperkeratoses were associated with ulcers hidden underneath in 10% of cases [12]. The loss of tissue was usually hidden below the hyperkeratotic layers and was easily suspected because of the inflammation and oedema of the perilesional skin (Fig. 3.10). Spontaneous pain was often present. These ulcers were deeper than DU derived from DPS. However, they had benign course, analogously to what observed for ulcers derived from DPS in the upper limbs. In fact, bone and tendon exposure and autoamputation were never detected. The mean time to healing was 15 weeks which was longer than the time to healing of ulcers derived from DPS (around 4 weeks) [12].

(b) *Ulcers secondary to calcinosis*: These ulcers were caused by calcinosis erupting through the skin (Fig. 3.11). They occurred most frequently on pretibial area and had very large dimensions, irregular borders and inflamed perilesional skin. They were deep and painful. The rate of infection was higher compared to other types of ulcers, similarly to what observed by Amanzi in the fingers [5]. The mean time to healing was four times longer than the time to healing of the ulcers secondary to calcinosis in the upper limbs (390 vs 90 days) [12]. It was probably related to major extension and dimensions of calcinosis in the lower limbs.

(c) *Pure ulcers*: These ulcers were defined as loss of soft tissue not occurring in association with hyperkeratosis or in association with calcinosis (Fig. 3.8). Pure ulcers were observed most frequently on toes and in the perimalleolar lateral areas. They were deep and painful and their time to healing was around 5 months (25.6 ± 23.5 weeks) [12]. Infection rate was 48% [12].

Since in the lower limbs macrovascular arterial and/or venous involvement may overlap SSc-related microangiopathy, lower limb pure ulcers may be additionally classified into arterial, venous and microvascular ulcers, according to the criteria described in the literature [15, 16]. There are also mixed arterial-venous ulcers occurring in patients with concomitant arterial and venous macrovascular involvement. In SSc, macrovascular arterial disease may be the result of SSc-related involvement of large vessels [9, 17] and/or a result of accelerated atherosclerosis.

Venous ulcers often occur over the medial malleolus, have irregular, slightly sloping edges and are associated with concomitant signs of venous pathology as varicosities, oedema and venous dermatitis (Fig. 3.12). Arterial ulcers occur frequently on bony prominences of the foot as toes and heels and have well-demarcated edges and cold surrounding skin (Fig. 3.13). They are usually associated with intermittent claudication, worsening pain following leg elevation and reduced or abolished peripheral pulses. Microvascular ulcers have morphological characteristics of arterial ulcers in the absence of signs of macrovascular arterial impairment. Mixed arterial-venous ulcers present with features of a venous ulcer in combination with signs of macrovascular arterial impairment (as abolished peripheral pulses). Microvascular and venous ulcers may coexist in the lower limbs of SSc patients with venous insufficiency.

In our cohort of patients, half of the subjects with pure ulcers did not present macrovascular involvement [12]. Therefore, in these patients pure ulcers were most likely due to isolated SSc-related microangiopathy. Thirty percent of these lesions were proximal (above ankle, including ankle),

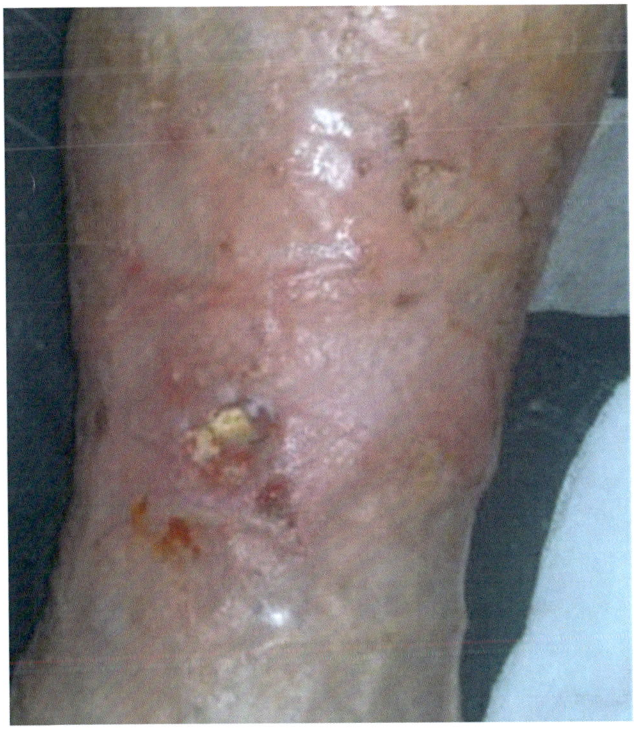

Fig. 3.11 Ulcer secondary to calcinosis in the lower limbs (leg)

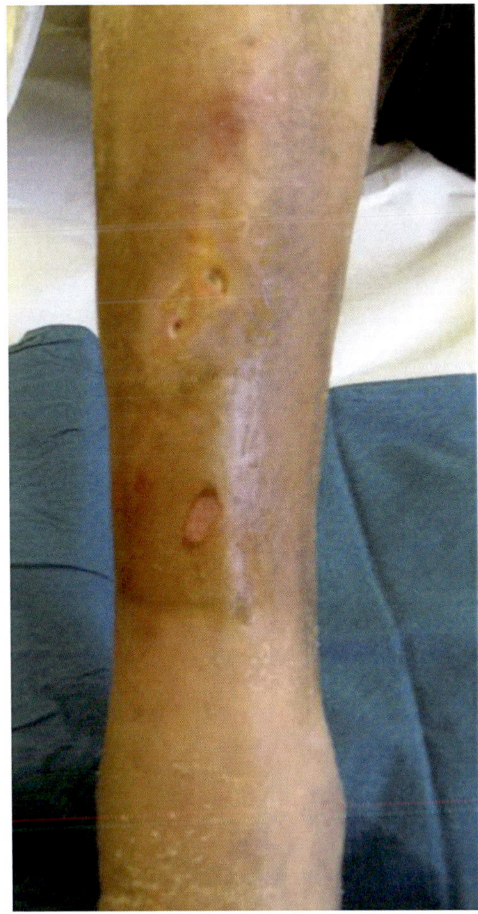

Fig. 3.12 Leg ulcers in SSc patient with venous insufficiency

while 70% were distal (below ankle) [12]. Proximal lesions were observed more frequently in the lateral malleolar region, pretibial region and medial malleolar region, while distal lesions were observed on toes and soles [12]. These pure ulcers had morphological characteristics of arterial ulcers, but were not associated with absent pulses and/or intermittent claudication [12].

In five cases dry gangrene of the fingertips was observed as an initial presentation. It was secondary to microvascular involvement in 20% and to critical macrovascular arterial disease in 80% cases [12].

Since macrovascular arterial and/or venous involvement may frequently overlap SSc-related microangiopathy, clinical signs of macrovascular disease (absent or diminished pulses, varicosities, oedema and/or venous dermatitis) should always be searched in SSc patients with lower limb lesions. If macrovascular disease is suspected, based on anamnesis and on clinical examination, echo Doppler is recommended to rule out the macrovascular involvement.

Although lower limb ulcers seem to be less frequent, they are much more difficult to manage and specifically treat than DU. They have longer time to healing and higher rates of infection and amputation than superior limb DU of corresponding type. Table 3.1 highlights similarities and differences between the classifications of the upper and lower limb lesions in SSc.

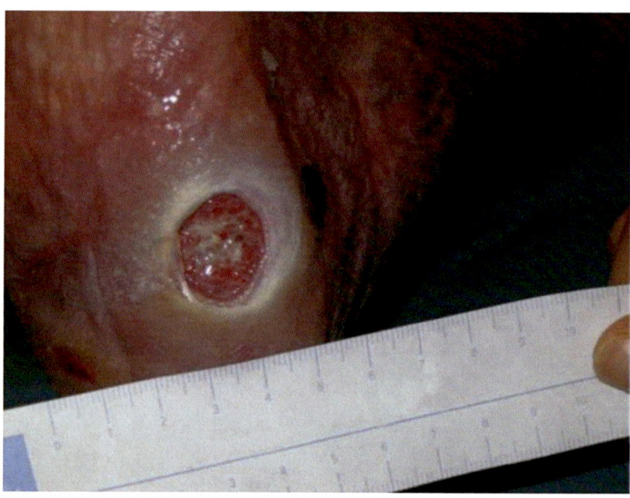

Fig. 3.13 Heel ulcer in SSc patients with arterial macrovascular disease

Table 3.1 Lower limb lesions vs upper limb digital ulcers

	Lower limbs lesions (60 patients/554 cutaneous lesions)	Upper limb digital ulcers (100 patients/1614 cutaneous lesions)
Type of lesions	Hyperkeratoses: 61.6% Ulcers: 37.5% Calcinosis 11.1% Gangrene: 0.9%	Hyperkeratoses: 44.1% Digital ulcers: 48.7% Calcinosis: 6.8% Gangrene: 0.4%
Classification of lower limb ulcers/ digital ulcers	Associated with hyperkeratosis Pure ulcers Secondary to calcinosis	Derived from DPS Pure ulcers Secondary to (derived from) calcinosis Derived from gangrene
Limited vs diffuse subset	66.7% vs 33.3%	47% vs 60.9%

Data from [5, 12]

State of Healing

Another important issue regarding DU is a definition of a state of healing. The ulcer is healed once it has been completely re-epithelialized. The ulcer can cause permanent loss of tissue, but when it is healed, it is always covered by the epithelialized skin (Fig. 3.14). It is not always easy to define the state of healing, since the eschar (crust) can persist after the healing process has occurred. It is very important to distinguish between healed and non-healed DU; thus the removal of the eschar and dead tissue covering DU is mandatory in order to verify the state of healing and to promote the healing itself. Terms as active, not active and indeterminate ulcer should be avoided, as they may create confusion and they do not reflect the real state of healing.

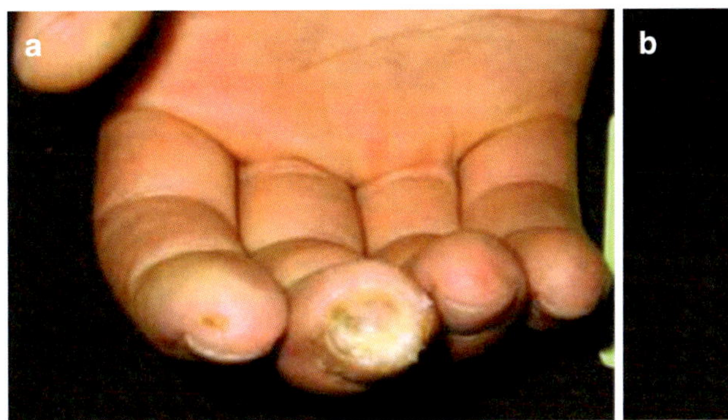
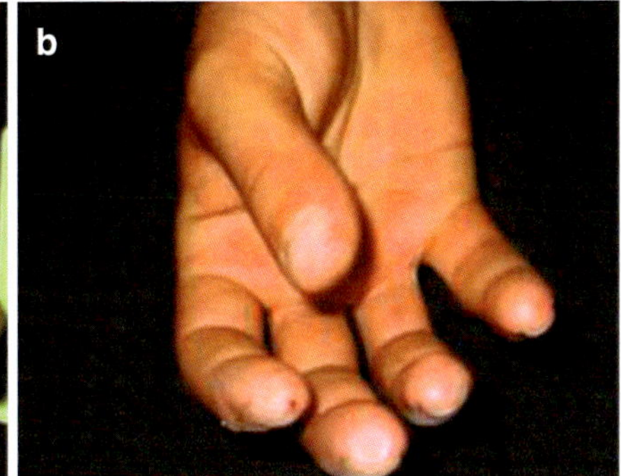

Fig. 3.14 Healing. (**a**) Digital ulcer. (**b**) Healed DU

Conclusion

In conclusion, different types of cutaneous lesions can be observed in SSc both in the upper and in the lower limbs. It is very important to classify properly cutaneous lesions in SSc because different lesions may require different treatment. The classification is also needed for the purposes of the guidelines and in order to design and interpret clinical trials.

We reviewed the existing classification of the upper limb DU and proposed the classification of the lower limb cutaneous lesions. These classifications can be very easily applied both in clinical practice and in clinical trials, and their performance requires a minimal training. However, their inter- and intra-observer variability has not been tested, and they have still to be validated in large prospective multicentre studies.

References

1. Dealey C, Lindholm C. Pressure ulcer classification. In: Romanelli M, Michael Clark M, Cherry G, Colin D, Defloor T, editors. Science and practice of pressure ulcer management. London: Springer; 2006. p. 37–41.
2. Steen V, Denton CP, Pope JE, Matucci-Cerinic M. Digital ulcers: overt vascular disease in systemic sclerosis. Rheumatology (Oxford). 2009;48(Suppl 3):S9–24.
3. Galuccio F, Matucci-Cerinic M. Two faces of the same coin: Raynaud phenomenon and digital ulcers in systemic sclerosis. Autoimmun Rev. 2011;10(5):241–3.
4. Park JH, Sung YK, Bae SC, Song SY, Seo HS. Jun JB Ulnar artery vasculopathy in systemic sclerosis. Rheumatol Int. 2009;29(9):1081–6.
5. Amanzi L, Braschi F, Fiori G, Galluccio F, Miniati I, Guiducci S, et al. Digital ulcers in scleroderma: staging, characteristics and subsetting through observation of 1614 digital lesions. Rheumatology (Oxford). 2010;49:1374–82.
6. Maeda M, Matubara K, Hirano H, Watabe H, Ichiki Y, Mori S. Pitting scars in progressive systemic sclerosis. Dermatology. 1993;187(2):104–8.
7. Dissemond J, Körber A, Grabbe S. Differential diagnoses in leg ulcers. J Dtsch Dermatol Ges. 2006;4:627–34.
8. Tuffanelli DL, Winkelmann RK. Systemic scleroderma: a clinical study of 727 cases. Arch Dermatol. 1961;84:359–7.
9. Youssef P, Brama T, Englert H, Bertouch J. Limited scleroderma is associated with increased prevalence of macrovascular disease. J Rheumatol. 1995;22:469–72.
10. Hafner J, Schneider E, Burg G, Cassina PC. Management of leg ulcers in patients with rheumatoid arthritis or systemic sclerosis: the importance of concomitant arterial and venous disease. J Vasc Surg. 2000;32:322–9.
11. Shanmugam VK, Price P, Attinger CE, Steen VD. Lower extremity ulcers in systemic sclerosis: features and response to therapy. Int J Rheumatol. 2010;2010:747946.
12. Blagojevic J, Piemonte G, Benelli L, Braschi F, Fiori G, Bartoli F, et al. Assessment, definition and classification of lower limb ulcers in systemic sclerosis: a challenge for the rheumatologist. J Rheumatol. 2016;43(3):592–8.
13. Silva I, Almeida J, Vasconcelos C. A PRISMA-driven systematic review for predictive risk factors of digital ulcers in systemic sclerosis patients. Autoimmun Rev. 2015;142:140–52.
14. Edmonds ME, Foster AV. Diabetic foot ulcers. BMJ. 2006;18(332):407–10.
15. Mekkes JR, Loots MA, Van Der Wal AC, Bos JD. Causes, investigation and treatment of leg ulceration. Br J Dermatol. 2003;148:388–401.
16. Grey JE, Harding KG, Enoch S. Venous and arterial leg ulcers. BMJ. 2006;11:347–50.
17. Hettema ME. Bootsma H, Kallenberg CG Macrovascular disease and atherosclerosis in SSc. Rheumatology (Oxford). 2008;47:578–83.

Pathobiology of Digital Ulcers

Vascular Mechanisms of Systemic Sclerosis

4

Janine Schniering, Britta Maurer, and Oliver Distler

Introduction

Systemic sclerosis (SSc) is a systemic autoimmune connective tissue disease in which the combination of microvasculopathy, inflammation, and autoimmunity leads to fibrosis of the skin and the internal organs. Microvascular abnormalities are one of the earliest hallmarks of the disease, clinically manifesting in Raynaud's phenomenon and ischemic complications including digital ulcers [1, 2], which contribute substantially to the high disease morbidity of SSc (Fig. 4.1a) [3, 4].

In SSc, microvascular injury is characterized by a progressive reduction of capillary density, the formation of an irregular and chaotic capillary architecture (Fig. 4.1b) [5–7], and a proliferative vasculopathy with intimal hyperplasia, extracellular matrix (ECM) deposition, luminal narrowing, and finally vessel occlusion [8–10].

So far, the initiating events leading to the vascular dysfunction in SSc have not been elucidated. However, endothelial cell (EC) injury and apoptosis are regarded as one of the earliest and most central events in the initiation of SSc microvasculopathy [11, 12]. Furthermore, an impaired angiogenic and vasculogenic response were identified to be involved in the disease pathophysiology. An overview about the pathophysiologic mechanisms leading to the SSc vascular disease is illustrated in Fig. 4.2.

In the following, we will discuss the cellular and molecular key players as well as animal models of the SSc microvasculopathy. We will focus on the peripheral vascular mechanisms, whereas the mechanisms underlying pulmonary arterial hypertension (PAH) and scleroderma renal crisis are discussed elsewhere.

J. Schniering · B. Maurer · O. Distler (✉)
Department of Rheumatology, University Hospital Zurich,
Zurich, Switzerland
e-mail: oliver.distler@usz.ch

© Springer Nature Switzerland AG 2019
M. Matucci-Cerinic, C. P. Denton (eds.), *Atlas of Ulcers in Systemic Sclerosis*, https://doi.org/10.1007/978-3-319-98477-3_4

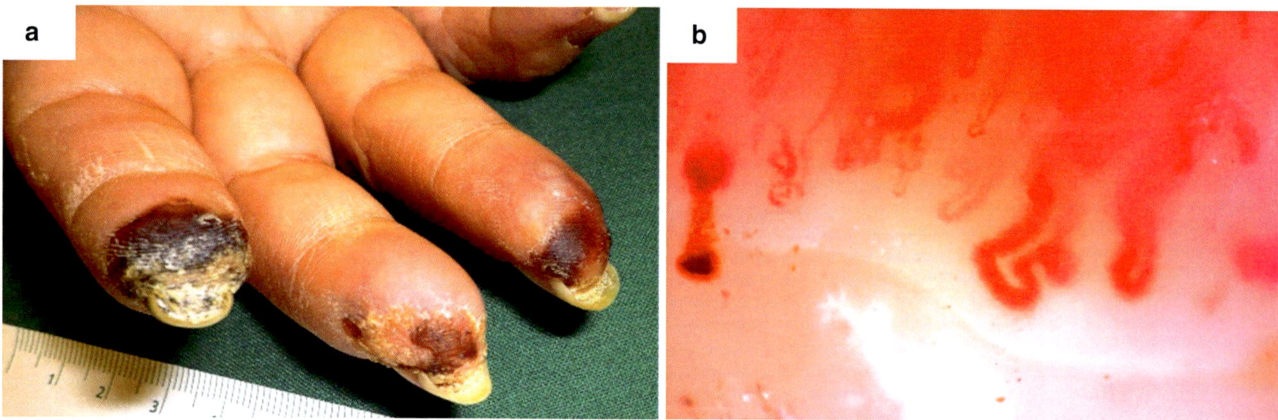

Fig. 4.1 Clinical manifestations of the SSc microvascular disease. (**a**) Fingertip ulcers with signs of necrosis. (**b**) Nailfold capillaroscopy showing the formation of irregularly shaped dilated and bushy capillaries

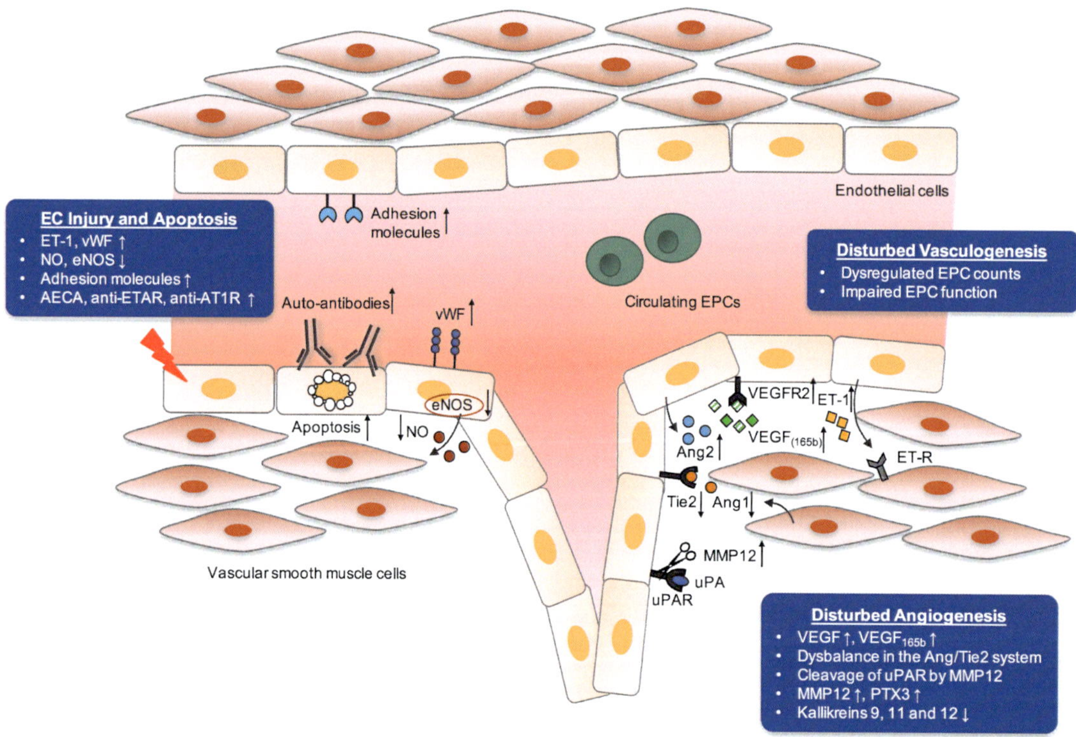

Fig. 4.2 Overview of the vascular mechanisms of the SSc microvasculopathy. This figure summarizes the molecular and cellular mechanisms of the peripheral SSc microvasculopathy (see text for explanation). AECA (anti-endothelial antibodies), Ang1/2 (angiopoietin 1/2), anti-AT1R (anti-angiotensin receptor type-1), anti-ETAR (anti-endothelin receptor type A), eNOS (endothelial nitric oxide synthase), EPC (endo-thelial progenitor cell), ET-1 (endothelin-1), ET-R (endothelin recep-tor), NO (nitric oxide), PTX3 (pentraxin 3), uPA (urokinase-type plasminogen activator), uPAR (urokinase-type plasminogen activator receptor), MMP12 (matrix metalloproteinase 12), VEGF (vascular endothelial growth factor), VEGFR2 (vascular endothelial growth fac-tor receptor 2), vWF (von Willebrand factor)

Role of the Endothelium

Apart from functioning as a barrier, the endothelium exerts major physiological effects including endocrine functions, regulation of vascular tone, platelet aggregation and leucocyte adhesion, inhibition of deposition of ECM proteins, and regulation of proliferation of vascular smooth muscle cells (VSMC) [1]. Given the pleiotropic effects, endothelial dysfunction can have severe pathological consequences.

In SSc, endothelial dysfunction is morphologically reflected by the formation of large gaps between ECs, vacuolization of EC cytoplasm, and the thickening of the capillary basement membrane [10, 13, 14]. Additionally, it manifests in increased serum levels of von Willebrand factor (vWF) and endothelin-1 (ET-1) as well as reduced levels of nitric oxide (NO) and endothelial NO synthase (eNOS) gene expression, changing the endothelial functional profile from a protective vasodilating to a vasoconstrictive cell type [1, 14]. ET-1 is a potent VSMC and fibroblast mitogen [15–17], whereas NO strongly inhibits VSMC proliferation [18]. Thus, in the presence of EC injury, the proliferation of VSMC is favored causing neointimal hyperplasia with luminal narrowing and ultimately vessel obliteration [10, 19].

Furthermore, the expression of cell adhesion molecules is significantly increased on the EC surface, facilitating the adhesion of inflammatory cells and subsequent tissue invasion [19], eventually leading to the characteristic histopathological feature of perivascular tissue infiltrates observed in SSc patients [20].

In addition to EC dysfunction, EC apoptosis is a central event in the pathogenesis of vasculopathy in SSc, which was firstly described in the University of California at Davis (UCD) lines 200/206 chicken model [12]. The triggering events causing EC cell death are not yet identified; however many possible pathogenic mechanisms are proposed including viral triggers, cytotoxic T cells, antibody-dependent cellular cytotoxicity, anti-endothelial antibodies (AECAs), and ischemia-reperfusion injury [11].

Depending on patient selection and detection techniques, AECAs can be detected in 22–86% of sera from SSc patients [21, 22]. These autoantibodies were shown to induce EC apoptosis in vitro and in vivo. Incubation of ECs with AECAs positive sera from SSc patients resulted in induction of apoptosis, whereas incubation with sera from healthy donors did not show an effect [23, 24]. In vivo confirmation was performed using the UCD-200/206 chicken model. AECA isolated from sera from UCD-200 animals were able to bind to ECs and to induce apoptosis in normal chicken embryos [25]. However, the molecular mechanism leading to EC apoptosis are widely unknown and need to be further elucidated. Sgonc et al. proposed that EC apoptosis is mediated via the FAS (CD95) pathway as evidenced by the inhibition of apoptosis induction using an anti-Fas ligand antibody [24]. In contrast, Bordron et al. reported that EC apoptosis occurs via FAS-independent pathways [23].

Underscoring the role of AECA in digital ulcers, the presence of AECA antibodies in SSc patients correlates significantly with an increase in the incidence of digital ischemia [26, 27]. However, the epitopes targeted by AECA are still unknown, and the presence of these autoantibodies is not restricted exclusively to SSc. AECA are additionally detected in other autoimmune diseases including systemic vasculitis and systemic lupus erythematosus (SLE) [28]. Currently, it is under debate whether the occurrence of AECA is an epiphenomenon associated with vascular injury or whether AECA have a pathogenic role in SSc [21, 29].

Apart from AECA, stimulating autoantibodies targeting the endothelin receptor type A (ETAR) and the angiotensin receptor type-1 (AT1R) expressed on ECs were implicated in the disease pathophysiology, especially in the development of pulmonary vasculopathy and digital ulcers, and also predicted survival [30, 31]. Becker et al. found evaluated levels of these autoantibodies in patients with SSc-PAH and connective tissue disease (CTD)-PAH as compared to other PAH types. Pathophysiological effects favoring the pathogenesis of SSc were analyzed using microvascular endothelial cells, fibroblasts, peripheral blood mononuclear cells, and IgG transfer into mice. As a smaller study could partially not reproduce some of the findings in SSc-PAH, further confirmation in other cohorts will be important [32, 33].

Angiogenesis and Vasculogenesis

By limiting the vascular supply, EC injury and apoptosis with resulting loss of capillaries are known to trigger tissue hypoxia [19]. Hypoxia is a potent inducer of vascular repair mechanisms including angiogenesis and vasculogenesis.

Angiogenesis

Angiogenesis, the formation of new blood vessels from pre-existing ones, is known to be impaired in SSc. Paradoxically to the severe reduction in the capillary density in SSc, there is an insufficient angiogenic response in SSc [7, 19, 34]. To ensure an effective angiogenesis, the expression of pro- and anti-angiogenic factors needs to be regulated strictly in a temporal and spatial manner. In SSc, this control is disturbed [19]. Vascular endothelial growth factor A (VEGF-A, hereafter referred to as VEGF), one of the key physiological pro-angiogenic factors, is drastically upregulated in different cell types of the skin from SSc patients including keratinocytes, endothelial cells, and dermal fibroblasts [35]. Additionally, the expression of its receptors, especially VEGFR2, is significantly increased on ECs in skin biopsies derived from SSc patients [2, 35]. In line with the results obtained from tissue biopsies, increased VEGF levels were also detected in sera from SSc patients compared to healthy controls [36, 37].

In addition, patients with fingertip ulcers showed increased VEGF serum levels than healthy controls. However, VEGF levels were lower as compared to patients without digital ulcerations, revealing that VEGF has a protective role against ischemic complications once a threshold serum level of VEGF is exceeded [37]. Under normal physiologic conditions, VEGF is involved in many steps of the angiogenic process by increasing vascular permeability, stimulation of EC proliferation and migration, and promotion of tube formation [7, 38, 39]. Therefore, a dysregulation of VEGF expression could have severe effects on the process of angiogenesis. Prolonged overexpression of VEGF causes an exaggerated angiogenic response with uncontrolled vessel fusion resulting in chaotic vessel architectures with giant capillaries. In addition to the overall upregulation of VEGF expression, the time kinetic of the VEGF overexpression is critical [7, 39] as a too short VEGF response results in an unstable vessel formation as well [40].

Recently, two different splice variants of VEGF were identified, $VEGF_{165}$ and $VEGF_{165}b$ possessing pro- or anti-angiogenic properties, respectively. Manetti et al. [41] showed that the elevated levels of VEGF in serum and skin of SSc patients are based on the overexpression of the anti-angiogenic $VEGF_{165b}$ isoform revealing that a switch from pro- to anti-angiogenic splice variants may be the main cause for the insufficient angiogenic response in SSc [2]. Manetti and coworkers could link this switch to the increased expression levels of transforming growth factor-beta 1 (TGF-β1) and the serine/arginine protein 55 (SrP55) VEGF splice factor [41, 42].

Recently, the angiopoietin (Ang)/Tie2 system was found to be involved in the disturbed angiogenesis in SSc. Tie2 is tyrosine kinase receptor expressed on the cell surface of ECs with Ang1 and Ang2 as the main ligands [43, 44]. Whereas Ang1 is expressed by many cell types, including pericytes, VSMCs, and fibroblasts, the expression of Ang2 seems to be restricted to ECs [45].

While Ang1 inherits vasoprotective and anti-inflammatory properties and is crucial for vessel maturation and vessel integrity, Ang2 occupies vessel-destabilizing properties and functions at a natural antagonist of Tie2 and Ang1 [46]. However, the functions of Ang2 are contextual and are regulated by VEGF [44, 47–49]. Furthermore, it was shown that VEGF induces shedding of membrane-bound Tie2. Soluble Tie2 (sTie2) can bind to Ang1 and 2 and inhibit Ang/Tie2 signaling [47].

In SSc, it was shown that Ang1 and Ang2 are differentially expressed in the sera from SSc patients with significantly decreased levels of Ang1 and increased levels of Ang2 [43]. The increased serum levels of Ang2 correlated significantly with disease severity and activity leading to the hypothesis that an altered expression of Ang1 and Ang2 might contribute to the vascular disease of SSc. Furthermore, also increased serum levels of sTie2 were detected in a sub-group of SSc patients and the elevated levels correlated with the occurrence of PAH and the frequency of microhemorrhages in nailfold capillaroscopy [50].

In line with the results obtained for serum levels of Ang2 and sTie2, Dunne et al. [45] measured increased plasma levels of these molecules. However, in contrast to Michalska-Jakubus et al. [43], they detected increased levels of Ang1. Nevertheless, taken all three studies together, there is strong evidence that an imbalance of angiopoietins and Tie2 might play a key role in the pathogenesis of the SSc microvasculopathy.

Interestingly, in dermal microvessels of SSc patients, an imbalance favoring the expression of Ang2 was observed. Additionally, the expression of membrane-bound Tie2 (mTie) was substantially reduced, since compared with healthy controls, only 5.5% vs. 90% of dermal microvessels expressed mTie2 [51]. Furthermore, in line with the results from Michalska-Jakubus et al. [43], a reduced Ang1/Ang2 ratio in patients' sera was detected, which was associated with an increase of sTie2, thus indicating that the loss of mTie2 occurred due to increased shedding. Notably, the results obtained in SSc patients were mirrored in VEGF transgenic (tg) mice [51]. In VEGF tg mice, chronically elevated levels of VEGF lead to the development of microvasculopathy and dermal fibrosis, reminiscent of SSc [52]. In contrast, nonvascular models of SSc such as the model of bleomycin-induced skin fibrosis or the TSK1 (tight skin 1) model did not show the same alterations of the Ang/Tie2 system underlining its importance for the vascular pathology. Thus, these studies suggest a complex interplay between VEGF and the Ang/Tie2 system in the pathogenesis of the SSc microvasculopathy.

In addition to VEGF and the Ang/Tie2 system, the urokinase-type plasminogen activator (uPA)-uPA receptor (uPAR) system plays an important role in the impaired angiogenesis in SSc. Activated by VEGF, uPAR is centrally involved in the angiogenic process by catalyzing the cleavage of plasminogen to plasmin, which in turn activates matrix metalloproteinases (MMPs) resulting in ECM proteolysis [53, 54]. This leads to the degradation of the basement membrane enabling EC migration and invasion during the process of angiogenesis [53]. Microvascular ECs (MVECs) derived from SSc patients show higher expression levels of uPAR on their cell surface as compared to healthy MVECs. However, in SSc uPAR functions are impaired due to MMP-12-dependent truncation of uPAR in between the binding domain of uPA [55]. Thus, the receptor loses its ability to bind uPA compromising MVECs proliferation and invasion and therefore the angiogenic process in SSc [55]. MMP-12 is constitutively overexpressed in SSc MVECS [55, 56]. Transfecting normal MVECs with MMP-12 led to similar results with loss of EC proliferation, and invasion, and disturbed capillary formation [57]. In addition to overexpression of MMP-12, MVECs express higher amounts of pentraxin 3 (PTX3), a multifunctional pattern recognition receptor suppressing fibroblast growth factor-2 (FGF-2)-dependent EC proliferation and neovascularization [58, 59]. Silencing of MMP-12 and PTX3 in SSc MVECs using small interfering RNAs (siRNAs) restored the angiogenic potential of these cells [57]. Recently, PTX3 was identified to be a useful biomarker predicting the presence and future occurrences of digital ulcerations [59]. Furthermore, downregulation of several pro-angiogenic factors, including tissue kallikreins 9, 11, and 12, is accompanied with the dysregulated angiogenic response in SSc [60].

Moreover, recently, we could show that micro-RNAs (miRNAs) might play a pivotal role in the microvasculopathy in SSc. Specifically, we could identify miR-139b as a key molecule involved in the pathogenesis of the microvascular disease in SSc [61]. MiR-139b was downregulated in SSc cultured fibroblasts and SSc skin biopsies, and this downregulation was associated with an overexpression of uPA. By inducing VSMC proliferation and inhibiting VSMC apoptosis, the increased levels of uPA contributed to the proliferative microvasculopathy characteristic for SSc in an uPAR-independent manner. These findings suggest a dual role of the uPA-uPAR system in the SSc vasculopathy, with (1) an impaired angiogenesis with decreased proliferation and migration capacity of MVECs due to the lack of functional uPAR on the cell surface of MVECs and (2) an increased VSMC proliferation and decreased apoptosis of VSMCs leading to intimal hyperplasia occurring independently of uPAR [61].

Vasculogenesis

Apart from an insufficient angiogenesis, a dysregulated vasculogenesis is an additional pathophysiologic mechanism of microvasculopathy in SSc [7]. Vasculogenesis describes the formation of new vessels from circulating precursor cells, including endothelial progenitor cells (EPCs) independent of pre-existing vessels mostly occurring during development [2]. EPCs, also termed late EPCs, are bone marrow-derived cells, which can also be detected to a lesser extent in the adult peripheral blood circulation. They can be characterized as CD14-, CD133+, CD34+, and VEGF2R+ cells [62–64]. Using this marker combination, conflicting results concerning the number of EPCs in peripheral blood from SSc patients were received. Whereas Kuwana et al. [63] detected reduced numbers of EPCs in SSc patients, Del Papa et al. [62] measured significantly increased numbers of EPCs. Subgroup analysis of the SSc patient cohort revealed a negative correlation between the EPCs counts and the disease duration [34, 62]. As the patient cohort of Kuwana et al. was mainly composed of late-stage SSc patients, the discrepancy observed between both studies may be referred to the diseases duration of the selected SSc patients [62]. In line with the results from Del Papa and coworkers, Avouac et al. [65] also measured increased circulating EPCs counts in SSc, proposing an increased mobilization of these cells from the bone marrow. Additionally, they found a positive correlation between low EPC numbers and diseases severity as well as the past occurrence and the presence of digital ulcers, suggesting an increased homing of EPCs in later diseases stages [65]. However, recently further conflicting results were reported by two additional studies [66, 67]. They detected significantly decreased circulating EPCs counts also in SSc patients with early disease stages.

These contradictory results might be based on the different methodologies used to analyze EPCs, the use of different combinations of surface markers for EPC characterization, and differences in the subsets of patients, medications, and disease durations between the study cohorts [34, 66–68].

In contrast to the conflicting results obtained for the cell numbers of EPCs, consistent results were reported for the functional defects of EPCs in the peripheral blood as well as bone marrow from SSc patients. It was found that the potential of SSc EPCs to differentiate to mature ECs is impaired [63]. Recently, Kuwana and Okazaki reported that the neovascularization capacity of SSc EPCs is affected in vivo as well [69]. Tumors from mice that received transplants of SSc-derived CD133+ cells showed fewer vessel formations with incorporation of human EPC-derived mature endothelial cells as compared to tumors from mice receiving transplants of CD133+ cells from healthy controls [69].

So far, the pathophysiologic mechanisms leading to the impaired EPC functions and numbers have not been fully elucidated. Recently, Zhu et al. [67] proposed that autoantibody-induced EPC apoptosis might be a potential cause. They could demonstrate that incubation of EPCs with SSc sera induced EPC apoptosis. Since the depletion of the IgG fractions in the sera prevented the apoptosis of EPC, these results indicate that autoantibodies might be involved in this process.

In addition, we found a link between EC apoptosis and reduced numbers of circulating angiogenic cells (CACs) [2, 70]. CACs, also termed as early EPCs, are a subpopulation of EPCs and are regarded as transdifferentiated CD14+ monocytes acquiring EC characteristics under defined culture conditions [34, 71]. CACs are strong promotors of the angiogenic response by inducing migration and sprouting of ECs without the capacity of forming blood vessels [72]. We could show that CACs phagocytize microparticles derived from apoptotic ECs leading to the initiation of the apoptotic cascade in this EPC subtype via sphingomyelinase-/ceramide-dependent pathways [70].

In conclusion, functional impairment as well as disturbed EPC counts might play a critical role in the SSc microvascular disease. However, EPC counts in SSc patients are still unresolved, and the underlying mechanisms leading to the impaired EPC numbers and functions remain enigmatic.

Animal Models of Microvasculopathy

To study the molecular basis of the SSc microvasculopathy and to serve as platforms for therapeutic proof of concept-studies, animal models reflecting the characteristic microvascular features of SSc are of outmost importance. An overview of the existing vascular SSc models is depicted in Table 4.1.

Table 4.1 SSc animal models of vasculopathy

Animal model	EC apoptosis	Peripheral vasculopathy		Visceral vasculopathy		References
		Destructive	Proliferative	Destructive	Proliferative	
UCD 200/206	+	+	−	+	−	[12, 72–75]
Fli-1−/−	−	+	−	−	−	[78, 81]
VEGF tg	−	−	+	−	−	[51, 88]
Modified Scl GVHD	−	−	+	−	+	[85]
uPAR −/−	+	+	−	−	−	[87]
TβRIIΔk-fib	+	−	−	+	+	[89–92]
Fra-2 tg	+	+	−	+	+	[94–98]

This table summarizes the key features of the SSc microvasculopathy and their representation by the vascular SSc animal models: University of California at Davis lines 200/206 chickens (UCD 200/206), Friend leukemia integration-1-deficient mice (Fli-1−/−), vascular endothelial growth factor transgenic mice (VEGF tg), modified sclerodermatous graft-versus-host disease mice (modified Scl GVHD), urokinase-type plasminogen activator receptor deficient mice (uPAR −/−) mice, fibroblasts expressing kinase-deficient type II transforming growth factor-beta receptor transgenic mice (TβRIIΔk-fib), fos-related antigen 2 transgenic mice (Fra-2 tg)

UCD-200/206 Chickens

UCD-200/206 chickens spontaneously develop inherited scleroderma covering the full spectrum of the SSc disease symptoms, including fibrosis of the skin and visceral organs, the presence of autoantibodies, and perivascular mononuclear infiltrates as well as obliterative vasculopathy [73–75]. These chickens develop the first symptoms 1 to 2 weeks post-hatch starting with the induction of EC apoptosis by AECA followed by the occurrence of perivascular infiltrates and the development of skin and organ fibrosis [12, 76]. Sgonc and coworkers showed that the primary event of the vascular disease in these chickens is AECA-dependent EC apoptosis resulting in severe capillary loss and chronic ischemia manifesting in necrosis of the combs and digits [12, 77].

Despite the fact that the UCD chickens display the entire hallmarks of the SSc pathophysiology, this model finds only relatively limited application in SSc research due to the clinical heterogeneity, the high costs of maintenance, the prolonged generation times, and the different genetic background as compared to humans [2]. Very recently, this model was applied to test the therapeutic efficacy of local administration of $VEGF_{121}$ bound to a fibrin matrix enabling the cell-demanded release of VEGF from the matrix, which is stopped as soon as it is no longer required. Upon $VEGF_{121}$-fibrin treatment, 79.3% of all lesions showed clinical improvement with prevention of digital ulcerations when applied early in the disease course. Simultaneously, the angiogenic response was increased reflecting in an increase microvascular density as well as increased numbers of ECs in the combs and neck lesions treated with $VEGF_{121}$-fibrin [78].

Friend Leukemia Integration-1 (Fli-1)-Deficient Mice

Fli-1 is a member of the Ets (E26 transformation-specific) transcription factor family. It is highly expressed in the endothelial cell and hematopoietic cell lineage and to a lesser extent in dermal fibroblasts [79]. Fli-1 is a negative regulator of type 1 collagen expression [80, 81]. In SSc skin biopsies, the expression of Fli-1 is significantly reduced in ECs and even undetectable in fibroblasts, and the observed downregulation correlates with the induction of collagen synthesis [81]. In order to assess the role of Fli-1 downregulation in the SSc vascular disease, Asano et al. generated conditional Fli-1 knockout mice with a deficiency of Fli-1 restricted to ECs [82]. These Fli-1 ECKO mice show severe abnormalities of the skin vasculature with arteriolar stenosis, formation of micro-aneurysms, and capillary dilation [79, 82]. In addition, vessel stability is compromised and vascular permeability is significantly increased [82] emphasizing the role of Fli-1 in the microvasculopathy observed in SSc.

Fli-1 deficiency in these mice is associated with a reduced expression of vascular endothelial cadherin (VE-cadherin), platelet/endothelial cell adhesion molecule (PECAM-1), platelet-derived growth factor (PDGF-B), and sphingosine 1 phosphate (S1P1) receptors, as well as an increased expression of MMP-9 in ECs [79, 82]. In accordance with the results in this animal model, reduced expression of VE-cadherins and PECAM-1 and increased levels of MMP-9 in ECs are also found in SSc patients revealing that this mouse model recapitulates important features of microvasculopathy in SSc and supports the hypothesis that Fli-1 is involved in the pathogenesis of the SSc vasculopathy [79].

Sclerodermatous Graft-Versus-Host Disease

The murine model of sclerodermatous graft-versus-host disease (Scl GVHD) displays important features of the SSc pathophysiology including dermal and pulmonary fibrosis, severe dermal mononuclear infiltration, and a significant upregulation of TGF-β1 and procollagen 1 mRNA levels in the dermis [83–85]. In the Scl GVHD model, lethally irradiated Balb/c mice are transplanted with B10.D2 bone marrow and spleen cells differing in minor histocompatibility antigens [84, 85]. The manifestations of the first SSc symptoms become apparent at day 21 after bone marrow transplantation [84]. However, signs of pulmonary and peripheral vasculopathy were not detectable in this model. In 2004, Ruzek and coworkers [86] introduced a modified Scl GVDH model, manifesting microvascular changes as well. In contrast to the original model, RAG-2 knockout mice lacking B and T cells are used as recipients for transfer B10.D2 spleen cells to induce the GVH SSc disease. Besides dermal and visceral fibrosis, these mice show a significant reduction in the ratio of total vessel to lumen area in skin and kidney indicating vasoconstriction. Intimal hyperplasia due to proliferation of VSMCs was identified as a major contributor to the observed vessel occlusion. Apart from luminal narrowing, these mice also show evaluated levels of ET-1 and an altered SMC morphology.

uPAR Deficient Mice

While originally constructed by Dewerchin and coworkers [87] to study the in vivo role of soluble versus receptor-bound uPA, Manetti and coworkers recently proposed uPAR-deficient mice as a novel model for SSc peripheral vasculopathy [88]. Apart from the development of dermal and lung fibrosis, these mice show a significant reduction in the dermal capillary density which was accompanied by a significant increase in EC apoptosis. However, signs of proliferative vasculopathy characterized by neointimal hyperplasia of dermal and pulmonary vessels were not detected in these knockout mice. Interestingly, uPAR expression was also significantly downregulated in skin biopsies from SSc patients revealing that inactivation of uPAR is recapitulating the SSc disease pathophysiology.

VEGF tg Mice

VEGF tg mice selectively overexpress VEGF under the control of the keratin 14 promotor in basal epidermal keratinocytes [89] leading to increased dermal levels of VEGF. As VEGF overexpression represents a key feature in the pathophysiology of the SSc vascular disease, these mice became interesting as a model of microvasculopathy in SSc. Recently, we reported that VEGF tg mice show an increase in the number of dermal microvessels as well as in the vessel wall thickness characteristic for a proliferative vasculopathy [52]. However, these changes were more pronounced in heterozygous than homozygous transgenic mice, suggesting that the pro-angiogenic effects of VEGF are dose-dependent and too high levels of VEGF, as in SSc patients, could have adverse effects. Notably, apart from vascular changes, homozygous VEGF overexpression led to the spontaneous development of skin fibrosis with dermal thickening and collagen accumulation [52].

TβRIIΔk-fib Mice

TβRIIΔk-fib mice selectively overexpress the kinase-deficient type II transforming growth factor-beta (TGF-β) receptor on fibroblasts under a pro-α2(I) collagen promoter [90, 91]. This overexpression leads to a ligand-dependent upregulation of TGF-β signaling inducing the spontaneous development of dermal and pulmonary fibrosis. These mice additionally show macrovascular changes with aortic adventitial fibrosis, VSMC attenuation, and altered vasoreactivity of isolated aortic rings [92]. Besides the macrovascular changes, these mice develop a constitutive pulmonary vasculopathy with neointimal hyperplasia, perivascular infiltration and collagen deposition, and a mild elevation in right ventricular systolic pressure (RVSP), resembling the chronic hypoxia model of PAH [93]. However, they do not show an endothelial phenotype characteristic for human PAH. Administrating the VEGF receptor tyrosine kinase inhibitor SU5416 aggravates the observed pulmonary vasculopathy with PAH, reflected in the obliteration of small and medium-sized pulmonary vessel and the upregulation of luminal cell proliferation. Furthermore, treatment with SU5416 induces EC apoptosis, which was followed by an apoptosis-resistant EC proliferation and a marked raise of the RVSP, and the development of a right ventricular hyper-

trophy, closely resembling human PAH [93, 94]. The manifestation of peripheral microvascular changes has not been reported yet. However, this mouse model represents a promising animal model for the SSc pulmonary vasculopathy and PAH.

Fos-Related Antigen 2 (Fra-2) tg Mice

Fra-2 tg mice, generated by Eferl and coworkers [95], ectopically express the transcription factor Fra-2 of the activator protein-1 (AP-1) family under the control of the ubiquitous major histocompatibility complex class I antigen H2Kb promotor. Fra-2 mice simultaneously develop microvascular alterations as well as dermal and visceral fibrosis closely resembling the pathophysiologic characteristics of human SSc [96].

Fra-2 tg mice display prominent features of the SSc vascular disease, including increased EC apoptosis, progressive vessel loss, and a severe proliferative pulmonary vasculopathy resembling PAH [96–98].

Starting at 12 weeks of age, Fra-2 tg mice show a significant reduction in the capillary density which is paralleled by the development of skin fibrosis characterized by a time-dependent increase in the dermal thickness reaching its peak at week 16 [97]. Of note, the manifestation of the peripheral vasculopathy in these mice is preceded by the appearance of EC apoptosis [97]. This is in accordance with the results obtained in SSc patients and in the UCD-200/206 chicken model, underscoring the hypothesis that EC apoptosis is one of the initiating events in the SSc vasculopathy [96].

Further emphasizing the role of the Fra-2 in the pathophysiology of microvasculopathy, Fra-2 is overexpressed in ECs and VSMCS in the skin from Fra-2 tg mice and SSc patients [97].

In addition to the pronounced peripheral vasculopathy, Fra-2 tg mice display a severe proliferative pulmonary vasculopathy with obliteration of pulmonary arteries characterized by a marked formation of neointima due to proliferation of VSMCS and especially myofibroblasts [95, 98]. Interestingly, these vascular alterations start to manifest at week 12 and precede the development of pulmonary fibrosis by 2 to 3 weeks [95, 98]. In contrast to the peripheral vasculopathy, elevated levels of EC apoptosis were not detected in the lungs [96]. Typical for PAH, this severe pulmonary vasculopathy was accompanied with an increased RVSP in Fra-2 tg mice as compared to wildtype littermates [99]. Manifesting at week 8, this raise in the RVSP steadily persisted in these mice and was not associated with an increase in the systemic arterial pressure [99].

So far, Fra-2 tg mice are the only murine SSc model displaying in a time-dependent manner the development of the destructive and proliferative vasculopathy characteristic for the human SSc microvascular disease.

Conclusion

In SSc, microvascular abnormalities become apparent at earliest diseases stages, clinically manifesting in ischemic complications including digital ulcers. Due to the high morbidity associated with these peripheral manifestations, the elucidation of the underlying molecular mechanism is of outmost importance in order to allow for the development of effective therapeutic interventions.

To date, the pathophysiologic mechanisms of the SSc vascular disease have not been fully clarified. Using in vitro and in vivo models, EC cell injury and apoptosis, an imbalance of pro- and anti-angiogenic factors, and an insufficient angiogenic and vasculogenic response have been identified as potential disease mechanisms. However, a comprehensive picture of the disease pathophysiology has not been obtained yet, and future research is needed to unravel the underlying connections.

Key Messages

- Microvascular changes are one of the earliest hallmarks of the SSc pathophysiology clinically manifesting in severe ischemic complications such as digital ulcers.
- In SSc, the destructive and proliferative vasculopathy precede the development of dermal and visceral fibrosis.
- Endothelial cell injury and apoptosis are regarded as one of the initiating events in the SSc microvasculopathy.
- Despite the severe loss of microvessels, there is an insufficient angiogenic response characterized by an imbalance between pro- and anti-angiogenic factors, as well as an insufficient vasculogenesis due to impaired EPCs functions and potentially numbers.
- To study the molecular basis of microvasculopathy in SSc, animal models, which cover distinct pathophysiologic aspects, are of outmost importance.

Acknowledgments This work was financially supported by the Swiss National Science Foundation (Grant: CRSII3_154490).

References

1. Abraham D, Distler O. How does endothelial cell injury start? The role of endothelin in systemic sclerosis. Arthritis Res Ther. 2007;9(Suppl 2):S2.
2. Suliman Y, Distler O. Novel aspects in the pathophysiology of peripheral vasculopathy in systemic sclerosis. Curr Rheumatol Rev. 2014;9:237–44.
3. Guiducci S, Giacomelli R, Cerinic MM. Vascular complications of scleroderma. Autoimmun Rev. 2007;6:520–3.
4. Steen V, et al. Digital ulcers: overt vascular disease in systemic sclerosis. Rheumatology (Oxford, England). 2009;48(Suppl 3):iii19–24.
5. Cutolo M, Matucci Cerinic M. Nailfold capillaroscopy and classification criteria for systemic sclerosis. Clin Exp Rheumatol. 2007;25:663–5.
6. Cutolo M, Sulli A, Smith V. Assessing microvascular changes in systemic sclerosis diagnosis and management. Nat Rev Rheumatol. 2010;6:578–87.
7. Distler JHW, Gay S, Distler O. Angiogenesis and vasculogenesis in systemic sclerosis. Rheumatology (Oxford, England). 2006;45(Suppl 3):iii26–7.
8. D'Angelo WA, et al. Pathologic observations in systemic sclerosis (scleroderma). Am J Med. 1969;46:428–40.
9. Fleming JN, et al. Is scleroderma a vasculopathy? Curr Rheumatol Rep. 2009;11:103–10.
10. Pattanaik D, Brown M, Postlethwaite AE. Vascular involvement in systemic sclerosis (scleroderma). J Inflamm Res. 2011;4:105–25.
11. Kahaleh B. The microvascular endothelium in scleroderma. Rheumatology (Oxford, England). 2008;47(Suppl 5):v14–5.
12. Sgonc R, et al. Endothelial cell apoptosis is a primary pathogenetic event underlying skin lesions in avian and human scleroderma. J Clin Invest. 1996;98:785–92.
13. Fleischmajer R, et al. Skin capillary changes in early systemic sclerodermaelectron microscopy and "in vitro" autoradiography with tritiated thymidine. Arch Dermatol. 1976;112:1553–7.
14. Kahaleh MB. Vascular involvement in systemic sclerosis (SSc). Clin Exp Rheumatol. 2004;22:S19–23.
15. Alberts GF, et al. Constitutive endothelin-1 overexpression promotes smooth muscle cell proliferation via an external autocrine loop. J Biol Chem. 1994;269:10112–8.
16. Gallelli L, et al. Endothelin-1 induces proliferation of human lung fibroblasts and IL-11 secretion through an ETA receptor-dependent activation of map kinases. J Cell Biochem. 2005;96:858–68.
17. Piacentini L, et al. Endothelin-1 stimulates cardiac fibroblast proliferation through activation of protein kinase C. J Mol Cell Cardiol. 2000;32:565–76.
18. Ahanchi SS, Tsihlis ND, Kibbe MR. The role of nitric oxide in the pathophysiology of intimal hyperplasia. J Vasc Surg. 2007;45(Suppl A):A64–73.
19. Guiducci S, et al. Mechanisms of vascular damage in SSc–implications for vascular treatment strategies. Rheumatology (Oxford, England). 2008;47(Suppl 5):v18–20.
20. Varga J, Abraham D. Systemic sclerosis: a prototypic multisystem fibrotic disorder. J Clin Invest. 2007;117:557–67.
21. Mihai C, Tervaert JWC. Anti-endothelial cell antibodies in systemic sclerosis. Ann Rheum Dis. 2010;69:319–24.
22. Renaudineau Y, et al. Anti-endothelial cell antibodies in systemic sclerosis. Clin Diagn Lab Immunol. 1999;6(2):156–60.
23. Bordron A, et al. The binding of some human antiendothelial cell antibodies induces endothelial cell apoptosis. J Clin Invest. 1998;101:2029–35.
24. Sgonc R, et al. Endothelial cell apoptosis in systemic sclerosis is induced by antibody-dependent cell-mediated cytotoxicity via CD95. Arthritis Rheum. 2000;43(11):2550–62.
25. Worda M, et al. In vivo analysis of the apoptosis-inducing effect of anti-endothelial cell antibodies in systemic sclerosis by the chorionallantoic membrane assay. Arthritis Rheum. 2003;48:2605–14.
26. Negi VS, et al. Antiendothelial cell antibodies in scleroderma correlate with severe digital ischemia and pulmonary arterial hypertension. J Rheumatol. 1998;25:462–6.
27. Pignone A, et al. Anti-endothelial cell antibodies in systemic sclerosis: significant association with vascular involvement and alveolocapillary impairment. Clin Exp Rheumatol. 1998;16:527–32.
28. Belizna C, Tervaert JW. Specificity, pathogenecity, and clinical value of antiendothelial cell antibodies. Semin Arthritis Rheum. 1997;27:98–109.
29. Belizna C, et al. Antiendothelial cell antibodies in vasculitis and connective tissue disease. Ann Rheum Dis. 2006;65:1545–50.

30. Becker MO, et al. Vascular receptor autoantibodies in pulmonary arterial hypertension associated with systemic sclerosis. Am J Respir Crit Care Med. 2014;190(7):808–17.

31. Riemekasten G, et al. Involvement of functional autoantibodies against vascular receptors in systemic sclerosis. Ann Rheum Dis. 2011;70(3):530–6.

32. Bourji KI, et al. Vascular receptor autoantibodies in pulmonary arterial hypertension. Am J Respir Crit Care Med. 2015;191(5):602.

33. Distler O. Vascular receptor autoantibodies in pulmonary arterial hypertension associated with systemic sclerosis. J Club. [cited 2017 07.03.2017]; Available from: https://www.thoracic.org/members/assemblies/assemblies/pc/journal-club/vascular-receptor-autoantibodies-in-pulmonary-arterial-hypertension-associated-with-systemic-sclerosis.php.

34. Distler JHW, et al. Endothelial progenitor cells: novel players in the pathogenesis of rheumatic diseases. Arthritis Rheum. 2009;60:3168–79.

35. Distler O, et al. Uncontrolled expression of vascular endothelial growth factor and its receptors leads to insufficient skin angiogenesis in patients with systemic sclerosis. Circ Res. 2004;95:109–16.

36. Choi J-J, et al. Elevated vascular endothelial growth factor in systemic sclerosis. J Rheumatol. 2003;30:1529–33.

37. Distler O, et al. Angiogenic and angiostatic factors in systemic sclerosis: increased levels of vascular endothelial growth factor are a feature of the earliest disease stages and are associated with the absence of fingertip ulcers. Arthritis Res. 2002;4:R11.

38. Byrne AM, Bouchier-Hayes DJ, Harmey JH. Angiogenic and cell survival functions of Vascular Endothelial Growth Factor (VEGF). J Cell Mol Med. 2005;9:777–94.

39. Müller-Ladner U, et al. Mechanisms of vascular damage in systemic sclerosis. Autoimmunity. 2009;42:587–95.

40. Dor Y, et al. Conditional switching of VEGF provides new insights into adult neovascularization and pro-angiogenic therapy. EMBO J. 2002;21:1939–47.

41. Manetti M, et al. Overexpression of VEGF165b, an inhibitory splice variant of vascular endothelial growth factor, leads to insufficient angiogenesis in patients with systemic sclerosis. Circ Res. 2011;109:e14–26.

42. Manetti M, et al. Impaired angiogenesis in systemic sclerosis: the emerging role of the antiangiogenic VEGF(165)b splice variant. Trends Cardiovasc Med. 2011;21:204–10.

43. Michalska-Jakubus M, et al. Angiopoietins-1 and -2 are differentially expressed in the sera of patients with systemic sclerosis: high angiopoietin-2 levels are associated with greater severity and higher activity of the disease. Rheumatology (Oxford). 2011;50(4):746–55.

44. Yancopoulos GD, et al. Vascular-specific growth factors and blood vessel formation. Nature. 2000;407(6801):242–8.

45. Dunne J, Keen K, Van Eeden S. Circulating angiopoietin and Tie-2 levels in systemic sclerosis. Rheumatol Int. 2013;33(2):475–84.

46. Maisonpierre PC, et al. Angiopoietin-2, a natural antagonist for Tie2 that disrupts in vivo angiogenesis. Science. 1997;277(5322):55–60.

47. Findley CM, et al. VEGF induces Tie2 shedding via a phosphoinositide 3-kinase/Akt dependent pathway to modulate Tie2 signaling. Arterioscler Thromb Vasc Biol. 2007;27(12):2619–26.

48. Lobov IB, Brooks PC, Lang RA. Angiopoietin-2 displays VEGF-dependent modulation of capillary structure and endothelial cell survival in vivo. Proc Natl Acad Sci U S A. 2002;99(17):11205–10.

49. Augustin HG, et al. Control of vascular morphogenesis and homeostasis through the angiopoietin-Tie system. Nat Rev Mol Cell Biol. 2009;10(3):165–77.

50. Noda S, et al. Serum Tie2 levels: clinical association with microangiopathies in patients with systemic sclerosis. J Eur Acad Dermatol Venereol. 2011;25(12):1476–9.

51. Moritz F, et al. Tie2 as a novel key factor of microangiopathy in systemic sclerosis. Arthritis Res Ther. 2017;19(1):105.

52. Maurer B, et al. Vascular endothelial growth factor aggravates fibrosis and vasculopathy in experimental models of systemic sclerosis. Ann Rheum Dis. 2014;73:1880–7.

53. Breuss JM, Uhrin P. VEGF-initiated angiogenesis and the uPA/uPAR system. Cell Adhes Migr. 2012;6:535–615.

54. Smith HW, Marshall CJ. Regulation of cell signalling by uPAR. Nat Rev Mol Cell Biol. 2010;11:23–36.

55. D'Alessio S, et al. Matrix metalloproteinase 12-dependent cleavage of urokinase receptor in systemic sclerosis microvascular endothelial cells results in impaired angiogenesis. Arthritis Rheum. 2004;50:3275–85.

56. Margheri F, et al. Domain 1 of the urokinase-type plasminogen activator receptor is required for its morphologic and functional, beta2 integrin-mediated connection with actin cytoskeleton in human microvascular endothelial cells: failure of association in systemic sclerosis. Arthritis Rheum. 2006;54:3926–38.

57. Margheri F, et al. Modulation of the angiogenic phenotype of normal and systemic sclerosis endothelial cells by gain-loss of function of pentraxin 3 and matrix metalloproteinase 12. Arthritis Rheum. 2010;62:2488–98.

58. Rusnati M, et al. Selective recognition of fibroblast growth factor-2 by the long pentraxin PTX3 inhibits angiogenesis. Blood. 2004;104:92–9.

59. Shirai Y, et al. Elevated levels of pentraxin 3 in systemic sclerosis: associations with vascular manifestations and defective vasculogenesis. Arthritis Rheumatol (Hoboken, NJ). 2015;67:498–507.

60. Giusti B, et al. The antiangiogenic tissue kallikrein pattern of endothelial cells in systemic sclerosis. Arthritis Rheum. 2005;52:3618–28.

61. Iwamoto N, et al. Downregulation of miR-193b in systemic sclerosis regulates the proliferative vasculopathy by urokinase-type plasminogen activator expression. Ann Rheum Dis. 2016;75(1):303–10.

62. Del Papa N, et al. Bone marrow endothelial progenitors are defective in systemic sclerosis. Arthritis Rheum. 2006;54:2605–15.

63. Kuwana M, et al. Defective vasculogenesis in systemic sclerosis. Lancet. 2004;364:603–10.

64. Brunasso AMG, Massone C. Update on the pathogenesis of Scleroderma: focus on circulating progenitor cells. F1000Research. 2016;5:F1000 Faculty Rev-723.

65. Avouac J, et al. Circulating endothelial progenitor cells in systemic sclerosis: association with disease severity. Ann Rheum Dis. 2008;67:1455–60.

66. Andrigueti FV, et al. Decreased numbers of endothelial progenitor cells in patients in the early stages of systemic sclerosis. Microvasc Res. 2015;98:82–7.

67. Zhu S, et al. Transcriptional regulation of Bim by FOXO3a and Akt mediates scleroderma serum-induced apoptosis in endothelial progenitor cells. Circulation. 2008;118:2156–65.

68. Distler JH, et al. EULAR Scleroderma Trials and Research group statement and recommendations on endothelial precursor cells. Ann Rheum Dis. 2009;68(2):163–8.

69. Kuwana M, Okazaki Y. Brief report: impaired in vivo neovascularization capacity of endothelial progenitor cells in patients with systemic sclerosis. Arthritis Rheumatol (Hoboken, NJ). 2014;66:1300–5.

70. Distler JHW, et al. Induction of apoptosis in circulating angiogenic cells by microparticles. Arthritis Rheum. 2011;63:2067–77.

71. Rehman J, et al. Peripheral blood "endothelial progenitor cells" are derived from monocyte/macrophages and secrete angiogenic growth factors. Circulation. 2003;107:1164–9.

72. Mukai N, et al. A comparison of the tube forming potentials of early and late endothelial progenitor cells. Exp Cell Res. 2008;314:430–40.

73. Gershwin ME, et al. Characterization of a spontaneous disease of white leghorn chickens resembling progressive systemic sclerosis (scleroderma). J Exp Med. 1981;153:1640–59.

74. van de Water J, Gershwin ME. Animal model of human disease. Avian scleroderma. An inherited fibrotic disease of white Leghorn chickens resembling progressive systemic sclerosis. Am J Pathol. 1985;120:478–82.

75. van de Water J, et al. Identification of T cells in early dermal lymphocytic infiltrates in avian scleroderma. Arthritis Rheum. 1989;32:1031–40.

76. Nguyen VA, et al. Endothelial injury in internal organs of University of California at Davis line 200 (UCD 200) chickens, an animal model for systemic sclerosis (Scleroderma). J Autoimmun. 2000;14:143–9.

77. Beyer C, et al. Animal models of systemic sclerosis: prospects and limitations. Arthritis Rheum. 2010;62:2831–44.

78. Allipour Birgani S, et al. Efficient therapy of ischaemic lesions with VEGF121-fibrin in an animal model of systemic sclerosis. Ann Rheum Dis. 2016;75(7):1399–406.

79. Asano Y, Bujor AM, Trojanowska M. The impact of Fli1 deficiency on the pathogenesis of systemic sclerosis. J Dermatol Sci. 2010;59:153–62.

80. Czuwara-Ladykowska J, et al. Fli-1 inhibits collagen type I production in dermal fibroblasts via an Sp1-dependent pathway. J Biol Chem. 2001;276:20839–48.

81. Kubo M, et al. Persistent down-regulation of Fli1, a suppressor of collagen transcription, in fibrotic scleroderma skin. Am J Pathol. 2003;163:571–81.

82. Asano Y, et al. Endothelial Fli1 deficiency impairs vascular homeostasis: a role in scleroderma vasculopathy. Am J Pathol. 2010;176:1983–98.

83. Jaffee BD, Claman HN. Chronic graft-versus-host disease (GVHD) as a model for scleroderma. I. Description of model systems. Cell Immunol. 1983;77(1):1–12.

84. McCormick LL, et al. Anti-TGF-beta treatment prevents skin and lung fibrosis in murine sclerodermatous graft-versus-host disease: a model for human scleroderma. J Immunol. 1999;163(10):5693–9.

85. Zhang Y, et al. Murine sclerodermatous graft-versus-host disease, a model for human scleroderma: cutaneous cytokines, chemokines, and immune cell activation. J Immunol. 2002;168(6):3088–98.

86. Ruzek MC, et al. A modified model of graft-versus-host–induced systemic sclerosis (scleroderma) exhibits all major aspects of the human disease. Arthritis Rheum. 2004;50(4):1319–31.

87. Dewerchin M, et al. Generation and characterization of urokinase receptor-deficient mice. J Clin Invest. 1996;97(3):870–8.

88. Manetti M, et al. Inactivation of urokinase-type plasminogen activator receptor (uPAR) gene induces dermal and pulmonary fibrosis and peripheral microvasculopathy in mice: a new model of experimental scleroderma? Ann Rheum Dis. 2014;73(9):1700–9.

89. Detmar M, et al. Increased microvascular density and enhanced leukocyte rolling and adhesion in the skin of VEGF transgenic mice. J Investig Dermatol. 1998;111(1):1–6.

90. Denton CP, et al. Activation of key profibrotic mechanisms in transgenic fibroblasts expressing kinase-deficient type II Transforming growth factor-{beta} receptor (T{beta}RII{delta}k). J Biol Chem. 2005;280(16):16053–65.

91. Denton CP, et al. Fibroblast-specific expression of a kinase-deficient type II transforming growth factor beta (TGFbeta) receptor leads to paradoxical activation of TGFbeta signaling pathways with fibrosis in transgenic mice. J Biol Chem. 2003;278(27):25109–19.

92. Derrett-Smith EC, et al. Systemic vasculopathy with altered vasoreactivity in a transgenic mouse model of scleroderma. Arthritis Res Ther. 2010;12(2):R69.

93. Derrett-Smith EC, et al. Endothelial injury in a transforming growth factor β–dependent mouse model of scleroderma induces pulmonary arterial hypertension. Arthritis Rheum. 2013;65(11):2928–39.

94. Gilbane AJ, et al. Impaired bone morphogenetic protein receptor II signaling in a transforming growth factor-β–dependent mouse model of pulmonary hypertension and in systemic sclerosis. Am J Respir Crit Care Med. 2015;191(6):665–77.

95. Eferl R, et al. Development of pulmonary fibrosis through a pathway involving the transcription factor Fra-2/AP-1. Proc Natl Acad Sci. 2008;105:10525–30.

96. Maurer B, Distler JHW, Distler O. The Fra-2 transgenic mouse model of systemic sclerosis. Vasc Pharmacol. 2013;58:194–201.

97. Maurer B, et al. Transcription factor fos-related antigen-2 induces progressive peripheral vasculopathy in mice closely resembling human systemic sclerosis. Circulation. 2009;120:2367–76.

98. Maurer B, et al. Fra-2 transgenic mice as a novel model of pulmonary hypertension associated with systemic sclerosis. Ann Rheum Dis. 2012;71:1382–7.

99. Biasin V, et al. Meprin β, a novel mediator of vascular remodelling underlying pulmonary hypertension. J Pathol. 2014;233(1):7–17.

Introduction to Wound Healing and Tissue Repair

5

Sabine A. Eming

Restoration of tissue integrity and homeostasis following injury is a fundamental property of all organisms. The repair response is a dynamic, interactive response to tissue damage that involves complex interactions of different classes of resident cells and multiple infiltrating leukocyte subtypes, extracellular matrix molecules, and soluble mediators [1]. The immediate goal in repair is to achieve tissue integrity and homeostasis [2]. To achieve this goal, in most tissues the healing process follows in different organs the principle of sequential phases that overlap in time and space: hemostasis, inflammation, tissue formation, and tissue remodeling (Fig. 5.1).

In humans most organs heal with the end result of a scar that replaces the damaged tissue. Although scar formation is in principle an efficient mechanism to rapidly restore tissue integrity in most organs, it is associated with significant loss of tissue architecture and function. Ideally, wounds would heal by tissue regeneration, a process restoring tissue morphology and function. Fetal wound healing is the paradigm for scarless wound healing; however in most organs this regenerative capacity is lost postnatally. One of the few remarkable examples of postnatal tissue regeneration is the phenomenon of post-injury fingertip regeneration in early childhood [3]. Clinical reports describe that conservatively managed amputation injuries in children restore the digit contour, the fingerprint, normal sensibility, and digit function and heal with minimal scarring [4, 5]. Yet, this regenerative response is restricted to amputation within the terminal phalangeal bone. The underling molecular mechanisms for this process are unresolved.

Cellular responses to injury involve direct cell-cell and cell-matrix interactions, as well as the indirect crosstalk between different tissue resident and recruited cell populations by soluble mediators. Indeed, complex interactions between the epidermal and dermal compartment are essential. During the past decade, numerous factors have been identified that are engaged in a complex reciprocal dialogue between epidermal and dermal cells to facilitate wound repair [6]. Furthermore, more recent evidence revealed the importance and engagement of the adjacent fat layer in tissue repair and regenerative responses [7]. The sensitive balance between stimulating and inhibitory mediators between neighboring tissue compartments is crucial for achieving tissue homeostasis following injury.

In most organs tissue injury causes immediate leakage of blood constituents into the wound area as well as release of vasoactive factors resulting in the activation of the coagulation cascade. The hemostatic blood clot provides the provisional extracellular matrix (ECM) that facilitates cell adhesion and migration of invading cells. Fibrin, fibronectin, vitronectin, type III collagen, and tenascin among others are important components of the provisional ECM.

Platelets trapped into the initial matrix provide a rich source of cytokines and growth factors (e.g., platelet-derived growth factor, vascular derived growth factor, transforming growth factor-1) which bind to the ECM and together orchestrate the recruitment and activation of immune cells, endothelial cells, and fibroblasts at the wound site [8].

In addition to platelets also polymorphonuclear leukocytes (neutrophils) are entrapped in the clot releasing a wide spectrum of factors and chemoattractants that initiate and amplify the inflammatory phase. Neutrophils are essential effectors of host defense; they initiate the debridement of devitalized tissue and attack infectious agents. To perform this task, they release a variety of highly active antimicrobial substances (reactive oxygen species, eicosanoids) and proteases (elastase, cathepsin G, proteinase 3). Uncontrolled release of these factors can cause severe damage to the tissues of the host [9].

The function of this early inflammatory phase is not limited to combat invading microbes but also to promote the recruit-

S. A. Eming
Dermatology, University of Cologne, Cologne, Germany
e-mail: sabine.eming@uni-koeln.de

© Springer Nature Switzerland AG 2019
M. Matucci-Cerinic, C. P. Denton (eds.), *Atlas of Ulcers in Systemic Sclerosis*, https://doi.org/10.1007/978-3-319-98477-3_5

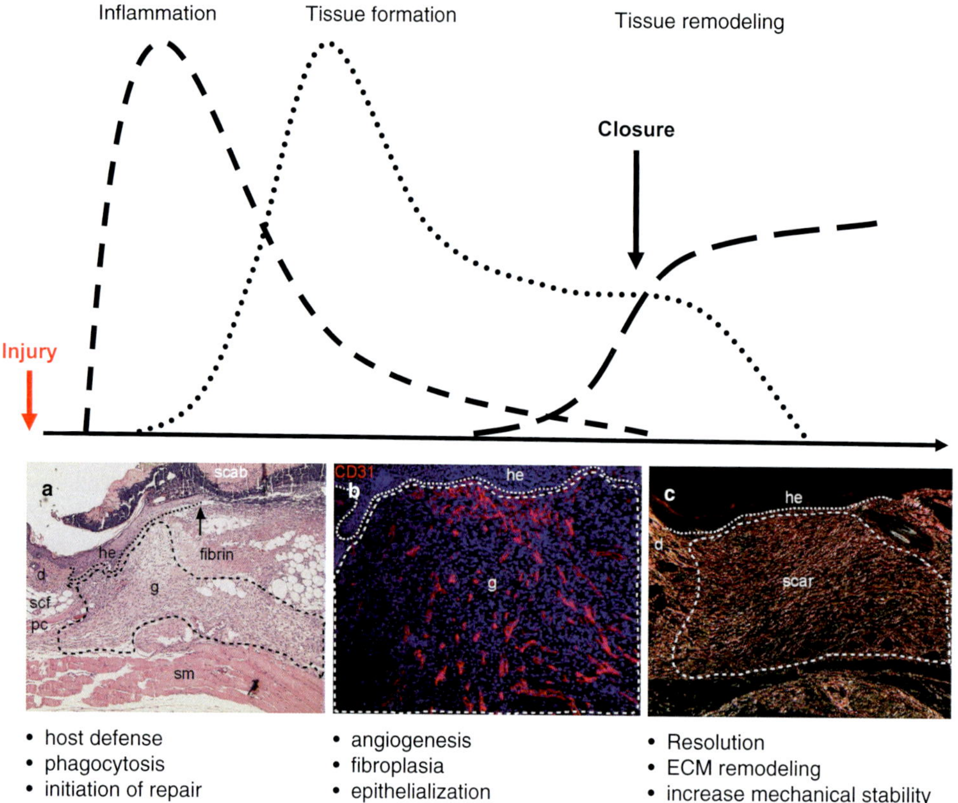

Fig. 5.1 Sequential phases of the healing response: hemostasis, inflammation, tissue formation and tissue remodeling

ment and activation of blood monocytes at the wound site. As monocytes extravasate from the blood vessel, they become activated and differentiate into wound macrophages [10]. This activation process implies major changes in macrophage gene expression which is fundamental to execute multiple functions at the wound site including debridement, induction of tissue growth, and resolution of inflammation [11, 12]. Recent evidence showed that beyond local environmental factors, macrophage functional plasticity is regulated at different levels including ontogeny and epigenetic changes [13].

During the phase of tissue formation, newly formed granulation tissue, consisting of macrophages, endothelial cells, and myofibroblasts, begins to cover and fill the wound area to restore tissue integrity. Fibroblasts differentiate into myofibroblasts, a critical process in the replacement of the provisional ECM in a collagenous matrix [14]. The spatiotemporal regulation of acquisition and maintenance of the myofibroblast phenotype is critical for the balance in ECM homeostasis and the ultimate outcome of the healing response. Biochemical and mechanical factors are fundamental in controlling myofibroblast function [15]. In parallel to granulation tissue maturation, epithelial cells at the wound edge are activated and undergo marked phenotypic and functional alterations, assuring epithelialization of the wound bed [6]. After completion of epithelialization, further remodeling of the ECM is critical for final progression into the healing state.

Phases of repair must occur in a proper sequence for optimal wound healing. Multiple systemic diseases and local factors can inhibit mechanisms of normal wound repair, which may lead to non-healing wounds. The non-healing wound is a result of an impairment in one or more of the healing mechanisms [16].

It is essential to consider which aspect of wound healing biology has been altered when analyzing a chronic non-healing wound. For example, disturbances in inflammation will interfere with all subsequent wound healing processes. Therefore, increased or impaired inflammation may manifest itself as inadequate angiogenesis, mesenchymal cell chemotaxis and proliferation, epithelialization, wound contraction, collagen synthesis, and remodeling.

The factors that lead to impaired healing can be classified as systemic and local factors. Local factors include necrotic tissue, senescent cells, bacterial components, local toxins, mechanical irritation, growth factor deficiency, increased proteolytic activity, and inadequate blood supply [16]. Systemic or constitutional factors are characterized by underlying internal conditions and/or diseases, including connective tissue diseases, vasculitis, age, and therapeutic interventions such as immunosuppressant drugs [17, 18]. When a therapeutic regime is discussed, each of these factors has to be critically considered, and an accurate diagnosis of the factors impairing healing is a prerequisite for the successful treatment of a non-healing wound (Fig. 5.2).

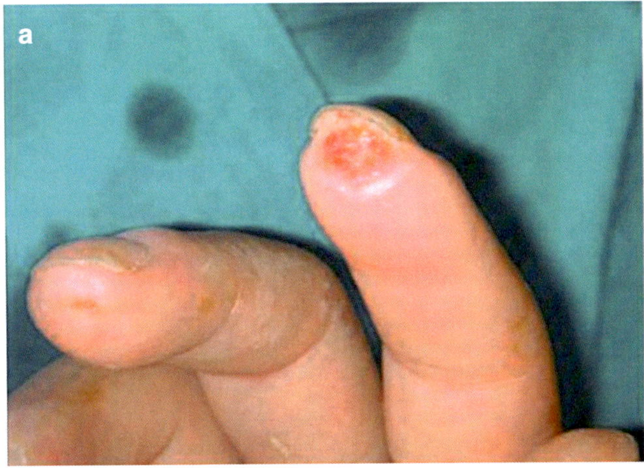

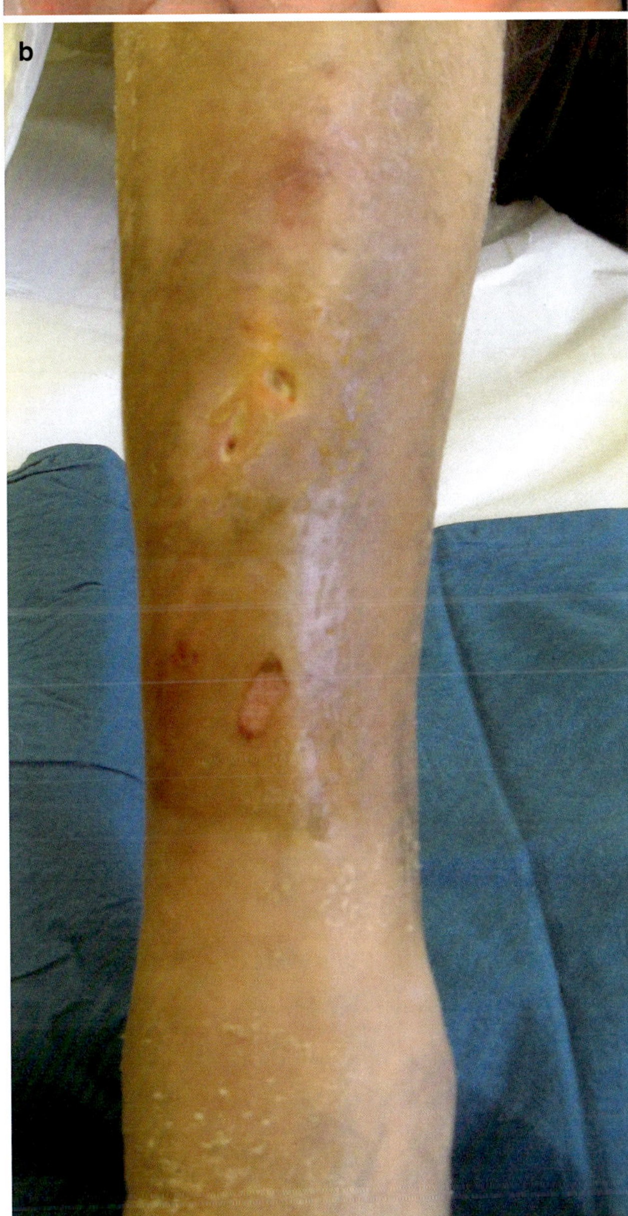

Fig. 5.2 Patient with systemic scleroderma representing (**a**) digital ulcer and (**b**) leg ulcer

References

1. Martin P. Wound healing – aiming for perfect skin regeneration. Science. 1997;276:75–81.
2. Gurtner GC, Werner S, Barrandon Y, Longaker MT. Wound repair and regeneration. Nature. 2008;453:314–21.
3. Eming SA, Hammerschmidt M, Krieg T, Roers A. Interrelation of immunity and tissue repair or regeneration. Semin Cell Dev Biol. 2009;20(5):517–27.
4. Vidal P, Dickson MG. Regeneration of the distal phalanx. J Hand Surg. 1993;18(2):230–3.
5. Lee LP, Lau PY, Chan CW. A simple and efficient treatment for fingertip injuries. J Hand Surg. 1995;20(1):63–71.
6. Werner S, Krieg T, Smola H. Keratinocyte-fibroblast interactions in wound healing. J Invest Dermatol. 2007;127(5):998–1008.
7. Rivera-Gonzalez G, Shook B, Horsley V. Adipocytes in skin health and disease. Cold Spring Harb Perspect Med. 2014;4(3):a015271.
8. Deppermann C, Cherpokova D, Nurden P, Schulz JN, et al. Gray platelet syndrome and defective thrombo-inflammation in Nbeal2-deficient mice. J Clin Invest. 2013;123:3331. pii: 69210.
9. Martin P, Leibovich SJ. Inflammatory cells during wound repair: the good, the bad and the ugly. Trends Cell Biol. 2005;15(11):599–607.
10. Lucas T, Waisman A, Ranjan R, Roes J, Krieg T, Müller W, Roers A, Eming SA. Differential roles of macrophages in diverse phases of skin repair. J Immunol. 2010;184(7):3964–77.
11. Willenborg S, Lucas T, van Loo G, Knipper J, Krieg T, Haase I, Brachvogel B, Hammerschmidt M, Nagy A, Ferrara N, Pasparakis M, Eming SA. CCR2 recruits an inflammatory macrophage subpopulation critical for angiogenesis in tissue repair. Blood. 2012;120:613–25.
12. Eming SA, Wynn TA, Martin P. Inflammation and metabolism in tissue repair and regeneration. Science. 2017;356(6342):1026–30.
13. Gomez Perdiguero E, Klapproth K, Schulz C, Busch K, et al. Tissue-resident macrophages originate from yolk-sac-derived erythro-myeloid progenitors. Nature. 2015;518(7540):547–51.
14. Tomasek JJ, Gabbiani G, Hinz B, Chaponnier C, Brown RA. Myofibroblasts and mechano-regulation of connective tissue remodelling. Nat Rev Mol Cell Biol. 2002;3(5):349–63.
15. Eckes B, Krieg T. Regulation of connective tissue homeostasis in the skin by mechanical forces. Clin Exp Rheumatol. 2004;22(3 Suppl 33):S73–6.
16. Eming SA, Martin P, Tomic-Canic M. Wound repair and regeneration: mechanisms, signaling, and translation. Sci Transl Med. 2014;6(265):265sr6.
17. Gabrielli A, Avvedimento EV, Krieg T. Scleroderma. N Engl J Med. 2009;360(19):1989–2003.
18. Denton CP, Khanna D. Systemic sclerosis. Lancet. 2017;S0140-6736(17)30933–9.

Part III

Microvascular Modifications and Ulcers

Raynaud's Phenomenon and Ulcers

6

Michael Hughes, Marina E. Anderson,
and Ariane L. Herrick

Introduction

Raynaud's phenomenon (RP) is a common vasospastic condition which manifests as an episodic colour change of the extremities (fingers and toes) in response to cold exposure and/or emotional stress. Other vascular beds can also be affected by attacks of RP including the lips, nose, ears and nipples. The skin colour (physiological rationale in parentheses) progresses from pallor (deoxygenation) to blue (cyanosis) and finally red (reactive hyperaemia). An example of an attack of RP is presented in Fig. 6.1. The hyperaemic phase can be associated with significant pain and discomfort. Patients may report mono- or biphasic colour change during attacks of RP. Symptoms usually resolve promptly (often within minutes) after rewarming. Although many individuals report sensitivity to the cold, in RP there must be an associated colour change.

The majority of patients with RP will have primary (idiopathic) Raynaud's phenomenon (PRP) in which vasospastic episodes are completely reversible and therefore are not associated with irreversible ischaemic tissue damage (e.g. digital pitting and ulcers). However RP can also occur due to an underlying aetiology (secondary RP; SRP) as presented in Table 6.1. RP is common in patients with autoimmune connective tissue diseases (CTD) and is often the presenting feature in systemic sclerosis (SSc) and therefore provides a window of opportunity (not to be missed) for early diagnosis [1–3].

Irrespective of the underlying aetiology, RP can be associated with significant morbidity. In an international online survey which included 443 responses from subjects with self-reported RP (originating from 15 countries), the majority of subjects with both PRP and SRP reported making at least one life adjustment due to RP (87% and 71%, respectively) [4]. Furthermore, the current perceived quality of life (where 10 was the best imaginable) with RP was impaired in both PRP and SRP (6.5 and 5.2, respectively). In patients with SSc, RP is responsible for much of the pain and disability associated with the disease. In a Canadian national survey which included 464 individuals with SSc, RP was the second highest-ranked symptom (out of 59) in terms of frequency and moderate to severe impact on the activities of daily living [5].

M. Hughes (✉)
Centre for Musculoskeletal Research, The University of
Manchester, Salford Royal NHS Foundation Trust, Manchester
Academic Health Science Centre, Manchester, UK
e-mail: michael.hughes-6@postgrad.manchester.ac.uk

M. E. Anderson
Institute of Ageing and Chronic Disease, University of Liverpool
and Aintree University Hospital NHS Foundation Trust, Liverpool,
UK

A. L. Herrick
NIHR Manchester Musculoskeletal Biomedical Research Unit,
Central Manchester NHS Foundation Trust, Manchester Academic
Health Science Centre, Manchester, UK

© Springer Nature Switzerland AG 2019
M. Matucci-Cerinic, C. P. Denton (eds.), *Atlas of Ulcers in Systemic Sclerosis*, https://doi.org/10.1007/978-3-319-98477-3_6

Fig. 6.1 Photographs of an attack of Raynaud's phenomenon taken by a patient with systemic sclerosis. (**a**) There is whiteness (pallor of the fingertips). (**b**) Normal colour has been restored to the fingers. The time between the two photographs was approximately 16 min. (Photographs provided courtesy of Dr. Graham Dinsdale, The University of Manchester)

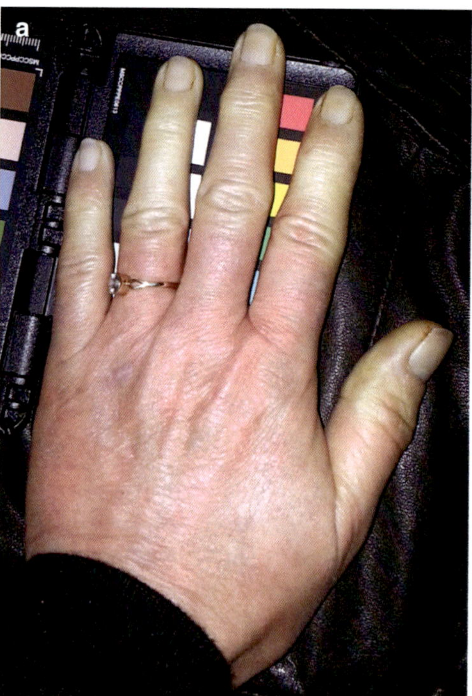
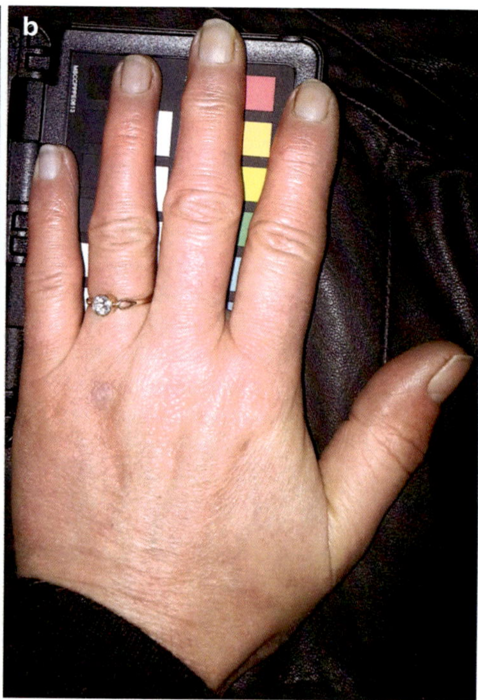

Table 6.1 The classification of Raynaud's phenomenon [105]

Primary (idiopathic) RP	Secondary RP
Vascular (usually proximal large vessel disease, often unilateral symptoms)	Compressive (e.g. cervical rib) Obstructive: noninflammatory (i.e. atherosclerosis) Inflammatory vascular disease (e.g. thromboangiitis obliterans [Buerger's disease])
Hand-arm vibration syndrome (vibration white finger)	
Autoimmune conditions	Systemic sclerosis Systemic lupus erythematosus Sjogren's syndrome Mixed connective tissue disease/overlap syndromes Undifferentiated connective tissue disease Idiopathic inflammatory myopathies
Drug-/chemical-related	Amphetamines Beta-blockers Bleomycin Cisplatin Clonidine Cyclosporine Interferons Methysergide Polyvinyl chloride
Conditions associated with increased plasma viscosity and reduced digital perfusion	Cryoglobulinaemia Cryofibrinogenaemia Paraproteinaemia Malignancy (including as a paraneoplastic phenomenon)
Other causes and associations	Carpal tunnel syndrome Frostbite Hypothyroidism

Epidemiology

The reported prevalence of RP has varied in previous studies, and this likely reflects differences in study design and geographical variations. In general, most studies have reported the prevalence of RP to be 3–5% [6]. RP is three to four times more common in females compared to males [7]. Patients with PRP (in particular females) often have an early onset and a family history (up to 50%) of RP in a first-degree relative [8, 9]. Conversely, late-onset RP (over the age of 40 years) is more likely to be SRP, and therefore the clinician must maintain a high index of suspicion.

As previously highlighted, RP often occurs in patients with autoimmune CTDs compared to the general population. For example, RP occurs in the majority (approximately 80–90%) of patients with mixed CTD [10, 11] and almost half of patients with systemic lupus erythematous [12]. In particular, RP almost invariably occurs in patients with SSc during the course of their disease. In an analysis (which included 7655 patients with SSc) from the European Scleroderma Trials and Research (EUSTAR) group, almost all (96.5%) patients had RP, with no difference in patients with limited or diffuse cutaneous subsets of the disease [13]. In patients with limited cutaneous SSc (lcSSc), there is often a long history of preceding RP (often decades) [14], whereas in diffuse cutaneous SSc (dcSSc), RP usually develops in close temporal relation (within a year before or after) of the onset of skin sclerosis [14].

Differential Diagnosis

The differential diagnosis is wide, and therefore the clinician must maintain a high index of diagnostic suspicion and perform a comprehensive clinical assessment with a key role for targeted investigations as discussed later. The conditions which can mimic RP are presented in Table 6.2 including a description of those clinical features which can help to differentiate from RP.

Table 6.2 The differential diagnosis of Raynaud's phenomenon

Condition	Description
Acrocyanosis	Presents as persistent, painless, symmetrical cyanotic colour of the hands, feet and knees. Like RP, acrocyanosis can be aggravated by cold exposure; however, unlike RP there is no pallor. Similar to RP, acrocyanosis typically occurs in young (aged 20–30 years) females. The condition can occur in isolation or secondary to a number of causes (e.g. haematological and malignant diseases)
Chilblains (primary pernio)	These present as palpable (often painful) inflammatory red/purple lesions after exposure to cold. Like RP the hands and feet (as well as the ears and nose) are typically affected and typically occurs in young females
Chilblain lupus	Characterised by painful erythematosus/purple colour change of the extremities (and often nose and ears) after cold exposure. Sporadic and familial forms are recognised. Can be associated with other cutaneous or systemic lupus features
Complex regional pain syndrome	This can mimic RP when patients present with blue/purple change of the extremities and pain
Erythromelalgia	Characterised by erythematous colour change and pain upon exposure to warmth. Can occur secondary to a wide range of secondary causes including myeloproliferative diseases
Frostbite	Cold-induced injury causing marked vasospasm resulting in tissue ischaemia, which can progress to necrosis and gangrene
Livedo reticularis and racemosa	Livedo reticularis presents as an erythematous/violaceous netlike network after cold exposure and resolves completely with warming. Livedo racemosa is characterised by an asymmetrical pattern of violaceous broken circles and does not reverse with rewarming. Whereas livedo reticularis is a normal physiological finding, livedo racemosa occurs secondary to an underlying inflammatory (e.g. SLE) or vascular disease (e.g. haematological malignancies and, in particular, antiphospholipid syndrome)
Thoracic outlet syndrome	Can present with pain, paraesthesia and discolouration of the fingers but not the feet (unlike RP)

Adapted from McMahan and Paik [106]

Pathogenesis

An understanding of the pathogenesis of RP is helpful for the clinician to understand the therapeutic rationale for the management (in particular drug therapies) of RP. Although the pathogenesis of RP will be considered under four discrete headings, it is important to be aware that these distinctions are somewhat arbitrary and that there is a complex interplay between the underlying pathogenic mechanisms. A schematic representation of the mechanisms implicated in the pathogenesis of RP is provided in Fig. 6.2.

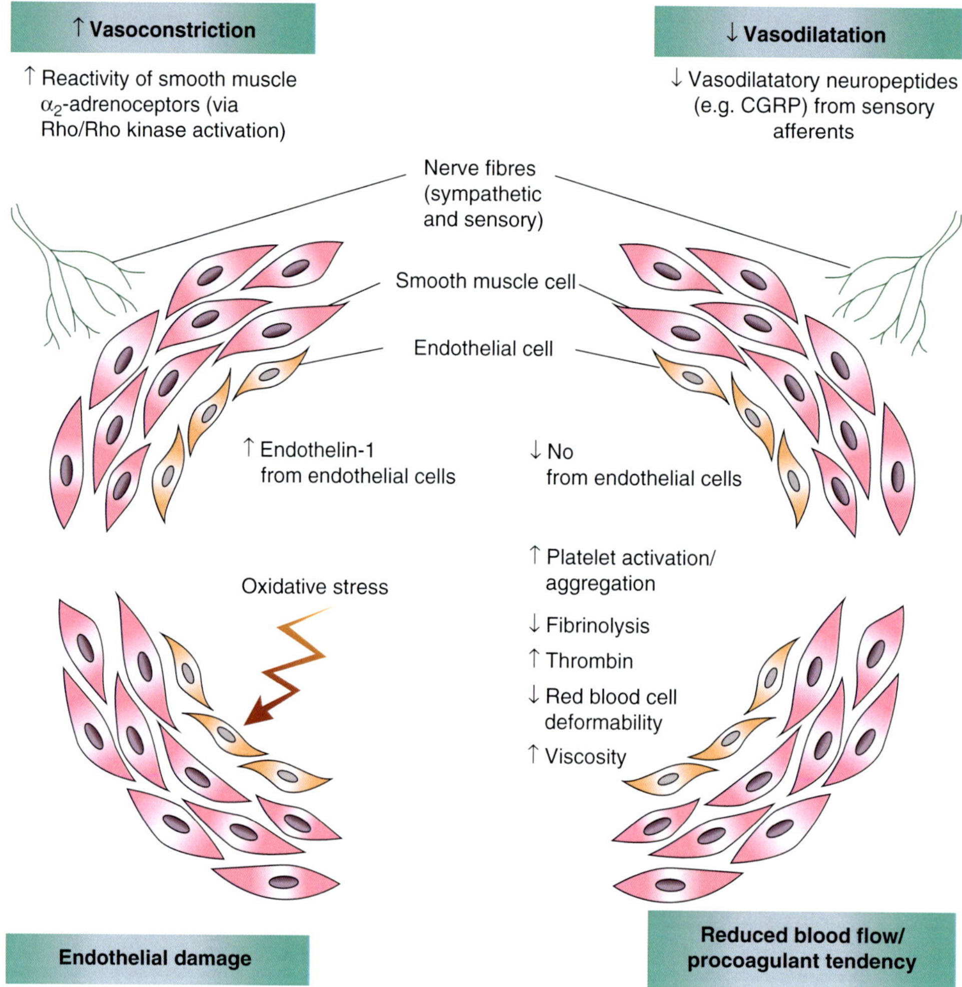

Fig. 6.2 The pathogenesis of Raynaud's phenomenon. CGRP calcitonin gene-related peptide, NO nitric oxide. (Reproduced from Herrick [24], with permission from Oxford University Press)

Vascular Abnormalities

Functional Vascular Abnormalities

In SSc, impaired endothelial-dependent and to a lesser extent endothelial-independent vasodilation have been reported in SSc [15–17]. Similar abnormalities have also been observed in patients with PRP [18]. Baseline finger blood flow in both PRP and SRP has been reported to be lower compared to healthy controls [19], with a greater sensitivity to cold exposure, in particular in SRP [20]. In patients with RP (unlike healthy controls), blood flow is reduced through both arterio-venous anastomoses and nutritional capillaries after cold exposure [19]. Furthermore, in patients with both PRP and SRP, there is marked constriction (vasospasm) of the digital arteries compared to healthy controls [21]. Vascular tone is the result of a complex interplay of vasoconstrictory and vasodilatory factors. For example, increased endothelin-1 and angiotensin II (both vasoconstrictors) have both been implicated in the pathogenesis of RP [22, 23], whereas, although the role of nitric oxide (a potent vasodilator) is complex and likely variable throughout the disease course in SSc, reduced nitric oxide from endothelial cells is likely to be a contributory mechanism in RP [24].

Structural Abnormalities

Abnormalities in both the microcirculation and the digital arteries have been well described in patients with RP. In SSc, the progressive microangiopathy that characterises the disease results in typical changes that include enlargement of capillaries with areas of avascularity that can easily be appreciated by capillaroscopy (Fig. 6.3). The nailfold capillaries are normal in patients with PRP, although slightly increased capillary dimensions compared to healthy controls have been reported [25]. Arterial disease is also well recognised in SSc, including abnormalities of the digital and ulnar arteries [26–29], the latter of which has been associated with digital ulcer (DU) disease [30, 31]. Furthermore, an increased risk of cardiovascular disease has been reported in patients with SSc [32, 33], although this remains a controversial topic requiring further research. Endothelial cell dysfunction and death [34, 35], including the presence of anti-endothelial antibodies [36, 37], have been postulated to be an early (and perhaps even initiating) mechanism in the aetiopathogenesis of SSc. In SSc, it is likely that episodes of ischaemia-reperfusion (with reduced nutritional blood flow during attacks of RP as previously described) result in local hypoxia which results in activation of inflammatory and fibrotic mechanisms.

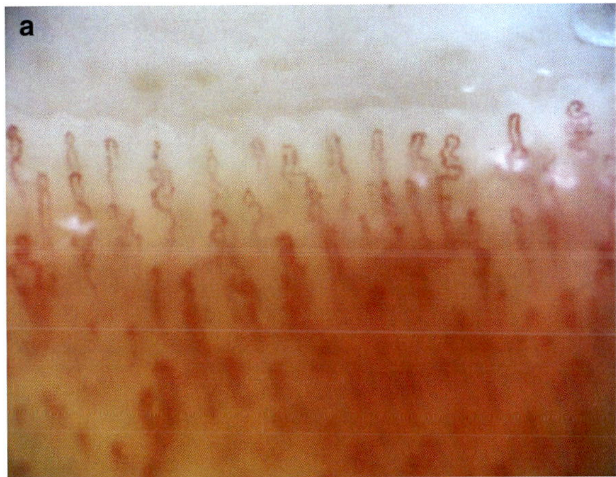

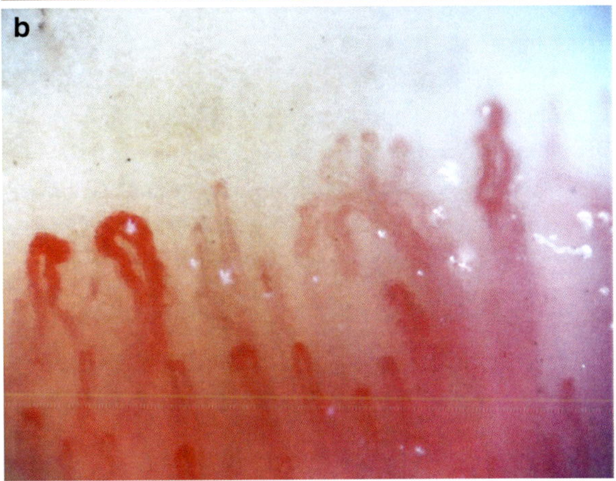

Fig. 6.3 Nailfold capillaroscopy. (**a**) Normal capillaroscopy images acquired by videocapillaroscopy. The capillaries are homogenous ('hairpin' like) in appearance, and this is reassuring in patients presenting with RP. (**b**) Abnormal nailfold capillaroscopy in a patient with SSc with capillary enlargement and areas of avascularity

Neural Abnormalities

Neural abnormalities may result in both increased vasoconstriction and reduced vasodilation in RP. In patients with PRP, and in particular SSc, reduced calcitonin gene-related peptide (which is vasodilatory) has been reported [38]. In RP, increased cold sensitivity is mediated through increased activity of smooth muscle alpha-2 adrenergic receptors [39, 40]. In particular, the alpha-2c receptor has been highly implicated in the mechanism of cold sensitivity, resulting in movement to the cell surface from the Golgi compartment [39, 40]. Vasoconstriction has been reported with increased activity of protein tyrosine kinase and tyrosine phosphorylation in both PRP- and SSc-related RP [41, 42]. Although many patients report attacks of RP resulting from stress, the role of the central nervous system in the pathogenesis of RP is little studied, and this is an area which requires future research.

Intravascular Abnormalities

Intravascular abnormalities can be both directly causative and contributory (e.g. in SSc) in the pathogenesis of RP. For example, in some conditions (Table 6.1), RP is likely directly driven by hyperviscosity and/or reduced digital microvascular perfusion (e.g. malignancy including through the presence of an associated cryoglobulin and/or paraprotein). In particular in SSc, increased platelet activation has been implicated in the pathogenesis of RP [43, 44]. Activated platelets produce a number of important molecules (e.g. vascular endothelial growth factor and transforming growth factor-β) [24], which can have a diverse range of effects on the vasculature as well as inflammatory and fibrotic pathways. The other intravascular abnormalities that have been described in the pathogenesis of RP are depicted in Fig. 6.2.

Other Factors

The importance of both genetic and hormonal factors has already been described in the epidemiology of RP. These likely have a range of important roles in the aetiopathogenesis of RP, including possibly through increased responsiveness of the alpha-2C adrenergic receptor [45].

Raynaud's Phenomenon and Digital Ulcers

Although there is a theoretical rationale to suspect that the severity of RP is associated with worse DU disease in SSc, at present there is little evidence to support such an association.

Nonetheless it seems likely that increased severity of RP attacks, including marked vasospastic disease of the digital artery, results in poor flow within the microcirculation, promoting digital ischaemia that can progress to tissue ulceration. In a multicentre study, patients with SSc living in the subtropical compared to tropical (warmer) climate were (5.4 times) more likely to develop DUs and had worse RP [46]. A key difference is that irreversible ischaemic tissue damage (e.g. DUs) is only observed in SRP and never PRP.

History and Examination

When assessing patients with RP, it is useful for the clinician to be aware of the classification criteria proposed by LeRoy and Medsger [47], which incorporate both clinical features and investigations and which have recently been revisited by Maverakis et al. [48].

It is useful for the clinician to consider the following two

> **Proposed Criteria for Primary Raynaud's Phenomenon [47]**
> Episodic attacks of acral pallor or cyanosis.
> Peripheral pulses should be strong and symmetrical.
> No evidence of digital pitting, ulceration or gangrene.
> Normal nailfold capillaries.
> Negative antinuclear antibody.
> Normal erythrocyte sedimentation rate.

questions when assessing the patient presenting with RP:

1. What is the aetiology of RP? In particular, could she/he have an autoimmune CTD?
2. What is the severity of RP? As this will dictate the need (and intensity) of treatment. For example, in patients with mild RP, symptoms may be sufficiently controlled with conservative measures alone, whereas in patients with more severe RP, drug therapies are often indicated, in particular, in the presence of digital ischaemic complications.

A full medical history should be elicited including those clinical features that could suggest the presence of an autoimmune CTD (e.g. aphthous mouth ulcers and UV photosensitivity). The impact of RP on the activities of daily living should be elicited including a history of DUs. A full systems enquiry and a drug history should be elicited with an awareness of the secondary causes of RP (Table 6.1). The patients occupational history should be explored as this may be contributory (e.g. vibratory tool use) and various occupational exposures (e.g. exposure to epoxy resins and vinyl chloride) have been associated with the development of SSc-like disorders. In addition, any potentially relevant family history should be documented, specifically of autoimmune CTDs.

A full physical examination must be completed in all patients with RP, in particular, focussing on the fingers and toes looking for signs of digital ischaemia (pitting scars and ulcers), skin sclerosis (sclerodactyly) and any visible nailfold changes. The peripheral pulses must be palpated, abnormalities of which indicate proximal (large) vessel disease. The clinician should carefully examine for associated signs which could indicate the presence of an autoimmune CTD (e.g. bibasal inspiratory crepitations that could indicate the presence of interstitial lung disease).

Investigations

The main purpose of investigating the patient presenting with Raynaud's phenomenon (RP) is to establish whether or not there is an underlying cause, i.e. to differentiate between primary (idiopathic) RP and RP secondary to an underlying disease/disorder, because this has major implications for management. Most patients with PRP may be reassured and discharged from follow-up, whereas if a diagnosis is made of, for example, a SSc-spectrum disorder, then the patient will require further investigation and long-term follow-up.

Investigations generally performed in the patient with RP are summarised below. In the patient with PRP, the full blood count, erythrocyte sedimentation rate (ESR), antinuclear antibody (ANA) and nailfold capillaroscopy will all be normal/negative (see Chap. 7). In the context of a patient in whom PRP is strongly suspected (onset of RP in the late teens or in the twenties in a patient who is otherwise well and with no abnormalities on examination), then no other investigations are required. Many clinicians, however, will in addition request a biochemical profile with thyroid function and a thoracic inlet radiograph to look for a bony cervical rib. Other investigations will depend on the clinical context. For example, if a diagnosis of a connective tissue disease is suspected, then other immunological investigations will be indicated, for example, SSc-specific autoantibodies.

> **Investigations Commonly Performed in the Patient Presenting with Raynaud's Phenomenon**
>
> *Basic set (for all patients)*
>   Full blood count
>   Erythrocyte sedimentation rate (ESR)
>   Antinuclear antibody (ANA)
>   Nailfold capillaroscopy
>
> *Other commonly requested investigations*
> Biochemical profile
> Thyroid function tests
>   Thoracic outlet radiograph (to look for a bony cervical rib)
> (Thermography – available in certain specialist centres)
>
> *Other investigations will depend on the clinical context and may include:*
> SSc-specific autoantibodies
> Complement levels
> Cryoglobulin and cryofibrinogen
> Immunoglobulins with protein electrophoresis
>   Lupus anticoagulant, anticardiolipin antibodies and anti-β2 glycoprotein 1 antibodies
>   Arterial Dopplers (if any suggestion that there may be a large [proximal] vessel component)

Nailfold capillaroscopy is discussed in Chap. 7. Normal nailfold capillaries (Fig. 6.3) are reassuring in patients with RP. Many rheumatologists will not have access to high-magnification videocapillaroscopy (the 'gold standard') or to a stereomicroscope: in this instance, an ophthalmoscope [49], dermatoscope [50–54] or USB microscope may be used (the dermatoscope or USB microscope is preferable to the ophthalmoscope because of their wider field of view). The dermatoscope is very portable being a hand-held device. A recent study suggested that dermoscopy compared favourably to videocapillaroscopy [54], although videocapillaroscopy images were more likely to be classifiable (and were graded more severely) than dermoscopy images.

Thermography (Fig. 6.4), which measures surface temperature, can help to differentiate between PRP- and SSc-related RP. Most thermography protocols incorporate a temperature challenge, usually a cold challenge [55–57]. We have found that the persistence of a temperature gradient of ≥ 1 °C along one or more fingers at a room temperature of 30 °C (Fig. 6.4) is a useful discriminator between PRP- and SSc-related RP [58, 59]. Thermography, however, requires specialist equipment and therefore at present is only available in certain specialist centres.

Although there are a number of other techniques that help to differentiate between PRP and SRP, at present these are primarily research tools [60]. These include laser Doppler imaging (using a laser-based system to measure blood flow over a defined area) and finger systolic pressure measurement [60].

Investigation for large (proximal) vessel disease If there is any question of large (proximal) vessel disease, for example, asymmetry of RP symptoms, or difficulty in detecting the peripheral pulses, then arterial Doppler ultrasound should be performed [61]. If large vessel disease is suspected, then large vessel imaging (discussed in Chap. 16) will be required.

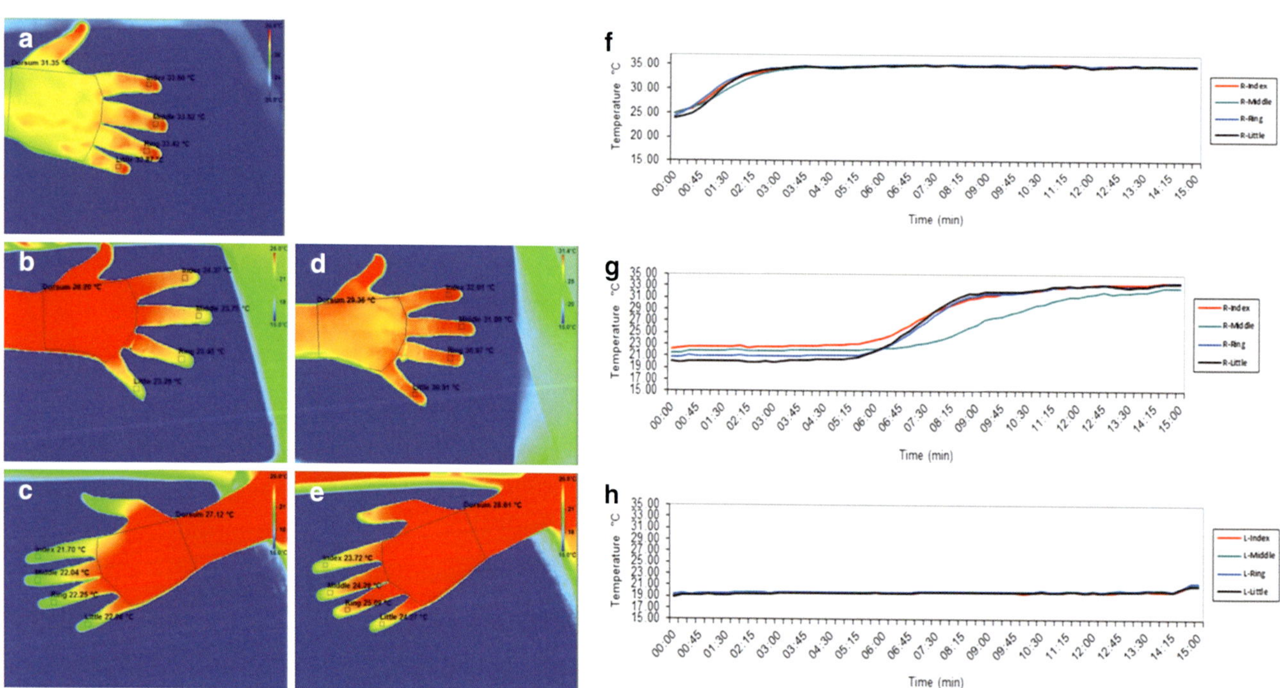

Fig. 6.4 Thermographic imaging of the hands during a dynamic temperature challenge. Left column, thermal images at 23 °C; middle column, thermal images at 30 °C; right column, rewarming curves after cold challenge. At 23 °C, the fingertips are cooler than the dorsum of the hand in patients with both primary RP (PRP) and secondary RP (SRP) (**b** and **c**), whereas, in healthy controls, the fingertips are warm (**a**). At 30 °C, unlike in PRP (**d**), there are persistent temperature gradients (fingers cooler than the dorsum of the hand) in SRP (**e**). Rewarming curves demonstrate prompt rewarming in a healthy control subject (top, **f**), whereas there is complete but delayed rewarming in a patient with PRP (middle, **g**) and no rewarming at all in a patient with SSc (bottom, **h**)

Management

The management of RP depends on its severity and on whether or not there is an underlying cause amenable to specific intervention. For example, the treatment of mild PRP, which does not progress to digital ulceration or to critical ischaemia, is very different from that of a patient with severe SSc-related RP and digital ulceration. The UK Systemic Sclerosis Study group has recently produced a 'consensus best practice pathway' for management of SSc-related digital vasculopathy [62]. This pathway includes three algorithms for management of (1) RP (relevant to RP not only due to SSc but also other causes), (2) digital ulceration in patients with SSc and (3) critical digital ischaemia in patients with SSc. Although these algorithms are all reproduced here (Figs. 6.5, 6.6, and 6.7) because they put the management of 'mild' and 'severe' RP into context, only treatment of 'uncomplicated' RP will be considered here. By 'uncomplicated' we mean RP which has not progressed to digital ulceration and/or critical ischaemia.

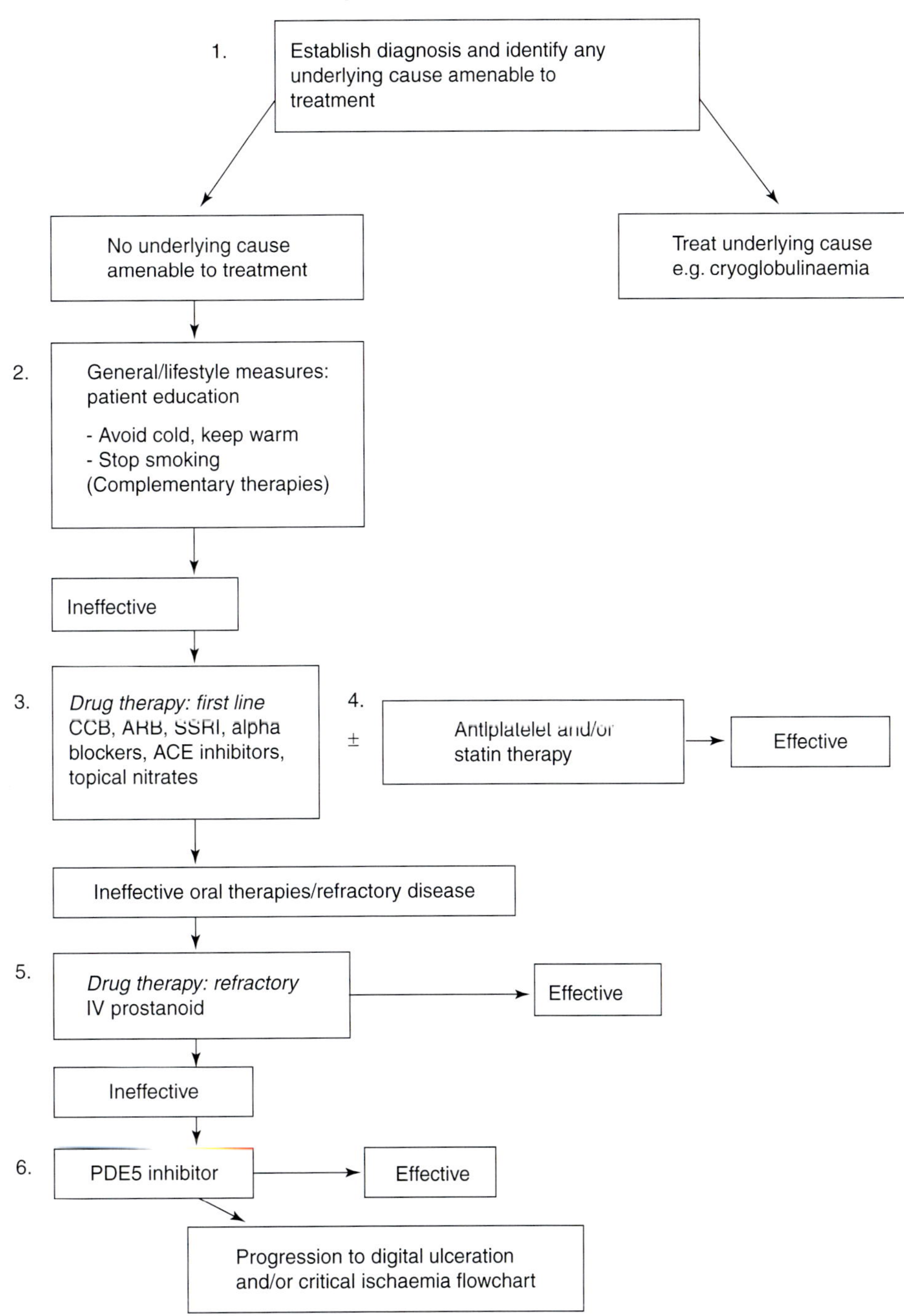

Fig. 6.5 The management of SSc-related Raynaud's phenomenon. If treatment of underlying or contributory causes is ineffective, further treatment should be commenced. Note that all patients with RP irrespective of aetiology (including patients with PRP) and who are symptomatic should be offered treatment. Clinicians who practise outside the United Kingdom might modify their approach depending on their access to drug therapies. ACE angiotensin-converting enzyme, ARB angiotensin receptor blocker, CCB calcium channel blocker, IV intravenous, PDE5 phosphodiesterase type 5, SSRI selective serotonin receptor inhibitor. (Reproduced with permission [62])

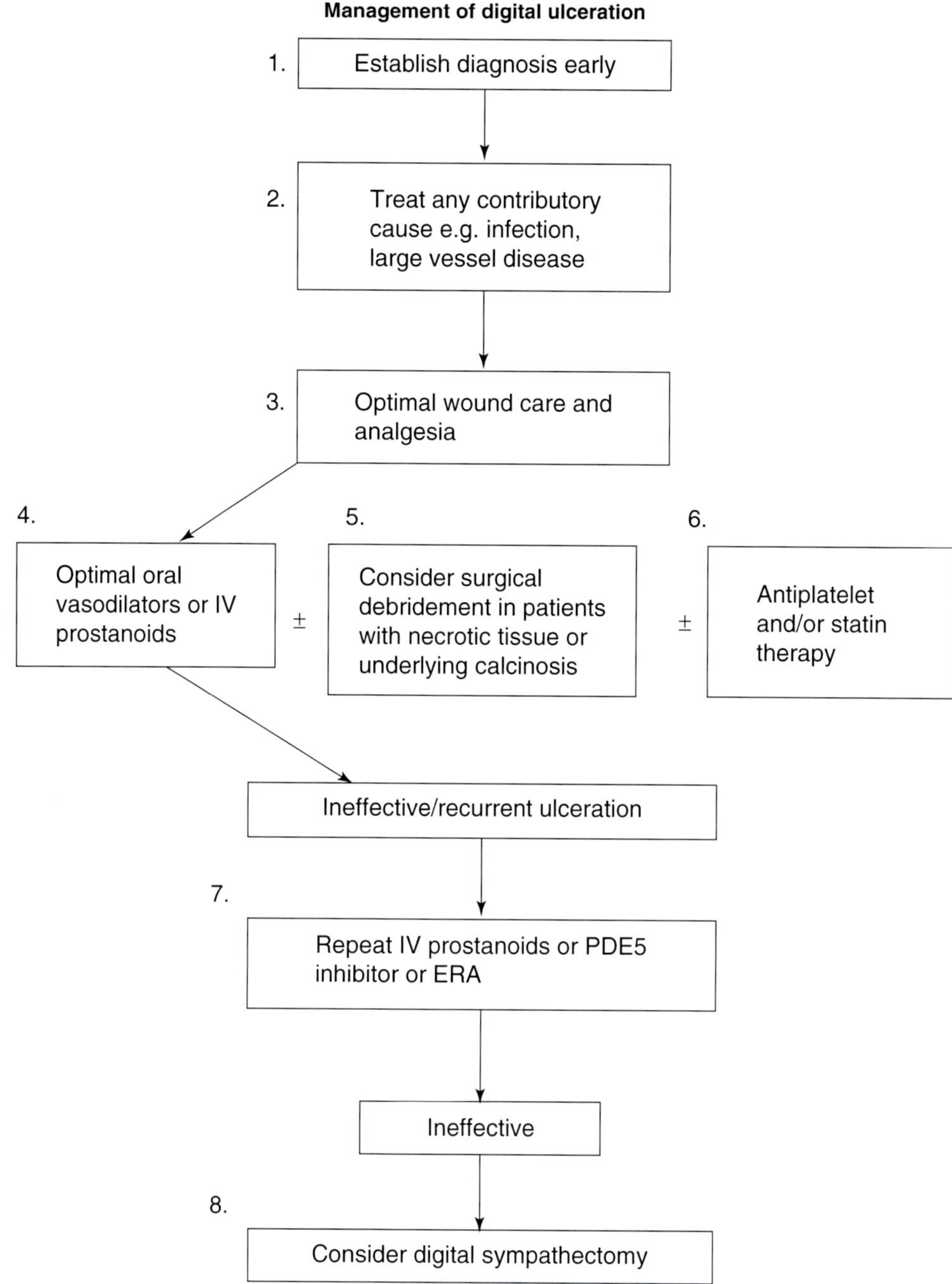

Fig. 6.6 The management of SSc-related digital ulceration. ERA endothelin-1 receptor antagonist, IV intravenous, PDE5 phosphodiesterase type 5. (Reproduced with permission [62])

Fig. 6.7 The management of SSc-related critical digital ischaemia. IV intravenous, PDE5 phosphodiesterase type 5. (Reproduced with permission [62])

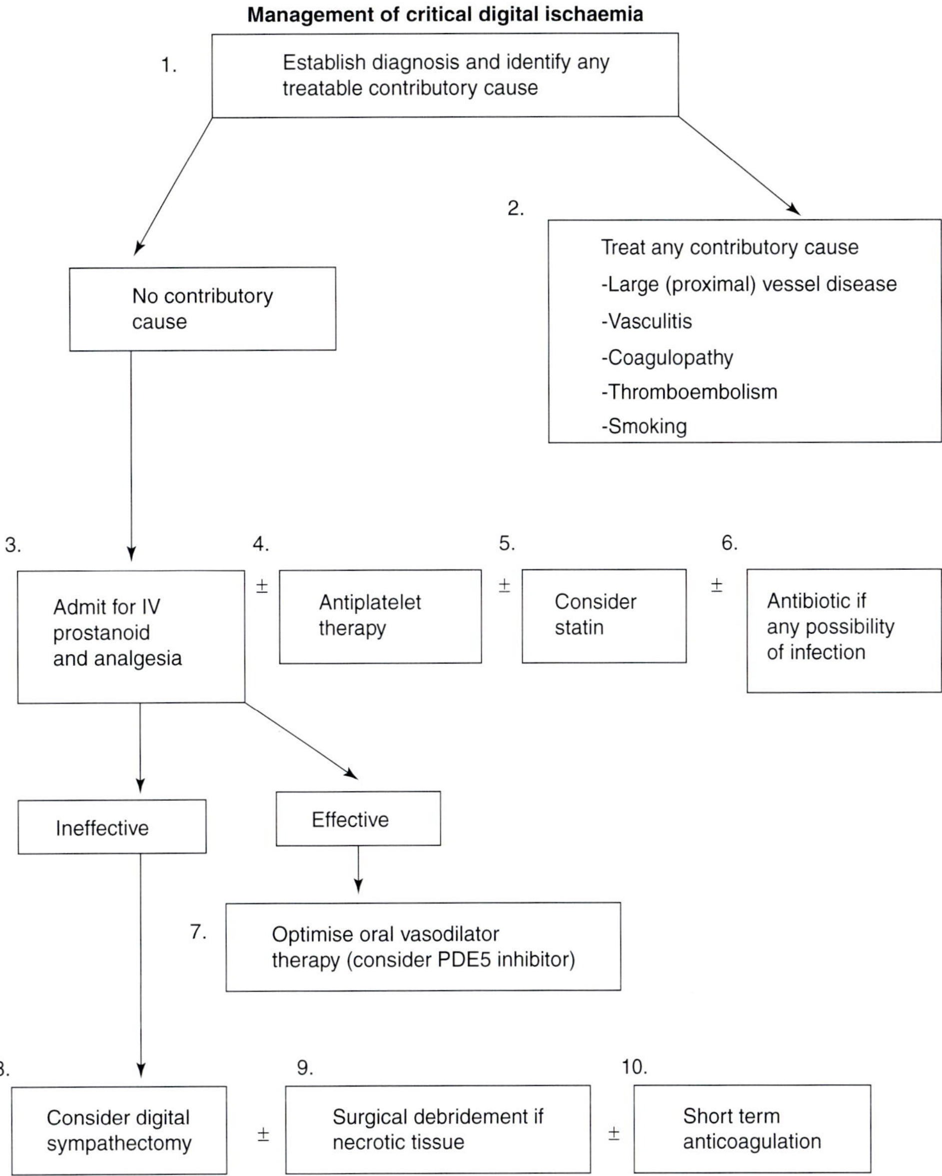

Treatment of Any Underlying Cause

To identify and treat (if possible) any underlying cause is the first principle of management in all patients with RP. Examples include (but are not limited to) treatment of paraproteinaemia or of a subclavian stenosis.

Patient Education/General Measures

This is a key aspect of management of all patients with RP that is often overlooked. Patients should try to avoid the impact of (even slight) temperature changes and dress warmly (including multiple layers), including wearing hat, socks and gloves. Hand warmers may be helpful or electrically heated gloves. Patient support groups provide excellent information leaflets. Patients should be strongly encouraged to stop smoking [63–65].

Drug Treatment

Drug therapy, RP should be offered to those patients who remain symptomatic despite the 'general' measures outlined above. Most patients with SSc-related RP will require drug treatment, as their RP is generally more severe than in those patients with PRP. The general approach to drug treatment for SSc-related RP is presented in Fig. 6.5 (although as previously highlighted, this is also relevant to RP due to other causes). Examples of drug doses are provided in Table 6.3.

It is worth highlighting that as a generalisation, the evidence base for drug treatment of RP is weak, because the number of randomised controlled trials is relatively small. This is in part due to the difficulty in conducting trials of RP that tend to be of short duration and run over the winter months [66]. However, on a positive note, there are now increasing numbers of clinical trials in patients with RP, including in patients with SSc-related digital vasculopathy.

Calcium Channel Blockers

These are generally considered first-line drug treatment for both PRP and SRP [67, 68], as reflected by both the recent British Society of Rheumatology and European League Against Rheumatism treatment recommendations for SSc [69, 70]. Calcium channel blockers act on smooth muscle cells to produce vasodilation. Adverse effects are common, including vasodilatory effects such as headache, dizziness and flushing. It is best to commence in low dose and gradually increase. Many clinicians through experience of treating patients with RP consider that sustained release preparations (e.g. sustained release nifedipine or amlodipine) are better tolerated than short-acting preparations. A recent Cochrane review of calcium channel blockers in PRP [71] that included

Table 6.3 Examples of drugs used in the treatment of Raynaud's phenomenon [62]

Drug class	Drug	Usual dose range in adults
Calcium channel blockers	Nifedipine (sustained release)	10 mg bd → 40 mg bd
	Amlodipine	5 mg od →10 mg od
	Diltiazem	60 mg bd →120 mg bd
Angiotensin receptor blockers	Losartan	25 mg od → 100 mg od
Selective serotonin reuptake inhibitors	Fluoxetine	20 mg od
Alpha-blockers	Prazosin	500 micrograms bd → 2 mg bd
Angiotensin-converting enzyme inhibitors	Lisinopril	5 mg od → 20 mg od
Phosphodiesterase type 5 inhibitors	Sildenafil	20 mg/25 mg tds → 50 mg tds
	Tadalafil	10 mg alternate days → 20 mg od

7 randomised trials and 296 patients reported that calcium channel blockers were only minimally effective. Despite the relatively small number of patients included in this and other meta-analyses [67, 68], calcium channel blockers are nonetheless the group of drugs that has been most studied in RP: two fairly recent reviews have both highlighted the lack of evidence base for other classes of drugs [72, 73].

Angiotensin-Converting Enzyme (ACE) Inhibitors and Angiotensin II Receptor Blockers

There is a strong rationale for inhibition of the renin-angiotensin system in RP, especially secondary to SSc. In particular, angiotensin-converting enzyme (ACE) inhibitors prevent deleterious fibrous remodelling in myocardial infarction, and angiotensin II is a potent vasoconstrictor. The evidence base for ACE inhibitors and angiotensin II receptor blockers in SSc-related RP is however weak. Earlier studies of ACE inhibitors (captopril and enalapril) were limited and conflicting [74]. In a multicentre, double-blind, placebo-controlled trial of quinapril, which included 210 patients with either limited cutaneous SSc or antibody-positive RP, there was no reported benefit in peripheral vascular manifestations after 2–3 years' treatment [75]. The angiotensin II receptor blocker losartan has been reported to be more effective than nifedipine, but this was in a small open study, and the dose of nifedipine was relatively low (20 mg) [76].

Supplementation of the L-Arginine/Nitric Oxide Pathway, Including Phosphodiesterase Type 5 Inhibitors

For the practising clinician, the important recent change in the management of 'uncomplicated' RP is the increasing use of phosphodiesterase type 5 (PDE5) inhibitors for RP [69, 70, 77, 78]. NO is a potent vasodilator, and PDE5 inhibitors enhance the effect of NO by inhibiting degradation of cyclic guanosine monophosphate. Although earlier clinical trials of PDE5 inhibitors in RP including patients with SSc gave somewhat conflicting results, more recent studies have suggested that PDE5 inhibitors confer benefit in patients with SRP. In a recent meta-analysis which included 244 patients (almost all of whom had CTD and, in particular, SSc-related RP) from 6 randomised clinical trials (1 with sildenafil, 1 with modified-release sildenafil, 3 with tadalafil and 1 with vardenafil), treatment was associated with a 'significant but moderate efficacy in SRP' [79].

Topical (transdermal) NO donation is another approach to treatment of RP. Topically applied glyceryl trinitrate (GTN), an NO donor, produces both local [80] and systemic [81] vasodilation. When given by transdermal patch for its systemic effects [81], it is often poorly tolerated and is therefore seldom used, although a retrospective report from the United Kingdom suggested that this approach was beneficial in children [82]. What is required is a preparation that maximises local efficacy but minimises adverse systemic effects. Although there is currently no commercially available preparation for application to the fingers, it is encouraging that topical nitrate therapy is being revisited. In a multicentre, placebo-controlled trial of MCQ-503, a novel preparation of GTN, 4 weeks of treatment (applied to the fingers immediately before or up to 5 min after the onset of an attack of RP) was associated with a reduction in the Raynaud's condition score, but not the frequency or duration of attacks [83]. Subsequently, in a laboratory-based, multicentre, double-blind, randomised, placebo-controlled, crossover study [84] examining two different doses of gel (0.5% and 1.25%), the proportion of subjects achieving baseline blood flow after a cold challenge was higher with MCQ-503 (66.2% and 69%, respectively) compared to placebo (45.8%).

Serotonin Reuptake Inhibitors

Serotonin is a vasoconstrictor, and therefore drugs antagonising its effects or limiting its availability may prevent vasoconstriction and improve symptoms of RP. Fluoxetine, a selective serotonin reuptake inhibitor, was beneficial in an open-label study [85] including patients with both primary and secondary RP. Serotonin reuptake inhibitors are less likely to cause vasodilatory side effects than some of the other drugs discussed above and so may be helpful in patients intolerant of other medications. However, further research is warranted to establish their place in the treatment of RP.

α-Adrenergic Blockers

These block vasoconstriction and so are sometimes prescribed for RP. However, the evidence base for non-selective α-receptor blockade in RP is very weak [86], mirroring the situation for many other classes of drug.

Prostanoids

These are seldom used in 'uncomplicated' RP, although they may have a role in patients with severe attacks impacting on quality of life, especially in patients in whom RP is secondary to SSc. Prostanoids are thought to have multiple modes of action, including vasodilation, inhibition of platelet aggregation and vascular remodelling [87]. In patients with SSc, they are effective in reducing frequency and severity of Raynaud's attacks as well as in healing DUs [88, 89], and many clinicians prescribe intravenous prostanoids to patients with SSc and severe RP at the onset of winter, with the aim of reducing severity of Raynaud's attacks and preventing digital ulceration. However, patients require hospitalisation to receive intravenous drug therapies, including the associated expense and inconvenience for the patient. Experience with oral prostanoids has been disappointing [90, 91]; however, oral prostanoids are being revisited. In an open-label laboratory study that included 19 patients, treatment with oral treprostinil diethanolamine increased finger perfusion and temperature [92]. In a recent multicentre, randomised, double-blind, placebo-controlled trial, 20-week treatment with oral treprostinil was associated with a small but not statistically significant reduction in DU burden [93].

Antiplatelet Agents and Statins

There is a strong therapeutic rationale for antiplatelet agents for patients in whom RP is secondary to SSc, because, as previously described, platelet activation is well recognised. Many clinicians therefore give low-dose aspirin (or an alternative antiplatelet agent when there are concerns about upper gastrointestinal side effects) to patients with SSc and severe digital ischaemia: however at present, there is no good evidence base to support this approach.

Regarding statin therapy, Abou-Raya et al. reported improvements in both clinical and laboratory measurements in patients with SSc-related RP treated with atorvastatin for 4 months (including an improvement in RP severity compared to placebo treatment), indicating that statins deserve further research in RP [94]: at present there is insufficient evidence to recommend these routinely.

Antioxidants

The evidence base for antioxidant therapy is limited and conflicting, with only some studies reporting an improvement in SSc-associated RP. In a controlled trial, treatment with probucol (a synthetic antioxidant) was associated with a significant reduction in RP symptoms (frequency and severity) compared to nifedipine [95]. Intravenous [96, 97] but not oral [98] N-acetylcysteine has been reported to improve RP symptoms (frequency and severity of RP attacks), as well as to reduce DU burden [97]. In a placebo-controlled, double-blind, crossover study that included 33 patients, treatment with a combination of micronutrient antioxidants was not associated with any clinical benefit in RP compared to placebo [99].

Surgery

Surgery has no role to play in 'uncomplicated' RP. There is increasing international experience using botulinum toxin injection and/or digital sympathectomy in the content of severe RP (refractory to treatment strategies previously described) and DU disease [100–103]. However, at present there is only a limited evidence base to support these interventions. Trials of botulinum toxin are ongoing. Fat grafting is a novel surgical approach which is being used in some centres for the management of SSc-related digital vascular disease [104].

Summary and Conclusions

In conclusion, RP is a common condition that can be associated with significant pain and disability, irrespective of the underlying aetiology. In patients with SSc, RP exists within a spectrum of digital vascular disease and can progress to ischaemic tissue loss. The clinician must perform a comprehensive clinical assessment and request key investigations (in particular, nailfold capillaroscopy and SSc-associated autoantibodies) in patients with RP. The management of RP must be tailored to the individual, although patient education is mandatory in all patients with RP. Future research is required to inform the management of RP, including the role for drug therapies (e.g. statins and antiplatelet agents) used in other conditions, and to better understand the complex pathogenesis underlying RP, which could drive therapeutic advances.

References

1. LeRoy EC, Medsger TA. Criteria for the classification of early systemic sclerosis. J Rheumatol [Internet]. 2001 [cited 2016 Jun 20];28(7):1573–6. Available from: http://www.ncbi.nlm.nih.gov/pubmed/11469464.
2. Matucci-Cerinic M, Allanore Y, Czirjak L, Tyndall A, Muller-Ladner U, Denton C, et al. The challenge of early systemic sclerosis for the EULAR Scleroderma Trial and Research group (EUSTAR) community. It is time to cut the Gordian knot and develop a prevention or rescue strategy. Ann Rheum Dis [Internet]. 2009 [cited 2017 Mar 24];68(9):1377–80. Available from: http://www.ncbi.nlm.nih.gov/pubmed/19674983.
3. Avouac J, Fransen J, Walker UA, Riccieri V, Smith V, Muller C, et al. Preliminary criteria for the very early diagnosis of systemic sclerosis: results of a Delphi Consensus Study from EULAR Scleroderma Trials and Research Group. Ann Rheum Dis [Internet]. 2011 [cited 2016 Jun 18];70(3):476–81. Available from: http://www.ncbi.nlm.nih.gov/pubmed/21081523.
4. Hughes M, Snapir A, Wilkinson J, Snapir D, Wigley FM, Herrick AL. Prediction and impact of attacks of Raynaud's phenomenon, as judged by patient perception. Rheumatology (Oxford). 2015;54(8):1443–7.
5. Bassel M, Hudson M, Taillefer SS, Schieir O, Baron M, Thombs BD. Frequency and impact of symptoms experienced by patients with systemic sclerosis: results from a Canadian National Survey. Rheumatology (Oxford) [Internet]. 2011 [cited 2016 Jun 21];50(4):762–7. Available from: http://www.ncbi.nlm.nih.gov/pubmed/21149249.
6. Maundrell A, Proudman SM. Epidemiology of Raynaud's phenomenon. In: Wigley FM, Herrick AL, Flavahan NA, editors. Raynaud's phenomenon. New York: Springer Science+Buisness Media; 2015. p. 21–35.
7. Silman A, Holligan S, Brennan P, Maddison P. Prevalence of symptoms of Raynaud's phenomenon in general practice. BMJ [Internet]. 1990 [cited 2017 Mar 9];301(6752):590–2. Available from: http://www.ncbi.nlm.nih.gov/pubmed/2242457.

8. Planchon B, Pistorius M-A, Beurrier P, De Faucal P. Primary Raynaud's phenomenon. Angiology [Internet]. 1994 [cited 2017 Mar 9];45(8):677–86. Available from: http://www.ncbi.nlm.nih.gov/pubmed/8048777.

9. Freedman RR, Mayes MD. Familial aggregation of primary Raynaud's disease. Arthritis Rheum [Internet]. 1996 [cited 2017 Mar 9];39(7):1189–91. Available from: http://www.ncbi.nlm.nih.gov/pubmed/8670329.

10. Sharp GC, Irvin WS, Tan EM, Gould RG, Holman HR. Mixed connective tissue disease--an apparently distinct rheumatic disease syndrome associated with a specific antibody to an extractable nuclear antigen (ENA). Am J Med [Internet]. 1972 [cited 2017 Mar 9];52(2):148–59. Available from: http://www.ncbi.nlm.nih.gov/pubmed/4621694.

11. Burdt MA, Hoffman RW, Deutscher SL, Wang GS, Johnson JC, Sharp GC. Long-term outcome in mixed connective tissue disease: longitudinal clinical and serologic findings. Arthritis Rheum [Internet]. 1999 [cited 2017 Mar 9];42(5):899–909. Available from: http://doi.wiley.com/10.1002/1529-0131%28199905%2942%3A5%3C899%3A%3AAID-ANR8%3E3.0.CO%3B2-L.

12. Hoffman IEA, Peene I, Meheus L, Huizinga TWJ, Cebecauer L, Isenberg D, et al. Specific antinuclear antibodies are associated with clinical features in systemic lupus erythematosus. Ann Rheum Dis [Internet]. 2004 [cited 2017 Mar 9];63(9):1155–8. Available from: http://www.ncbi.nlm.nih.gov/pubmed/15308527.

13. Meier FMP, Frommer KW, Dinser R, Walker UA, Czirjak L, Denton CP, et al. Update on the profile of the EUSTAR cohort: an analysis of the EULAR Scleroderma Trials and Research group database. Ann Rheum Dis [Internet]. 2012 [cited 2016 Jun 18];71(8):1355–60. Available from: http://www.ncbi.nlm.nih.gov/pubmed/22615460.

14. LeRoy EC, Black C, Fleischmajer R, Jablonska S, Krieg T, Medsger TA, et al. Scleroderma (systemic sclerosis): classification, subsets and pathogenesis. J Rheumatol [Internet]. 1988 [cited 2016 Jun 18];15(2):202–5. Available from: http://www.ncbi.nlm.nih.gov/pubmed/3361530.

15. Anderson ME, Moore TL, Hollis S, Clark S, Jayson MI, Herrick AL. Endothelial-dependent vasodilation is impaired in patients with systemic sclerosis, as assessed by low dose iontophoresis. Clin Exp Rheumatol [Internet]. [cited 2016 Jun 28];21(3):403. Available from: http://www.ncbi.nlm.nih.gov/pubmed/12846066.

16. Gunawardena H, Harris ND, Carmichael C, McHugh NJ. Maximum blood flow and microvascular regulatory responses in systemic sclerosis. Rheumatology (Oxford) [Internet]. 2007 [cited 2016 Jun 28];46(7):1079–82. Available from: http://www.ncbi.nlm.nih.gov/pubmed/17494087.

17. Rossi M, Bazzichi L, Di Maria C, Franzoni F, Raimo K, Della Rossa A, et al. Blunted increase of digital skin vasomotion following acetylcholine and sodium nitroprusside iontophoresis in systemic sclerosis patients. Rheumatology [Internet]. 2008 [cited 2017 Mar 24];47(7):1012–7. Available from: https://academic.oup.com/rheumatology/article-lookup/doi/10.1093/rheumatology/ken117.

18. Khan F, Litchfield SJ, McLaren M, Veale DJ, Littleford RC, Belch JJ. Oral L-arginine supplementation and cutaneous vascular responses in patients with primary Raynaud's phenomenon. Arthritis Rheum [Internet]. 1997 [cited 2017 Mar 24];40(2):352–7. Available from: http://www.ncbi.nlm.nih.gov/pubmed/9041947.

19. Coffman JD, Cohen AS. Total and capillary fingertip blood flow in Raynaud's phenomenon. N Engl J Med [Internet]. 1971 [cited 2017 Mar 24];285(5):259–63. Available from: http://www.nejm.org/doi/abs/10.1056/NEJM197107292850505.

20. Engelhart M, Kristensen JK. Raynaud's phenomenon: blood supply to fingers during indirect cooling, evaluated by laser Doppler flowmetry. Clin Physiol [Internet]. 1986 [cited 2017 Mar 24];6(6):481–8. Available from: http://www.ncbi.nlm.nih.gov/pubmed/2947773.

21. Singh S, de Trafford JC, Baskerville PA, Roberts VC. Digital artery calibre measurement–a new technique of assessing Raynaud's phenomenon. Eur J Vasc Surg [Internet]. 1991 [cited 2017 Mar 24];5(2):199–203. Available from: http://www.ncbi.nlm.nih.gov/pubmed/2037091.

22. Pignone A, Rosso A Del, Brosnihan KB, Perfetto F, Livi R, Fiori G, et al. Reduced circulating levels of angiotensin-(1–7) in systemic sclerosis: a new pathway in the dysregulation of endothelial-dependent vascular tone control. Ann Rheum Dis [Internet]. 2007 [cited 2017 Mar 24];66(10):1305–10. Available from: http://ard.bmj.com/cgi/doi/10.1136/ard.2006.064493.

23. Vancheeswaran R, Azam A, Black C, Dashwood MR. Localization of endothelin-1 and its binding sites in scleroderma skin. J Rheumatol [Internet]. 1994 [cited 2017 Mar 24];21(7):1268–76. Available from: http://www.ncbi.nlm.nih.gov/pubmed/7525957.

24. Herrick AL. The pathogenesis, diagnosis and treatment of Raynaud phenomenon. Nat Rev Rheumatol [Internet]. 2012 [cited 2017 Mar 24];8(8):469–79. Available from: http://www.ncbi.nlm.nih.gov/pubmed/22782008.

25. Bukhari M, Hollis S, Moore T, Jayson MI, Herrick AL. Quantitation of microcirculatory abnormalities in patients with primary Raynaud's phenomenon and systemic sclerosis by video capillaroscopy. Rheumatology (Oxford) [Internet]. 2000 [cited 2017 Mar 24];39(5):506–12. Available from: http://www.ncbi.nlm.nih.gov/pubmed/10852981.

26. Rodnan GP, Myerowitz RL, Justh GO. Morphologic changes in the digital arteries of patients with progressive systemic sclerosis (scleroderma) and Raynaud phenomenon. Medicine (Baltimore) [Internet]. 1980 [cited 2015 Oct 2];59(6):393–408. Available from: http://www.ncbi.nlm.nih.gov/pubmed/7442530.

27. Hasegawa M, Nagai Y, Tamura A, Ishikawa O. Arteriographic evaluation of vascular changes of the extremities in patients with systemic sclerosis. Br J Dermatol [Internet]. 2006 [cited 2015 Sep 11];155(6):1159–64. Available from: http://www.ncbi.nlm.nih.gov/pubmed/17107383.

28. Allanore Y, Seror R, Chevrot A, Kahan A, Drapé JL. Hand vascular involvement assessed by magnetic resonance angiography in systemic sclerosis. Arthritis Rheum [Internet]. 2007 [cited 2016 Jun 20];56(8):2747–54. Available from: http://www.ncbi.nlm.nih.gov/pubmed/17665441.

29. Wang J, Yarnykh VL, Molitor JA, Nash RA, Chu B, Wilson GJ, et al. Micro magnetic resonance angiography of the finger in systemic sclerosis. Rheumatology (Oxford) [Internet]. 2008 [cited 2016 Jun 20];47(8):1239–43. Available from: http://www.ncbi.nlm.nih.gov/pubmed/18559373.

30. Taylor MH, McFadden JA, Bolster MB, Silver RM. Ulnar artery involvement in systemic sclerosis (scleroderma). J Rheumatol [Internet]. 2002 [cited 2016 Jun 20];29(1):102–6. Available from: http://www.ncbi.nlm.nih.gov/pubmed/11824945.

31. Park JH, Sung Y-K, Bae S-C, Song S-Y, Seo HS, Jun J-B. Ulnar artery vasculopathy in systemic sclerosis. Rheumatol Int [Internet]. 2009 [cited 2016 Jun 20];29(9):1081–6. Available from: http://www.ncbi.nlm.nih.gov/pubmed/19363679.

32. Au K, Singh MK, Bodukam V, Bae S, Maranian P, Ogawa R, et al. Atherosclerosis in systemic sclerosis: a systematic review and meta-analysis. Arthritis Rheum [Internet]. 2011 [cited 2016 Jun 19];63(7):2078–90. Available from: http://www.ncbi.nlm.nih.gov/pubmed/21480189.

33. Man A, Zhu Y, Zhang Y, Dubreuil M, Rho YH, Peloquin C, et al. The risk of cardiovascular disease in systemic sclerosis: a population-based cohort study. Ann Rheum Dis [Internet]. 2013 [cited 2015 Sep 11];72(7):1188–93. Available from: http://www.pubmedcentral.nih.gov/articlerender.fcgi?artid=4386728&tool=pmcentrez&rendertype=abstract.

34. Katsumoto TR, Whitfield ML. The pathogenesis of systemic sclerosis. Annu Rev Pathol. 2011;6:509–37.

35. Altorok N, Wang Y, Kahaleh B. Endothelial dysfunction in systemic sclerosis. Curr Opin Rheumatol [Internet]. 2014 [cited 2016 Jun 21];26(6):615–20. Available from: http://www.ncbi.nlm.nih.gov/pubmed/25191994.

36. Renaudineau Y, Revelen R, Levy Y, Salojin K, Gilburg B, Shoenfeld Y, et al. Anti-endothelial cell antibodies in systemic sclerosis. Clin Diagn Lab Immunol [Internet]. 1999 [cited 2016 Jun 21];6(2):156–60. Available from: http://www.ncbi.nlm.nih.gov/pubmed/10066646.

37. Mihai C, Tervaert JWC. Anti-endothelial cell antibodies in systemic sclerosis. Ann Rheum Dis [Internet]. 2010 Feb [cited 2016 Jun 21];69(2):319–24. Available from: http://www.ncbi.nlm.nih.gov/pubmed/20107031.

38. Bunker CB, Terenghi G, Springall DR, Polak JM, Dowd PM. Deficiency of calcitonin gene-related peptide in Raynaud's phenomenon. Lancet (London, England) [Internet]. [cited 2017 Mar 24];336(8730):1530–3. Available from: http://www.ncbi.nlm.nih.gov/pubmed/1979366.

39. Flavahan NA. Pathophysiological regulation of the cutaneous vascular system in Raynaud's phenomenon. In: Wigley FM, Herrick A, Flavahan NA, editors. Raynaud's phenomenon. New York: Springer Science+Buisness Media; 2015. p. 57–79.

40. Flavahan NA. A vascular mechanistic approach to understanding Raynaud phenomenon. Nat Rev Rheumatol [Internet]. 2015 [cited 2016 May 28];11(3):146–58. Available from: http://www.ncbi.nlm.nih.gov/pubmed/25536485.

41. Furspan PB, Chatterjee S, Freedman RR. Increased tyrosine phosphorylation mediates the cooling-induced contraction and increased vascular reactivity of Raynaud's disease. Arthritis Rheum [Internet]. 2004 [cited 2017 Mar 24];50(5):1578–85. Available from: http://doi.wiley.com/10.1002/art.20214.

42. Furspan PB, Chatterjee S, Mayes MD, Freedman RR. Cooling-induced contraction and protein tyrosine kinase activity of isolated arterioles in secondary Raynaud's phenomenon. Rheumatology (Oxford) [Internet]. 2005 [cited 2017 Mar 24];44(4):488–94. Available from: https://academic.oup.com/rheumatology/article-lookup/doi/10.1093/rheumatology/keh517.

43. Kallenberg CG, Vellenga E, Wouda AA, The TH. Platelet activation, fibrinolytic activity and circulating immune complexes in Raynaud's phenomenon. J Rheumatol [Internet]. [cited 2017 Mar 24];9(6):878–84. Available from: http://www.ncbi.nlm.nih.gov/pubmed/7161779.

44. Pamuk GE, Turgut B, Pamuk ON, Vural O, Demir M, Cakir N. Increased circulating platelet-leucocyte complexes in patients with primary Raynaud's phenomenon and Raynaud's phenomenon secondary to systemic sclerosis: a comparative study. Blood Coagul Fibrinolysis [Internet]. 2007 [cited 2017 Mar 24];18(4):297–302. Available from: http://content.wkhealth.com/linkback/openurl?sid=WKPTLP:landingpage&an=00001721-200706000-00001.

45. Eid AH, Maiti K, Mitra S, Chotani MA, Flavahan S, Bailey SR, et al. Estrogen increases smooth muscle expression of alpha2C-adrenoceptors and cold-induced constriction of cutaneous arteries. Am J Physiol Heart Circ Physiol [Internet]. 2007 [cited 2017 Mar 24];293(3):H1955–61. Available from: http://ajpheart.physiology.org/cgi/doi/10.1152/ajpheart.00306.2007.

46. Souza E, Muller C, Horimoto A, Rezende R, Guimarães I, Mariz H, et al. Geographic variation as a risk factor for digital ulcers in systemic sclerosis patients: a multicentre registry. Scand J Rheumatol [Internet]. 2016 [cited 2017 Mar 25];1–8. Available from: http://www.ncbi.nlm.nih.gov/pubmed/27996340.

47. LeRoy EC, Medsger TA. Raynaud's phenomenon: a proposal for classification. Clin Exp Rheumatol [Internet]. 1992 [cited 2016 Jun 18];10(5):485–8. Available from: http://www.ncbi.nlm.nih.gov/pubmed/1458701.

48. Maverakis E, Patel F, Kronenberg DG, Chung L, Fiorentino D, Allanore Y, et al. International consensus criteria for the diagnosis of Raynaud's phenomenon. J Autoimmun [Internet]. 2014 [cited 2017 Mar 24];48–49:60–5. Available from: http://www.ncbi.nlm.nih.gov/pubmed/24491823.

49. Anders HJ, Sigl T, Schattenkirchner M. Differentiation between primary and secondary Raynaud's phenomenon: a prospective study comparing nailfold capillaroscopy using an ophthalmoscope or stereomicroscope. Ann Rheum Dis [Internet]. 2001 [cited 2016 May 30];60(4):407–9. Available from: http://www.pubmedcentral.nih.gov/articlerender.fcgi?artid=1753600&tool=pmcentrez&rendertype=abstract.

50. Bergman R, Sharony L, Schapira D, Nahir MA, Balbir-Gurman A. The handheld dermatoscope as a nail-fold capillaroscopic instrument. Arch Dermatol [Internet]. 2003 [cited 2017 Mar 9];139(8):1027–30. Available from: http://archderm.jamanetwork.com/article.aspx?doi=10.1001/archderm.139.8.1027.

51. Baron M, Bell M, Bookman A, Buchignani M, Dunne J, Hudson M, et al. Office capillaroscopy in systemic sclerosis. Clin Rheumatol [Internet]. 2007 [cited 2016 May 30];26(8):1268–74. Available from: http://www.ncbi.nlm.nih.gov/pubmed/17160528.

52. Hudson M, Taillefer S, Steele R, Dunne J, Johnson SR, Jones N, et al. Improving the sensitivity of the American College of Rheumatology classification criteria for systemic sclerosis. Clin Exp Rheumatol [Internet]. 2007 [cited 2017 Mar 9];25(5):754–7. Available from: http://www.ncbi.nlm.nih.gov/pubmed/18078627.

53. Moore TL, Roberts C, Murray AK, Helbling I, Herrick AL. Reliability of dermoscopy in the assessment of patients with Raynaud's phenomenon. Rheumatology (Oxford) [Internet]. 2010 [cited 2016 May 30];49(3):542–7. Available from: http://www.ncbi.nlm.nih.gov/pubmed/20028729.

54. Hughes M, Moore T, O'Leary N, Tracey A, Ennis H, Dinsdale G, et al. A study comparing videocapillaroscopy and dermoscopy in the assessment of nailfold capillaries in patients with systemic sclerosis-spectrum disorders. Rheumatology (Oxford) [Internet]. 2015 [cited 2016 May 29];54(8):1435–42. Available from: http://www.ncbi.nlm.nih.gov/pubmed/25749623.

55. Darton K, Black CM. Pyroelectric vidicon thermography and cold challenge quantify the severity of Raynaud's phenomenon. Br J Rheumatol [Internet]. 1991 [cited 2017 Mar 9];30(3):190–5. Available from: http://www.ncbi.nlm.nih.gov/pubmed/2049579.

56. O'Reilly D, Taylor L, el-Hadidy K, Jayson MI. Measurement of cold challenge responses in primary Raynaud's phenomenon and Raynaud's phenomenon associated with systemic sclerosis. Ann Rheum Dis [Internet]. 1992 [cited 2016 May 30];51(11):1193–6. Available from: http://www.pubmedcentral.nih.gov/articlerender.fcgi?artid=1012453&tool=pmcentrez&rendertype=abstract

57. Pauling JD, Flower V, Shipley JA, Harris ND, McHugh NJ. Influence of the cold challenge on the discriminatory capacity of the digital distal-dorsal difference in the thermographic assessment of Raynaud's phenomenon. Microvasc Res [Internet]. 2011 [cited 2016 May 30];82(3):364–8. Available from: http://www.ncbi.nlm.nih.gov/pubmed/21420982.

58. Clark S, Hollis S, Campbell F, Moore T, Jayson M, Herrick A. The "distal-dorsal difference" as a possible predictor of secondary Raynaud's phenomenon. J Rheumatol [Internet]. 1999 [cited 2016 May 30];26(5):1125–8. Available from: http://www.ncbi.nlm.nih.gov/pubmed/10332978.

59. Anderson ME, Moore TL, Lunt M, Herrick AL. The "distal-dorsal difference": a thermographic parameter by which to differentiate between primary and secondary Raynaud's phenomenon. Rheumatology (Oxford) [Internet]. 2007 [cited 2016 May 30];46(3):533–8. Available from: http://www.ncbi.nlm.nih.gov/pubmed/17018538.

60. Murray A, Pauling J. Non-invasive methods of assessing Raynaud's phenomenon. In: Wigley FM, Herrick AL, Flavahan NA, editors.

Raynaud's phenomenon. New York: Springer Science+Buisness Media; 2015. p. 199–242.

61. White C. Clinical practice. Intermittent claudication. N Engl J Med [Internet]. 2007 [cited 2017 Mar 9];356(12):1241–50. Available from: http://www.nejm.org/doi/abs/10.1056/NEJMcp064483.

62. Hughes M, Ong VH, Anderson ME, Hall F, Moinzadeh P, Griffiths B, et al. Consensus best practice pathway of the UK Scleroderma Study Group: digital vasculopathy in systemic sclerosis. Rheumatology [Internet]. 2015 [cited 2015 Jun 29];54(11):2015–24. Available from: http://www.ncbi.nlm.nih.gov/pubmed/26116156.

63. Harrison BJ, Silman AJ, Hider SL, Herrick AL. Cigarette smoking as a significant risk factor for digital vascular disease in patients with systemic sclerosis. Arthritis Rheum [Internet]. 2002 [cited 2015 Sep 3];46(12):3312–6. Available from: http://www.ncbi.nlm.nih.gov/pubmed/12483737.

64. Suter LG, Murabito JM, Felson DT, Fraenkel L. Smoking, alcohol consumption, and Raynaud's phenomenon in middle age. Am J Med [Internet]. 2007 [cited 2017 Mar 9];120(3):264–71. Available from: http://www.ncbi.nlm.nih.gov/pubmed/17349450.

65. Hudson M, Lo E, Lu Y, Hercz D, Baron M, Steele R, et al. Cigarette smoking in patients with systemic sclerosis. Arthritis Rheum [Internet]. 2011 [cited 2017 Mar 9];63(1):230–8. Available from: http://www.ncbi.nlm.nih.gov/pubmed/20936633.

66. Wilkinson J. Design and reporting of randomized controlled trials for Raynaud's phenomenon. In: Wigley FM, Herrick AL, Flavahan NA, editors. Raynaud's phenomenon. New York: Springer Science+Buisness Media; 2015.

67. Thompson AE, Shea B, Welch V, Fenlon D, Pope JE. Calcium-channel blockers for Raynaud's phenomenon in systemic sclerosis. Arthritis Rheum [Internet]. 2001 [cited 2017 Mar 24];44(8):1841–7. Available from: http://www.ncbi.nlm.nih.gov/pubmed/11508437.

68. Thompson AE, Pope JE. Calcium channel blockers for primary Raynaud's phenomenon: a meta-analysis. Rheumatology [Internet]. 2005 [cited 2017 Mar 24];44(2):145–50. Available from: http://www.ncbi.nlm.nih.gov/pubmed/15546967.

69. Denton CP, Hughes M, Gak N, Vila J, Buch MH, Chakravarty K, et al. BSR and BHPR guideline for the treatment of systemic sclerosis. Rheumatology (Oxford) [Internet]. 2016.; [cited 2016 Jun 17]; Available from: http://www.ncbi.nlm.nih.gov/pubmed/27284161.

70. Kowal-Bielecka O, Fransen J, Avouac J, Becker M, Kulak A, Allanore Y, et al. Update of EULAR recommendations for the treatment of systemic sclerosis. Ann Rheum Dis [Internet]. 2016 [cited 2017 Mar 24];annrheumdis-2016-209909editorsnote. Available from: http://www.ncbi.nlm.nih.gov/pubmed/27941129.

71. Ennis H, Hughes M, Anderson ME, Wilkinson J, Herrick AL. Calcium channel blockers for primary Raynaud's phenomenon. In: Herrick AL, editor. Cochrane database systematic reviews [Internet]. Chichester, UK: John Wiley & Sons, Ltd; 2016 [cited 2017 Mar 24]. p. CD002069. Available from: http://www.ncbi.nlm.nih.gov/pubmed/26914257.

72. Stewart M, Morling JR. Oral vasodilators for primary Raynaud's phenomenon. In: Stewart M, editor. Cochrane database systematic reviews [Internet]. Chichester, UK: John Wiley & Sons, Ltd; 2012 [cited 2017 Mar 24]. p. CD006687. Available from: http://www.ncbi.nlm.nih.gov/pubmed/22786498.

73. Pope J. Overview – Raynaud's phenomenon (primary) [Internet]. [cited 2017 Mar 24]. Available from: http://clinicalevidence.bmj.com/x/systematic-review/1119/overview.html.

74. Hughes M, Herrick AL. Prophylactic ACE inhibitor therapy in Raynaud's phenomenon: helpful or harmful? In: Cutolo M, Smith V, editors. Novel insights into systemic sclerosis management. Future Medicine Ltd; 2011. p. 232–241.

75. Gliddon AE, Doré CJ, Black CM, McHugh N, Moots R, Denton CP, et al. Prevention of vascular damage in scleroderma and autoimmune Raynaud's phenomenon: a multicenter, randomized, double-blind, placebo-controlled trial of the angiotensin-converting enzyme inhibitor quinapril. Arthritis Rheum [Internet]. 2007 [cited 2015 Aug 7];56(11):3837–46. Available from: http://www.ncbi.nlm.nih.gov/pubmed/17968938.

76. Dziadzio M, Denton CP, Smith R, Howell K, Blann A, Bowers E, et al. Losartan therapy for Raynaud's phenomenon and scleroderma: clinical and biochemical findings in a fifteen-week, randomized, parallel-group, controlled trial. Arthritis Rheum [Internet]. 1999 [cited 2017 Mar 24];42(12):2646–55. Available from: http://doi.wiley.com/10.1002/1529-0131%28199912%2942%3A12%3C2646%3A%3AAID-ANR21%3E3.0.CO%3B2-T.

77. Pope J, Harding S, Khimdas S, Bonner A, Hudson M, Markland J, et al. Agreement with guidelines from a large database for management of systemic sclerosis: results from the Canadian Scleroderma Research Group. J Rheumatol [Internet]. 2012 [cited 2017 Mar 24];39(3):524–31. Available from: http://www.jrheum.org/cgi/doi/10.3899/jrheum.110121.

78. Walker KM, Pope J. Treatment of systemic sclerosis complications: what to use when first-line treatment fails—a consensus of systemic sclerosis experts. Semin Arthritis Rheum [Internet]. 2012 [cited 2017 Mar 24];42(1):42–55. Available from: http://linkinghub.elsevier.com/retrieve/pii/S0049017212000170.

79. Roustit M, Blaise S, Allanore Y, Carpentier PH, Caglayan E, Cracowski J-L. Phosphodiesterase-5 inhibitors for the treatment of secondary Raynaud's phenomenon: systematic review and meta-analysis of randomised trials. Ann Rheum Dis [Internet]. 2013 [cited 2017 Mar 24];72(10):1696–9. Available from: http://www.ncbi.nlm.nih.gov/pubmed/23426043.

80. Anderson ME, Moore TL, Hollis S, Jayson MI V, King TA, Herrick AL. Digital vascular response to topical glyceryl trinitrate, as measured by laser Doppler imaging, in primary Raynaud's phenomenon and systemic sclerosis. Rheumatology (Oxford) [Internet]. 2002 [cited 2015 Sep 9];41(3):324–8. Available from: http://www.ncbi.nlm.nih.gov/pubmed/11934971.

81. Teh LS, Manning J, Moore T, Tully MP, O'Reilly D, Jayson MI. Sustained-release transdermal glyceryl trinitrate patches as a treatment for primary and secondary Raynaud's phenomenon. Br J Rheumatol [Internet]. 1995 [cited 2017 Mar 24];34(7):636–41. Available from: http://www.ncbi.nlm.nih.gov/pubmed/7670782.

82. Gargh K, Baildam EM, Cleary GA, Beresford MW, McCann LJ. A retrospective clinical analysis of pharmacological modalities used for symptomatic relief of Raynaud's phenomenon in children treated in a UK paediatric rheumatology centre. Rheumatology [Internet]. 2010 [cited 2017 Mar 24];49(1):193–4. Available from: http://www.ncbi.nlm.nih.gov/pubmed/19797310.

83. Chung L, Shapiro L, Fiorentino D, Baron M, Shanahan J, Sule S, et al. MQX-503, a novel formulation of nitroglycerin, improves the severity of Raynaud's phenomenon: a randomized, controlled trial. Arthritis Rheum [Internet]. 2009 [cited 2016 May 30];60(3):870–7. Available from: http://www.ncbi.nlm.nih.gov/pubmed/19248104.

84. Hummers LK, Dugowson CE, Dechow FJ, Wise RA, Gregory J, Michalek J, et al. A multi-centre, blinded, randomised, placebo-controlled, laboratory-based study of MQX-503, a novel topical gel formulation of nitroglycerine, in patients with Raynaud phenomenon. Ann Rheum Dis [Internet]. 2013 [cited 2016 May 30];72(12):1962–7. Available from: http://www.ncbi.nlm.nih.gov/pubmed/23268365.

85. Coleiro B, Marshall SE, Denton CP, Howell K, Blann A, Welsh KI, et al. Treatment of Raynaud's phenomenon with the selective serotonin reuptake inhibitor fluoxetine. Rheumatology (Oxford) [Internet]. 2001 [cited 2017 Mar 24];40(9):1038–43. Available from: http://www.ncbi.nlm.nih.gov/pubmed/11561116.

86. Harding SE, Tingey PC, Pope J, Fenlon D, Furst D, Shea B, et al. Prazosin for Raynaud's phenomenon in progressive systemic sclerosis. In: Pope J, editor. Cochrane database of systematic reviews [Internet]. Chichester, UK: John Wiley & Sons, Ltd; 1998 [cited 2017 Mar 24]. p. CD000956. Available from: http://www.ncbi.nlm.nih.gov/pubmed/10796398.

87. Fishman AP. Pulmonary Hypertension — Beyond Vasodilator Therapy. N Engl J Med [Internet]. 1998 [cited 2017 Mar 24];338(5):321–2. Available from: http://www.ncbi.nlm.nih.gov/pubmed/9445414.

88. Wigley FM, Seibold JR, Wise RA, McCloskey DA, Dole WP. Intravenous iloprost treatment of Raynaud's phenomenon and ischemic ulcers secondary to systemic sclerosis. J Rheumatol [Internet]. 1992 [cited 2015 Sep 3];19(9):1407–14. Available from: http://www.ncbi.nlm.nih.gov/pubmed/1279170.

89. Pope J, Fenlon D, Thompson A, Shea B, Furst D, Wells G, et al. Iloprost and cisaprost for Raynaud's phenomenon in progressive systemic sclerosis. In: Pope J, editor. Cochrane Database Syst Rev [Internet]. 2000 [cited 2017 Mar 24];(2):CD000953. Available from: http://doi.wiley.com/10.1002/14651858.CD000953.

90. Wigley FM, Korn JH, Csuka ME, Medsger TA, Rothfield NF, Ellman M, et al. Oral iloprost treatment in patients with Raynaud's phenomenon secondary to systemic sclerosis: a multicenter, placebo-controlled, double-blind study. Arthritis Rheum [Internet]. 1998 [cited 2016 Jul 24];41(4):670–7. Available from: http://www.ncbi.nlm.nih.gov/pubmed/9550476.

91. Vayssairat M. Preventive effect of an oral prostacyclin analog, beraprost sodium, on digital necrosis in systemic sclerosis. French Microcirculation Society Multicenter Group for the Study of Vascular Acrosyndromes. J Rheumatol [Internet]. 1999 [cited 2017 Mar 24];26(10):2173–8. Available from: http://www.ncbi.nlm.nih.gov/pubmed/10529135.

92. Shah AA, Schiopu E, Hummers LK, Wade M, Phillips K, Anderson C, et al. Open label study of escalating doses of oral treprostinil diethanolamine in patients with systemic sclerosis and digital ischemia: pharmacokinetics and correlation with digital perfusion. Arthritis Res Ther [Internet]. 2013 [cited 2017 Mar 24];15(2):R54. Available from: http://www.ncbi.nlm.nih.gov/pubmed/23597147.

93. Seibold J, Wigley F, Schiopu E, Denton C, Silver RM, Steen VD, et al. Digital ulcers in SSc treated with oral treprostinil: a randomized, double-blind, placebo-controlled study with open-label follow-up. J Scleroderma Relat Disord. 2017;2(1):1–68.

94. Abou-Raya A, Abou-Raya S, Helmii M. Statins: potentially useful in therapy of systemic sclerosis-related Raynaud's phenomenon and digital ulcers. J Rheumatol [Internet]. 2008 [cited 2015 Sep 9];35(9):1801–8. Available from: http://www.ncbi.nlm.nih.gov/pubmed/18709692.

95. Denton CP, Bunce TD, Dorado MB, Roberts Z, Wilson H, Howell K, et al. Probucol improves symptoms and reduces lipoprotein oxidation susceptibility in patients with Raynaud's phenomenon. Rheumatology (Oxford) [Internet]. 1999 [cited 2017 Mar 24];38(4):309–15. Available from: http://www.ncbi.nlm.nih.gov/pubmed/10378706.

96. Sambo P, Amico D, Giacomelli R, Matucci-Cerinic M, Salsano F, Valentini G, et al. Intravenous N-acetylcysteine for treatment of Raynaud's phenomenon secondary to systemic sclerosis: a pilot study. J Rheumatol [Internet]. 2001 [cited 2015 Sep 3];28(10):2257–62. Available from: http://www.ncbi.nlm.nih.gov/pubmed/11669166.

97. Rosato E, Borghese F, Pisarri S, Salsano F. The treatment with N-acetylcysteine of Raynaud's phenomenon and ischemic ulcers therapy in sclerodermic patients: a prospective observational study of 50 patients. Clin Rheumatol [Internet]. 2009 [cited 2015 Sep 3];28(12):1379–84. Available from: http://www.ncbi.nlm.nih.gov/pubmed/19690939.

98. Correa MJU, Mariz HA, Andrade LEC, Kayser C. [Oral N-acetylcysteine in the treatment of Raynaud's phenomenon secondary to systemic sclerosis: a randomized, double-blind, placebo-controlled clinical trial]. Rev Bras Reumatol [Internet]. 2014 [cited 2017 Mar 24];54(6):452–8. Available from: http://linkinghub.elsevier.com/retrieve/pii/S048250041400151X.

99. Herrick AL, Hollis S, Schofield D, Rieley F, Blann A, Griffin K, et al. A double-blind placebo-controlled trial of antioxidant therapy in limited cutaneous systemic sclerosis. Clin Exp Rheumatol [Internet]. [cited 2017 Mar 24];18(3):349–56. Available from: http://www.ncbi.nlm.nih.gov/pubmed/10895372.

100. Iorio ML, Masden DL, Higgins JP. Botulinum toxin A treatment of Raynaud's phenomenon: a review. Semin Arthritis Rheum [Internet]. 2012 [cited 2015 Sep 10];41(4):599–603. Available from: http://www.ncbi.nlm.nih.gov/pubmed/21868066.

101. Neumeister MW. Botulinum toxin type A in the treatment of Raynaud's phenomenon. J Hand Surg Am [Internet]. 2010 [cited 2015 Sep 10];35(12):2085–92. Available from: http://www.ncbi.nlm.nih.gov/pubmed/21134617.

102. Motegi S-I, Yamada K, Toki S, Uchiyama A, Kubota Y, Nakamura T, et al. Beneficial effect of botulinum toxin A on Raynaud's phenomenon in Japanese patients with systemic sclerosis: a prospective, case series study. J Dermatol [Internet]. 2016 [cited 2015 Sep 9];43(1):56–62. Available from: http://www.ncbi.nlm.nih.gov/pubmed/26173902.

103. Momeni A, Sorice SC, Valenzuela A, Fiorentino DF, Chung L, Chang J. Surgical treatment of systemic sclerosis-is it justified to offer peripheral sympathectomy earlier in the disease process? Microsurgery [Internet]. 2015 [cited 2015 Sep 9];35(6):441–6. Available from: http://www.ncbi.nlm.nih.gov/pubmed/25585522.

104. Bank J, Fuller SM, Henry GI, Zachary LS. Fat grafting to the hand in patients with Raynaud phenomenon: a novel therapeutic modality. Plast Reconstr Surg [Internet]. 2014 [cited 2015 Oct 6];133(5):1109–18. Available from: http://www.ncbi.nlm.nih.gov/pubmed/24445877.

105. Hughes M, Herrick AL. Raynaud's phenomenon. Best Pract Res Clin Rheumatol. 2016;30(1):112–32. Available from: https://www.ncbi.nlm.nih.gov/pubmed/27421220.

106. McMahan Z, Paik J. Raynaud's mimics. In: Wigley F, Herrick AL, Flavahan NA, editors. Raynaud's phenomenon. New York: Springer Science+Buisness Media; 2015. p. 163–85.

Maurizio Cutolo, Alberto Sulli, and Vanessa Smith

Introduction

Capillaroscopy: From the Beginning Up to Now

Literature concerning capillaroscopy has existed for several ages [1]. Capillaries in the nailfold were described in 1663 when Johan Christophorus Kolhaus used a primitive microscope to observe the small blood vessels surrounding the nails [1]. In the twentieth century, both specific morphologic changes in microcirculation in SSc were described as well as links with possible organ involvement in SSc [2–7]. Especially in the first half of the twenty-first century, the role of capillaroscopy in predicting digital ulcers has been established [2, 3, 8–14].

Techniques

What Is Nailfold Capillary Microscopy (Capillaroscopy)?

Capillaroscopy is a tool to look at the microcirculation of a patient [15]. Ideally, we look at the nailfold of the patient to the microcirculation as there the capillaries run parallel to the skin surface, and their whole longitudinal axis can be visualized [15].

As microangiopathy is a prominent feature in SSc, these microvascular morphological changes can be readily detected at the nailfold of the patients through nailfold capillary microscopy (Fig. 7.1). In fact, the essence of capillaroscopy is to examine noninvasively the morphology of nailfold dermal papillary capillaries. This is achieved by looking through the epidermis, after application of a drop of oil (Fig. 7.1) [16]. The nailfold and especially its distal capillary row are suitable for capillary examination as its papillae run parallel to the surface of the nail. Subsequently, the capillaries of the distal row are visible in their whole length and appear as red, hairpin-shaped loops (consisting of an afferent limb, a transitional [or apical] limb, and an efferent limb) that parallel the axis of the finger in a healthy subject (Fig. 7.2). In SSc and diseases of the scleroderma spectrum (([very] "early" SSc [see below]), mixed connective tissue disease, dermatomyositis, polymyositis)), there are characteristic changes of the microvascular morphology (see below), which can readily be detected by capillaroscopy [17, 18].

On behalf of the EULAR study group on microcirculation in rheumatic diseases
The EULAR centers for research and training on imaging (on capillaroscopy and laser)
The European Reference Network on Rare and Complex Connective Tissue and Musculoskeletal Diseases (ReCONNET)

M. Cutolo (✉) · A. Sulli
Research Laboratory and Academic Division of Clinical Rheumatology, Department of Internal Medicine, University of Genova, Genoa, Italy
e-mail: mcutolo@unige.it

V. Smith (✉)
Department of Internal Medicine, Ghent University, Ghent, Belgium

Department of Rheumatology, Ghent University Hospital, Ghent, Belgium
e-mail: vanessa.smith@ugent.be

© Springer Nature Switzerland AG 2019
M. Matucci-Cerinic, C. P. Denton (eds.), *Atlas of Ulcers in Systemic Sclerosis*, https://doi.org/10.1007/978-3-319-98477-3_7

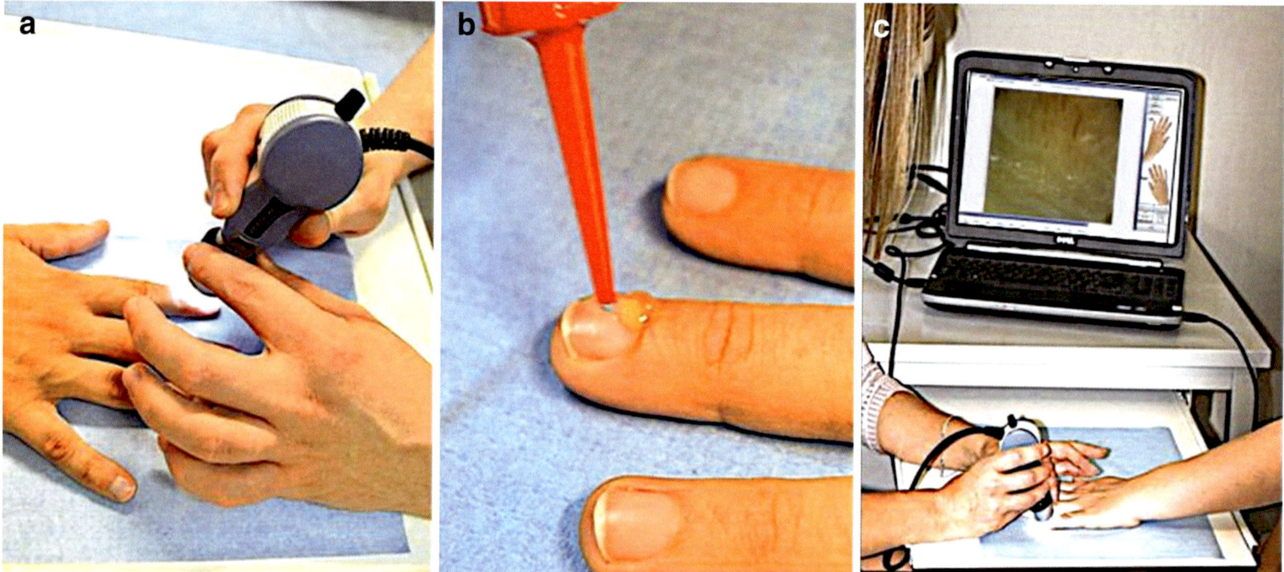

Fig. 7.1 (**a**) Capillaroscopy performed with a nailfold videocapillaroscope. The lens (magnification X200) which is incorporated in a contact probe rests on the nailfold of the patient. The contact probe makes it easy to explore the nail bed in all circumstances, even in patients with finger flexion contractures. (**b**) The operator puts a drop of oil on the nailfold of the patient to be able to better see through the epidermis. (**c**) After putting a drop of oil on the nailfold, the operator puts the probe in direct contact with the nailfold and is able to directly visualize the capillaries of the dermal papillae on the screen of the computer to which the nailfold capillaroscope is connected

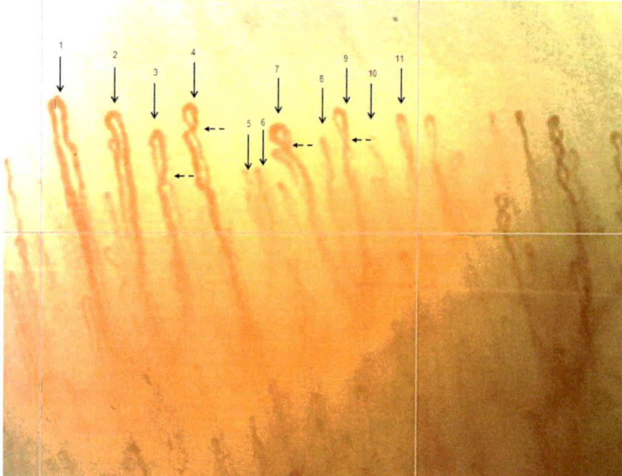

Fig. 7.2 A normal capillaroscopic image. Magnification X200. Morphology: open, hairpin, and crossed (horizontal dashed arrow). Dimension (measurement of diameter of a limb [black vertical line]): within normal limits. Architecture and distribution: capillaries are regularly arranged in a parallel fashion. Number: 11/mm (vertical arrows)

How to Perform Capillaroscopy

Magnification of Lens
Capillaroscopy may be performed with a lens with low and with high magnification. With a low magnification, a global evaluation of the entire nailfold area (wide-field capillaroscopy) is obtained. These instruments allow a panoramic vision of the whole nailfold microvascular network. In this way, prompt localization of abnormalities and analysis of architectural characteristics are performed (pattern recognition or qualitative assessment) [19].

One example of an optical instrument with low magnification is the stereomicroscope (magnification X14). Interestingly, already with this technique, the seminal descriptive papers concerning the scleroderma pattern were described by Maricq et al. in the last century (see below). Alternative choices are the dermatoscope and ophthalmoscope. The videocapillaroscope and stereomicroscope both allow not only low magnification but also the possibility to have sequential high magnifications (magnifications X100, X200, X600) which enable detailed observations of separate capillaries (Fig. 7.2). An advantage of the videocapillaroscope is that it consists of an optical probe which is moved to the finger of the patient and allows direct contact with the nailfold (Fig. 7.1) [15]. This facilitates examination of patients with SSc and severe flexion contractures, in which the probe can be moved to the nailfold of the contractured finger. When using the videocapillaroscope with a magnification of X200, two to four adjacent images of 1 mm per nailfold are being taken. Of note, the videocapillaroscope is available as a portable system which facilitates transport of the system.

Number of Fingers to Study
Different schools study different numbers of nailfolds. In this way, ten nailfolds, eight nailfolds and one nailfold (finger 4) have been studied [20, 21].

Screening a Patient with Raynaud's Phenomenon and Prediction of Digital Ulcers
Capillaroscopy is used in screening for SSc in patients with Raynaud's phenomenon (see below). As there may be a high variability in morphology in patients with SSc per nailfold (as not necessarily all nailfolds are affected by the scleroderma pattern), it may be opportune to screen every nailfold in a patient with Raynaud's phenomenon. In the prediction of digital ulcers, some studies evaluate several nailfolds, while others evaluate part of one nailfold [2, 3, 8–14].

Interpretation

The capillaroscopic images can be analyzed qualitatively and (semi)quantitatively.

Qualitative Assessment
In qualitative assessment (= pattern recognition, = "gestalt" assessment), an overall interpretation is given after commenting on the visibility of the image, the morphology of the capillaries, the density and dimensions "at sight" of the capillaries, and the architecture. Qualitative assessment readily allows to distinguish normal and non-specific changes in capillaroscopic image (Fig. 7.2) such as in a patient with primary Raynaud's phenomenon from an abnormal capillaroscopy due to a scleroderma spectrum disease (see below) [15, 16].

All of the abovementioned tools, even also the cheaper dermatoscopes, have in common that they have all testified reliability in discerning a normal capillaroscopy (in a healthy population) from the specific changes found in SSc through pattern recognition [22, 23]. Nevertheless, images captured by a dermatoscope might be hampered by visibility issues (up to 20% of unclassifiable images) [24]. Of note, prediction of digital ulcers based on capillaroscopy has been described mostly by nailfold videocapillaroscopy (see below).

(Semi)quantitative Assessment
Manual or (semi)automated measurements and countings can be made of certain characteristics of individual capillaries, in between others, of dimensions and density [21, 25]. Quantitation of certain characteristics of the capillaries in patients with SSc has been linked to clinical associations and more specifically to future development of digital ulcers in SSc (see below).

When to Perform Capillaroscopy

Investigation of a Patient with Raynaud's Phenomenon

Clinical rheumatologists frequently get patients with Raynaud's phenomenon referred. Prospective follow-up of patients with, as presenting symptom, merely Raynaud's phenomenon has attested that if a connective tissue disease is to appear after long-term follow-up, the key connective tissue disease which is to occur is SSc [26]. Consequently, the challenge is to distinguish patients with a primary Raynaud's phenomenon (not connected to any connective tissue disease) from patients with a secondary Raynaud's phenomenon (due to systemic sclerosis).

In 1992, LeRoy and Medsger proposed criteria to distinguish primary from secondary Raynaud's phenomenon due to systemic sclerosis [27]. These criteria have been prospectively validated (see below). Among other criteria, a "normal" capillaroscopy is obligatory to be able to speak of a "primary" Raynaud's phenomenon. Recently, also criteria for very early diagnosis of systemic sclerosis have been described, and capillaroscopy has been integrated in the 2013 American College of Rheumatology/European League Against Rheumatism classification criteria for systemic sclerosis (see below) [28, 29].

What Is Normal?

A normal capillaroscopic pattern, by qualitative assessment, is characterized by a homogeneous distribution of hairpin-shaped capillaries as a "comb-like structure," with a density of between 9 and 14 capillaries per mm in adults and not below 6 in children (Fig. 7.2) [30, 31]. Yet, there exists a wide intra- and inter-individual variety in a normal population. Andrade et al. extensively described the range of normal in 800 healthy adult subjects [32]. Apart from the stereotype hairpin-shaped open loop, there are common subtle morphological variations (non-specific variations) in the distal row capillaries such as tortuous (the limbs are curled but do not cross) (Fig. 7.2) and crossed capillaries (the limbs cross each other once or twice). Besides that certain anomalies, such as abnormal shapes (Fig. 7.3): meandering loops (the limbs are crossed upon themselves or with each other several times), bushy loops (the limbs originate small and have multiple buds) or abnormal dimensions, ectatic loops (the limbs are moderately enlarged, i.e., about four times the normal width or with the diameter of a limb >20 μm), and megacapillary (aneurysmatic loop, with the width of limbs ten times the normal one) and bizarre loops (striking atypical morphology, although not conforming to the four previously defined categories). In the healthy population, the prevalences of the mentioned anomalies are the following: meandering loops occur in 25% of healthy subjects, ectasia in 12%, bushy loops in 7%, bizarre loops in 2%, and megacapillaries in 0.3% and importantly in very low prevalence within a subject [32]. Of note, the EULAR study group on microcirculation in rheumatic diseases follows the definitions of Andrade to describe normal and non-specific morphological variations and for reasons of simplicity and standardization denotes all other shapes as "abnormal" (neoangiogenetic) shapes [33].

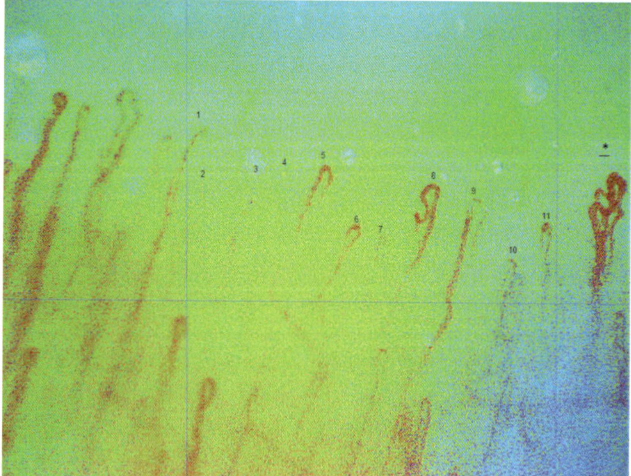

Fig. 7.3 A capillaroscopic image with morphological alterations. Magnification X200. Morphology: not only open, hairpin, and crossed but also abnormally shaped capillaries (underlined asterisk). An easy rule of thumb in defining morphology has been proposed by the EULAR study group on microcirculation in rheumatic diseases. In short, all shapes that are not "normal" ("open") or "non-specific" ("crossing" or "hairpin") are defined as "abnormal" shapes

What Is Pathognomonic Abnormal Due to SSc and Other Diseases of the Scleroderma Spectrum?

The majority of patients with clinically recognizable (= with skin involvement) SSc show a very characteristic combination of capillary abnormalities in the nailfold, which can easily be assessed through qualitative assessment (= pattern recognition). Maricq et al. described with the wide-field technique (magnification X12–X14) the scleroderma pattern. This pathognomonic combination contains the following: a striking widening of all three segments of the capillary loop (arterial, venous, and intermediate), loss of capillaries, and disorganization of the nailfold capillary bed [18]. Many abnormal morphologies such as branched "bushy" capillaries may also be observed. These scleroderma-type changes are also seen in diseases, "other than" clinically recognizable SSc such as patients with "(very) early" SSc (see below), dermatomyositis (DM), MCTD, and undifferentiated connective tissue disease (UCTD). Maricq et al. suggested that all these diseases may share some common pathogenetic factors and referred to these diseases as the family of scleroderma spectrum (SDS) disorders [18].

Through quantitative assessment, a decreased capillary density has been shown to be best predictive for a secondary Raynaud's phenomenon due to a scleroderma spectrum disease. More specifically, the loss of capillaries to a number of lower than 30 capillaries per 5 mm (= one nailfold) has a specificity of 92% [34].

In 2000, Cutolo et al. qualitatively assessed the nailfolds of an SSc cohort with patients fulfilling the former American College of Rheumatology (ACR) criteria for SSc with the nailfold videocapillaroscopy (NVC) technique (magnification X200) [35]. According to the different proportions of the hallmark parameters of the scleroderma pattern (giants, capillary loss, hemorrhages, and abnormal shapes, e.g., ramifications [definitions; see below]), Cutolo et al. defined three patterns: "early," "active," and "late" (Figs. 7.4, 7.5, 7.6, and 7.7) [16]. Of note, these scleroderma patterns are also associated with the development of digital ulcers (see below). The late pattern (with the most severe loss of capillaries) has the strongest odds ratio (OR) for future development of digital ulcers (see below) [2, 3].

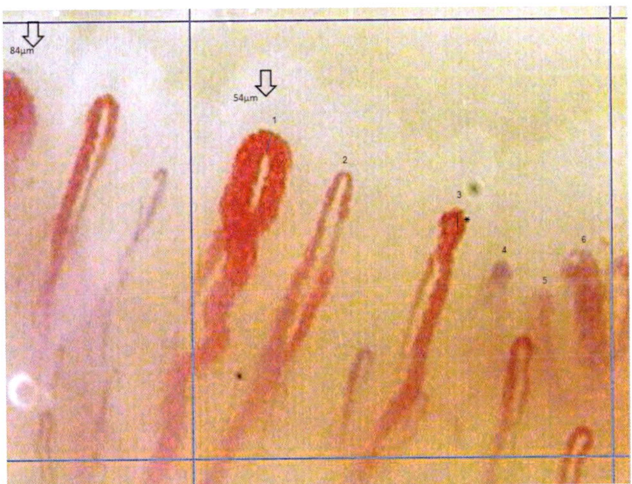

Fig. 7.4 An "early" scleroderma pattern. Description: magnification X200. Morphology: open, hairpin-shaped capillaries and crossed capillaries. Dimension: presence of giant capillaries (fat arrow) and ectasia (enlargement of diameter of capillary but below 50 μm [asterisk]). Number: six capillaries in the distal row

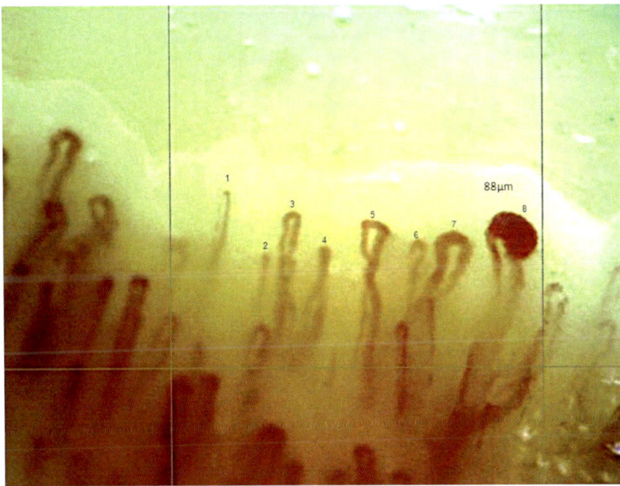

Fig. 7.5 Horseshoe-shaped giant capillary with an apical diameter of 88 μm

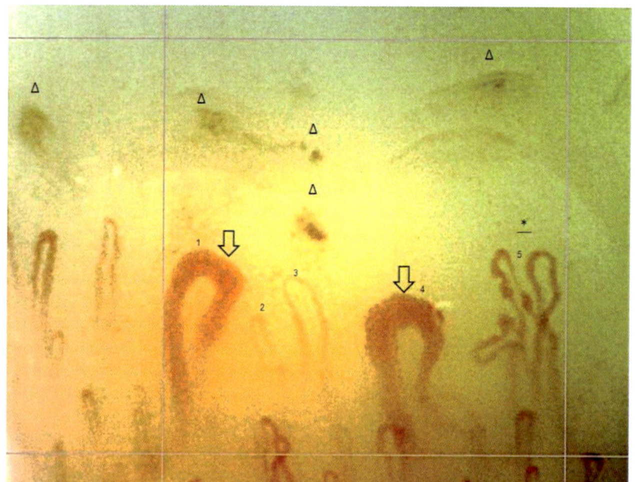

Fig. 7.6 An "active" scleroderma pattern. Description: magnification X200. Morphology: open, hairpin-shaped capillaries and abnormally shaped capillaries: (neo)angiogenesis (underlined asterisk). Dimension: presence of giant capillaries. Number: five capillaries in the distal row. Presence of hemorrhages (triangle)

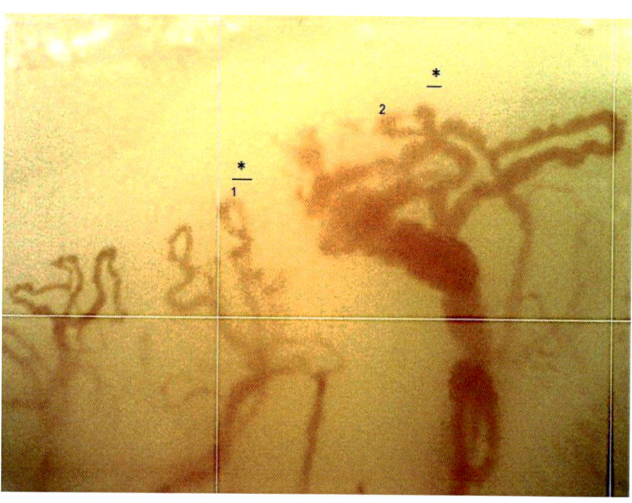

Fig. 7.7 A "late" scleroderma pattern. Description: magnification X200. Morphology: abnormally shaped capillaries: (neo)angiogenesis (underlined asterisk). Dimension: presence of dilations. Number: two capillaries in the distal row. The combination of loss of capillaries with abnormal form is representative of the "late" scleroderma pattern

"Early" and "Very Early" Diagnosis of SSc

When patients with SSc meet the former 1980 ACR criteria (Fig. 7.8), they already have "clinically recognizable" systemic sclerosis (skin involvement) that can be classified as belonging to either the limited cutaneous (lcSSc) or the diffuse cutaneous subset (dcSSc) [36]. Patients with "clinically recognizable" SSc undergo morbidity and mortality. As yet, no treatment has been proven, through randomized controlled trial, to halt the natural progression of the "clinically recognizable" disease. Consequently, efforts are being made to study the disease "early" or even "very early," before the "clinically recognizable" disease has set in and irreversible damage has occurred [28, 37].

Two recently proposed sets of criteria allow "early"/"very early" detection of SSc. On the one hand, there are the criteria LeRoy and Medsger proposed in 2001 for the "early" diagnosis of SSc, with Raynaud's phenomenon as the single major criterion. These criteria incorporate SSc-specific autoimmune antibodies and microvascular techniques, more specifically the "scleroderma-type" changes on capillaroscopy [38]. Like the ACR criteria, the LeRoy and Medsger criteria include patients with "clinically recognizable" SSc (with skin involvement), lcSSc, and dcSSc. But in addition

to that, they also allow patients to be included "earlier," before skin involvement has occurred. This third group of patients is classified as having limited systemic sclerosis (lSSc), identified by the presence of RP only (and no skin involvement yet) plus the presence of SSc-specific autoimmune antibodies (the anti-centromere, anti-topoisomerase I, anti-fibrillarin, anti-PM/Scl or anti-RNA polymerase I or III, and the Th/To antibodies) and/or typical "scleroderma-type" abnormalities on capillaroscopy. The third group is referred to as a "pre-scleroderma," as there is no skin involvement and subsequently as "early" systemic sclerosis. On the other hand, there is the recently published "very early" diagnosis of SSc (VEDOSS) criteria (Fig. 7.9) (which resulted from a Delphi consensus study) which also incorporate capillaroscopy as an important criterion in addition to the presence of antinuclear antibody positivity, puffy fingers, and SSc-specific antibodies. The validation process of these latter criteria is ongoing. Of note, next to the two sets of criteria for "early" and "very early" diagnosis of systemic sclerosis, the international SSc community has recently proposed updated ACR/EULAR criteria which have a higher sensitivity and specificity than the former 1980 ACR classification criteria and which also incorporate capillaroscopy as the main criterion [29].

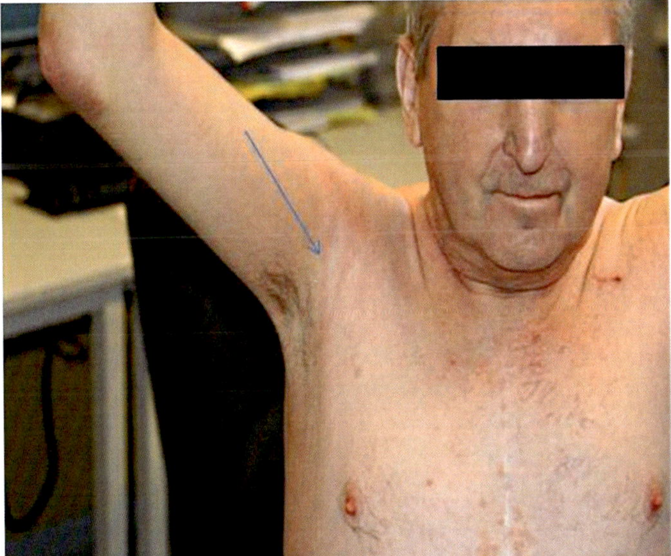

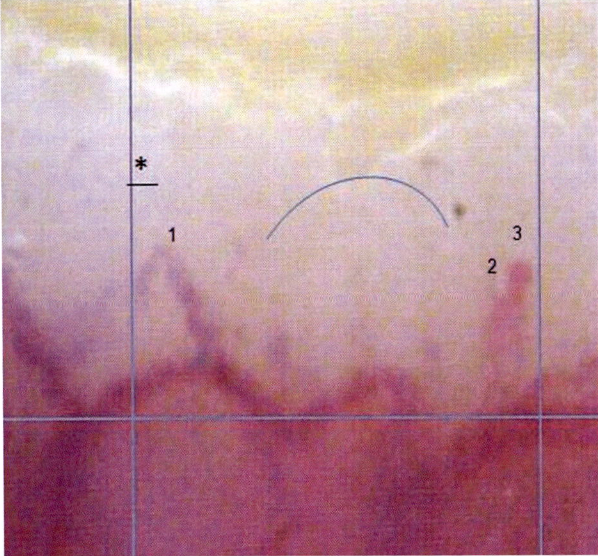

Fig. 7.8 Patient with the former ACR criteria for SSc. He is affected by diffuse skin involvement. Note the taut skin in the axillar region (arrow). A "late" scleroderma pattern. Description: magnification X200. Morphology: abnormally shaped capillary: (neo)angiogenesis (underlined asterisk). Dimension: presence of dilations. Number: three capillaries in the distal row. Note a large avascular area in between the two capillaries. This is also called desertification (bow)

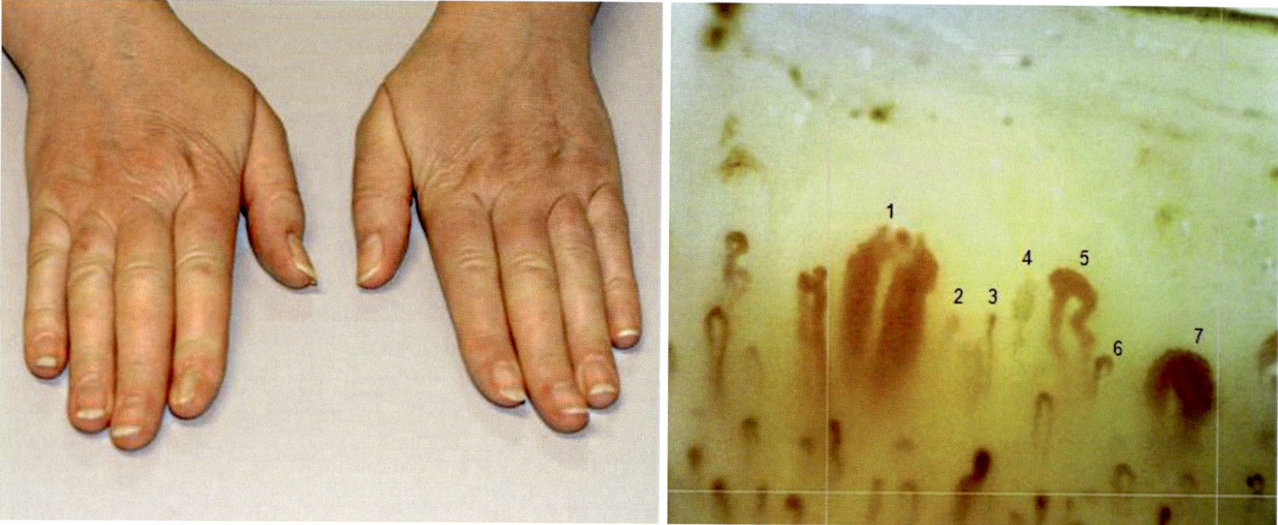

Fig. 7.9 Patient with Raynaud's phenomenon meeting the criteria for the very early diagnosis of systemic sclerosis (VEDOSS criteria): more specifically the presence of additionally puffy fingers and an early scleroderma pattern on capillaroscopy (presence of giants and hemorrhages without significant loss of capillaries)

How to Interpret Nailfold Capillaroscopy in Clinical Practice in SSc

Qualitative Assessment in SSc: The "Early," "Active," and "Late" Patterns

As mentioned previously, peripheral microangiopathy in SSc can be easily recognized and studied early in the disease course by the detection of characteristic capillaroscopic changes associated with the presence of secondary Raynaud's phenomenon due to SSc [39, 40].

These microvascular SSc alterations appear dynamically and reflect the pathophysiology of the disease. The morphological parameters that characterize SSc are the giant capillaries, the microhemorrhages, and the loss of capillaries and abnormal shapes, referred to as neovascularization or neoangiogenesis.

Giant Capillaries and Role of Dilations

Homogeneously enlarged microvascular loops (giant capillaries) are the earliest and most striking feature of secondary Raynaud's phenomenon. The enlargements show a characteristic symmetrical shape involving both afferent and efferent branches of the capillary (Fig. 7.4) or a horseshoe shape (with the diameter of the transitional limb being wider than the other two limbs) (Fig. 7.5). The detection of even a single loop with a homogeneous increase in diameter to more than 50 μm at the level of the nailfold should be considered a potential marker of microangiopathy related to a scleroderma spectrum disorder [41]. The capillary dilatations represent the first sign of microvessel wall damage (altered endothelial cell array). Of note, a frequently asked question is the role of dilations in the evaluation of subjects with Raynaud's phenomenon. The key question here is whether a dilation should alert the clinician to more frequent follow-up of the patient in the screening for SSc. A recent study could attest that dilations below the cutoff of 30 μm have a high negative predictive value in a Raynaud's population, attesting a low risk to develop SSc [42]. Subsequently, dilations below 30 μm may be considered as non-specific alterations and should not warn the capillaroscopist.

Microhemorrhages

Nailfold microhemorrhages are also linked to the altered endothelial cell array and appear as an easily detectable dark spot (Fig. 7.6). They arise from microvascular extravasation of red blood cells from the capillary loop and bridge the appearance of giant capillaries their subsequent collapse and disappearance [40].

Capillary Loss and Avascular Areas

A decreased number of capillary loops are specific for SSc [34]. The extensive disappearance of capillaries can generate large avascular areas, which have a desertlike appearance in the nail bed microvascular array (Fig. 7.8). Loss of capillaries seems to be related to tissue hypoxia that is linked to digital skin ulcers and other clinical complications in SSc.

(Neo)vascularization (= abnormal shapes, e.g., bushy shapes, ramifications)

Capillary loss creates tissue hypoxia and local production of vessel growth factors (such as non-exhaustively, vascular endothelial growth factor), which in turn stimulates the formation of new capillaries—(neo)angiogenesis. The main morphological hallmark of angiogenesis is the clustering of twisted capillaries, with pronounced heterogeneity in shape and size, winding together with bushy capillaries (Fig. 7.7). Highly convoluted and branched capillary loop clusters, surrounded by a dropout of normal capillary loops, are characteristic features of neoangiogenesis in the "late" SSc pattern.

The above discussed microvascular alterations that characterize the scleroderma pattern have been recently classified by Cutolo et al. into three defined and different NVC patterns (Figs. 7.4, 7.5, 7.6, and 7.7) that include an "early" pattern (few giant capillaries, few capillary microhemorrhages, no evident loss of capillaries, and relatively well-preserved capillary distribution), an "active" pattern (frequent giant capillaries, frequent capillary microhemorrhages, moderate loss of capillaries, and absent or mild ramified (abnormally shaped) capillaries with mild disorganization of the capillary architecture), and a "late" pattern (almost absent giant capillaries and microhemorrhages, severe loss of capillaries with extensive avascular areas, abnormal shapes (neovascularization) with ramified/bushy capillaries, and intense disorganization of the normal capillary array) (Fig. 7.7) [16, 22]. These patterns have been recently validated [2, 3, 10].

Semiquantitative Assessment in SSc

Counting or scoring of capillary abnormalities per unit of quantity, e.g., one linear mm, has become of great importance for several reasons. In this way, microvascular abnormalities can be correlated with other (clinical) variables (organ involvement and angiogenic/static factors) of the disease and might be used to evaluate pharmacological effects on the microvasculature [43–47]. For example, long-term effects of endothelin receptor antagonism on microvascular damage evaluated by nailfold capillaroscopic analysis in systemic sclerosis have been recently assessed in open study design setting [48].

Recently, practical systems to score the capillaroscopic alterations in patients with SSc have been proposed and validated [10, 13, 21, 22].

At least the following four major capillaroscopic parameters should be counted/scored at each capillaroscopic examination: number of capillaries, presence of giant capillaries, hemorrhages, and abnormally shaped capillaries (neoangiogenetic, e.g., ramified capillaries).

Practically, for each field of analysis (1 millimeter) at the level of the nailfold, usually two to four fields for each finger are analyzed (Fig. 7.9) [49].

Next to just counting the number of capillaroscopic characteristics per linear mm, also a semiquantitative rating scale (score 0–3) to score each abovementioned capillary parameter has been described [49]. These counting (=quantitative) systems have been applied in predictive associations of digital ulcers (see below) (Fig. 7.10).

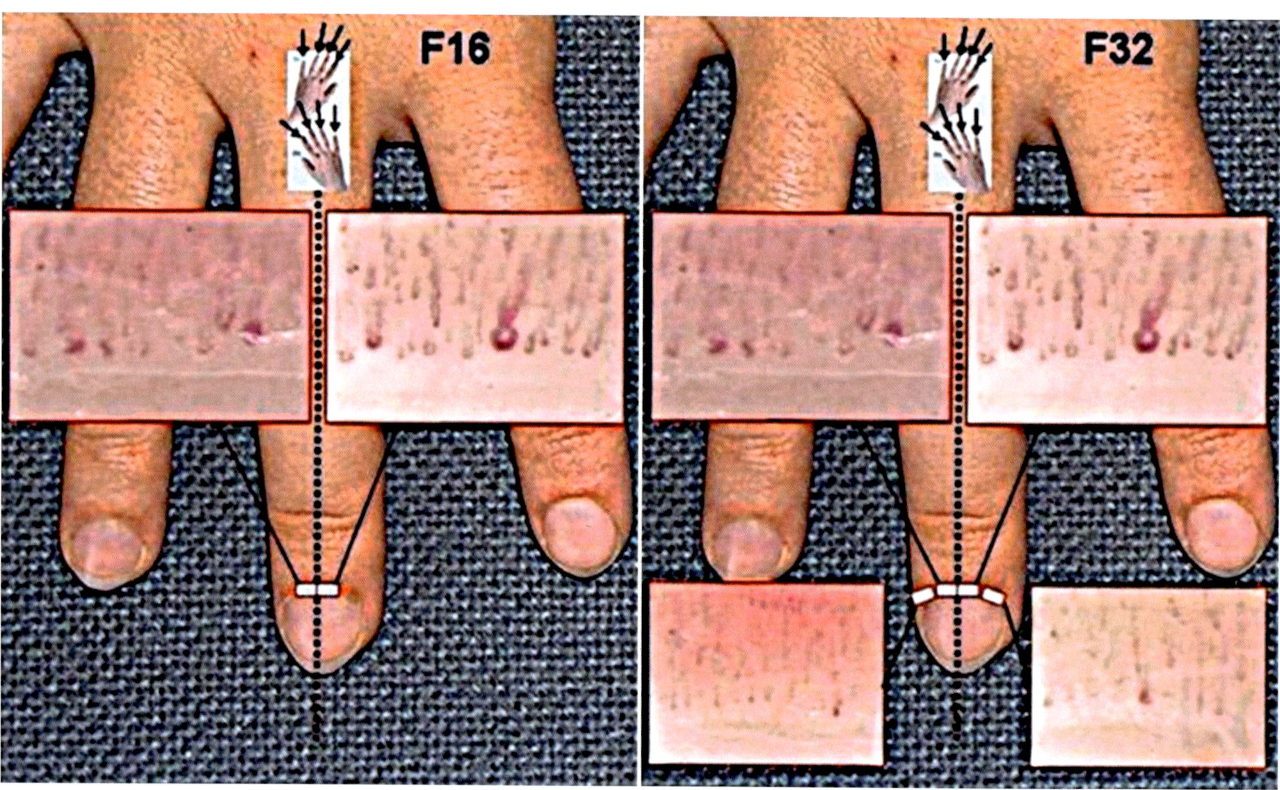

Fig. 7.10 The (semi)quantitative assessment. Eight fingers are being evaluated and two to four images per finger are being capitated. Capillaroscopic characteristics can be counted over a linear mm or can be translated into a score [10]

Association Between Capillaroscopy and Digital Ulcers in SSc

Especially since the beginning of the twenty-first century, the eyes are geared to the investigation of capillaroscopy as a tool to predict organ-specific complications [2, 3]. Two assessment types are being used to assess the biomarker properties of capillaroscopy. On the one hand, there is "qualitative" assessment (=pattern recognition on sight) with which capillaroscopic images are classified into "normal" or "early" and "active" or "late" scleroderma pattern (see above) [16]. The definitions of these patterns are based on the relative prevalence of scleroderma-type changes (see above) in the capillaroscopic images. On the other hand, there is the quantitative assessment in which scleroderma-type changes (lowered number of capillaries, giants, abnormally shaped capillaries (=[neo]angiogenesis) are quantitated over a linear millimeter [13, 21]. Both cross-sectional and prospective associations have been made between capillaroscopy and clinical complications in SSc.

In this way cross-sectional or retrospective associations have been made not only in small pilot but also in cohort studies between the scleroderma patterns and digital ulcers, interstitial lung disease, pulmonary (arterial) hypertension, cardiac involvement, skin involvement, and death [3–11, 13]. In line with this, these clinical associations have also been made with the quantitatively assessed number of capillaries (Fig. 7.11) [5, 7].

Some pilot studies described indici to predict digital ulcers (Table 7.1) [2, 3, 8–14, 50]. The common and logical (as SSc is a disease with progressive obliteration of the microcirculation) denominator is that loss of capillaries (qualitatively described as "late" scleroderma pattern or quantitatively as "lowered" number of capillaries) is a key criterion in prospective indici to predict new digital ulcers in an SSc population (Figs. 7.11 and 7.12).

The most noteworthy initiative though was a recent pan-European (59 centers) study which produced a risk chart to predict new DU within 6 months of the baseline visit in a patient population with a history of DU (most prone to develop new DU) [13]. This latter index is characterized by a high negative predictive value allowing the clinician to reassure the patients who will not develop new DU. In fact, a simple model consisting of merely counting the numbers of capillaries in the middle finger of the dominant hand, counting the number of digital ulcers at the baseline visit, and attesting the (non)-presence of critical digital ischemia has a negative predictive value of more than 80%. Subsequently, based on three simple obtainable parameters, the rheumatologist can with a high certainty reassure patients who will not develop digital ulcers within 6 months of the clinical visit. Further prospective studies should be aimed at producing indici which not only identify patients who will or will not develop digital ulcers but identify patients at risk for other organ involvement or infaust outcome such as death [2]. To this end a joint collaboration between the EULAR Scleroderma Trials and Research group (EUSTAR) and the EULAR study group on microcirculation in rheumatic diseases was set up. Extensive analysis of capillaroscopic data in a prospectively followed-up cohort of patients with SSc will be analyzed with the aim to provide an index based on capillaroscopic and SSc-related characteristics to identify patients with severe evolution of SSc disease.

Of note, a monocentric study also associated digital ulcers in a VEDOSS population with NVC scleroderma patterns. External validation through multicentric corroboration of these data is being awaited [51].

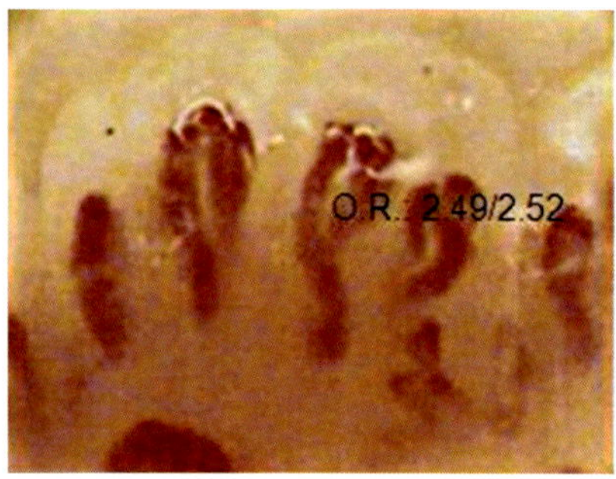

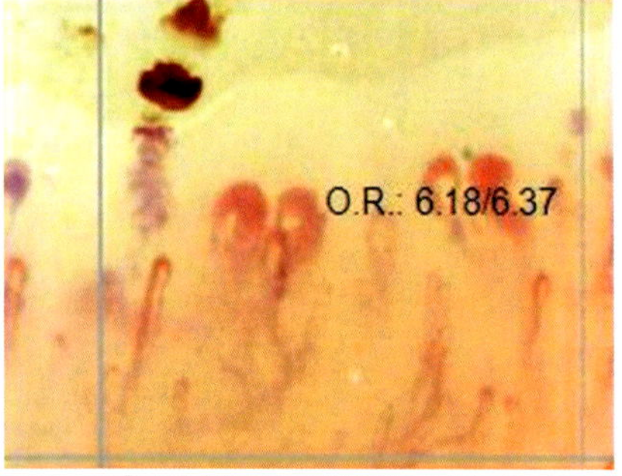

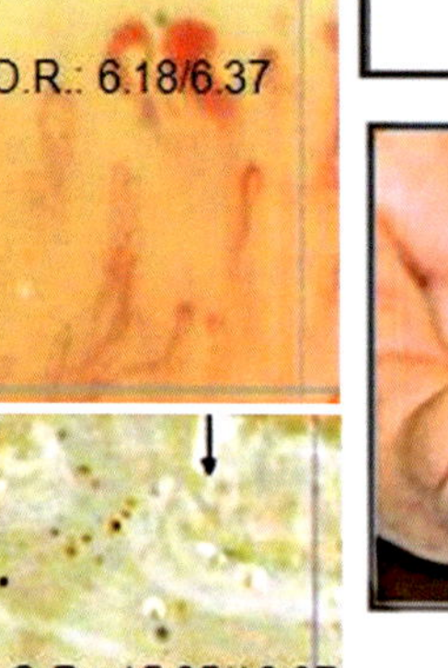

2 (moderate)	3 (severe)	4 (endstage)
Digital pitting scars	Digital tip ulcerations	Digital gangrene

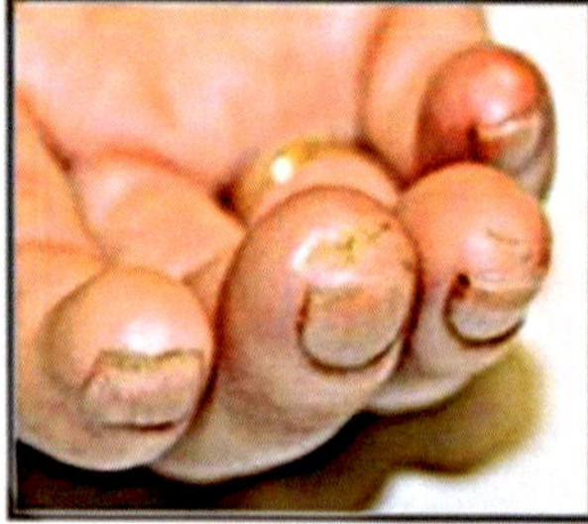

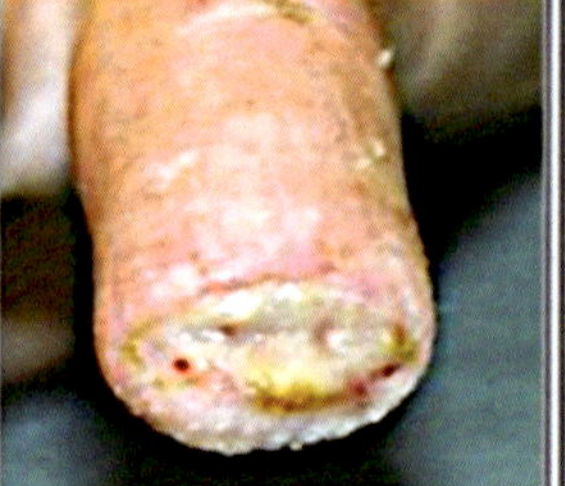

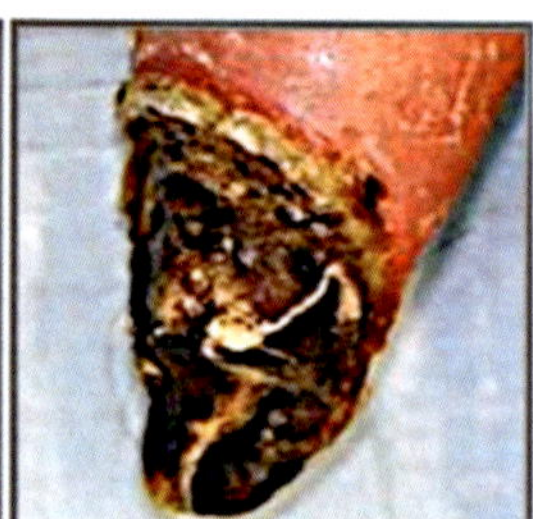

Fig. 7.11 Pilot proof-of-concept study in which qualitative assessment was associated with future development of digital trophic lesions in systemic sclerosis. Odds ratios (OR) are presented per qualitative scleroderma pattern. This study attested that the late scleroderma pattern (lower left image) had the highest OR after single and multiple logistic regression analysis to predict future digital trophic lesions [2]

Table 7.1 Prospective associations between capillaroscopy and clinical complications in SSc

Author	Quantitative assessment	Qualitative assessment	Results
Sebastiani et al. (2009) [8]	+		Prognostic index (based on the number of capillaries, number of giants, maximum capillary diameter) to predict digital ulcers within 3 months of baseline capillaroscopic visit (capillaroscopic skin ulcer risk index, CSURI)
Sebastiani et al. (2012) [9]	+		Multicenter validation of Sebastiani (2009) CSURI
Smith et al. (2011) [10]	+		Prognostic index (for the day-to-day practice) based on merely counting the number of capillaries over eight fingers (one field per finger) to predict digital trophic lesions within 6–12 months after the baseline capillaroscopic visit
Smith et al. (2012) [2]		+	Prognostic association between baseline capillaroscopic scleroderma patterns and future (12–24 months) development of digital trophic lesions. The "late" nailfold capillaroscopic scleroderma pattern heralding the strongest odds ratio
Smith et al. (2013) [11]		+	Bicenter validation of Smith (2012)
Ingegnoli et al. (2013) [3]		+	EUSTAR multicenter study corroboration of Smith (2012)
Manfredi et al. (2015) [12]	+		Italian multicenter risk chart to predict DU within 6 months of baseline visit in patients without endothelin receptor antagonist use at baseline

Table 7.1 (continued)

Cutolo et al. (2016) [13]	+	Pan-European multicenter prognostic index based on merely counting the number of capillaries in the middle finger of the dominant hand, having a high negative predictive value to pinpoint those patients who will not develop a DU within 6 months after the baseline capillaroscopic visit. Validation of the day-to-day Smith et al. (2011) index
Sebastiani et al. (2015) [14]	+	Monocenter Italian study showing only moderate performance of CSURI to predict digital ulcers in patients in daily clinical setting, more specifically, in patients allowed to be on endothelin receptor antagonist therapy at baseline
Avouac et al. (2017) [50]	+	Monocentric French study attesting association between reduction of the number of capillaries over time and occurrence of DU

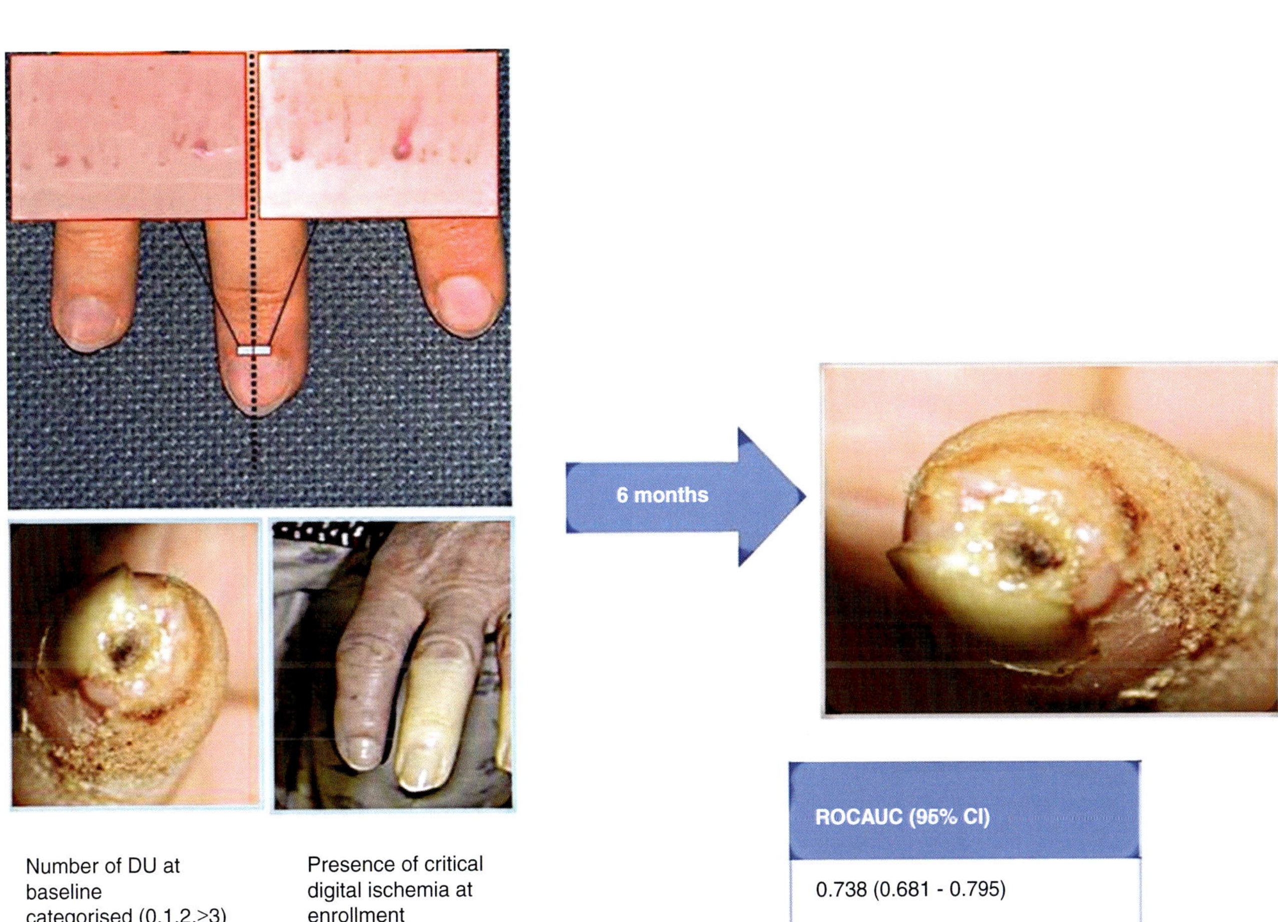

Fig. 7.12 The CAP study was the first large (59 centers) prospective study to evaluate capillaroscopy and clinical covariables in the assessment of future development of DU. This study produced a model (based on a mean number of capillaries in the middle finger of the dominant hand, number of DU at baseline visit, presence or absence of critical digital ischemia) with a high negative predictivity. In this way, for example, a patient with no critical digital ischemia at baseline and no digital ulcers at baseline is associated with a low risk to develop future DU

Capillaroscopy Versus Other Commonly Used Tools to Evaluate the Microcirculation: Laser

Capillaroscopy generally provides static information on microvascular involvement (morphologic alterations). Morphology in SSc evolves relatively slow in time, and the rate of change is inhomogeneous over the SSc population [21, 52]. On the other hand, laser provides dynamic information on microvascular involvement as it measures reactivity (flow [perfusions] alterations) [53]. These characteristics may potentiate high-performance models to predict peripheral vascular disease in SSc and especially allow laser to be a sensitive outcome measure.

Flow in SSc patients can be measured on a single point at the digits (single-point flowmetry) with the laser Doppler and recently also over a set area (e.g., the volar side of the fingertips) with the laser speckle contrast analysis (LASCA) [54–56]. Both laser techniques have been correlated with nailfold capillaroscopy and are significantly correlated [57, 58]. Logically, a lower skin perfusion is related to more extensive microvascular involvement either qualitatively (late scleroderma pattern) or quantitatively (higher microangiopathy evolution score) [58]. Both laser techniques have been used in open and randomized controlled peripheral vascular therapy trials in SSc. Notably, the LASCA has attested to reliably quantitate flow in a SSc population and has been recently used to follow up ulcer evolution after topical therapy in scleroderma and may seem to monitorize in an excellent manner the improvements [57–64].

Key Points

- Nailfold capillaroscopy is a noninvasive imaging technique that is used for in vivo morphological assessment of the microcirculation.
- Nailfold capillaroscopy is able to distinguish a primary Raynaud's phenomenon from a secondary Raynaud's phenomenon due to SSc and the diseases belonging to the scleroderma spectrum.
- The capillaroscopic images can be assessed qualitatively and (semi)quantitatively.
- Predictive associations have been made between the qualitative assessment (normal versus scleroderma patterns ["early," "active," "late"]) and quantitative indici and peripheral SSc microangiopathy, in particular the prediction of new digital ulcers.
- Proof-of-concept studies in the evaluation of microcirculatory therapies/digital ulcer follow-up have been described with nailfold videocapillaroscopy and/or laser.

References

1. Cutolo M. Capillaroscopy in rheumatic diseases. From the XVIII to the XXI century. In: Cutolo M, editor. Atlas of capillaroscopy in rheumatic diseases, vol. 1. Elsevier Srl: Milano; 2010. p. 3–5.
2. Smith V, Decuman S, Sulli A, Bonroy C, Piettte Y, Deschepper E, et al. Do worsening scleroderma capillaroscopic patterns predict future severe organ involvement? a pilot study. Ann Rheum Dis. 2012;71(10):1636–9.
3. Ingegnoli F, Ardoini I, Boracchi P, Cutolo M, EUSTAR co-authors. Nailfold capillaroscopy in systemic sclerosis: DATA from the EULAR scleroderma trials and research (EUSTAR) database. Microvasc Res. 2013;89:122–8.
4. Caramaschi P, Canestrini S, Martinelli N, Volpe A, Pieropan S, Ferrari M, et al. Scleroderma patients nailfold videocapillaroscopic patterns are associated with disease subset and disease severity. Rheumatology (Oxford). 2007;46(10):1566–9.
5. Bredemeier M, Xavier RM, Capobianco KG, Restelli VG, Rohde LE, Pinotti AF, et al. Nailfold capillary microscopy can suggest pulmonary disease activity in systemic sclerosis. J Rheumatol. 2004;31(2):286–94.
6. Kayser C, Sekiyama J, Próspero L, Camargo C, Andrade L. Nailfold capillaroscopy abnormalities as predictors of mortality in patients with systemic sclerosis. Clin Exp Rheumatol. 2013;31(2 Suppl 76):103–8.
7. Hofstee HM, Serne EH, Roberts C, Hesselstrand R, Scheja A, Moore TL, et al. A multicentre study on the reliability of qualitative and quantitative nail-fold videocapillaroscopy assessment. Rheumatology (Oxford). 2012;51(4):749–55.
8. Sebastiani M, Manfredi A, Colaci M, D'Amico R, Malagoli V, Giuggioli D, et al. Capillaroscopic skin ulcer risk index: a new prognostic tool for digital skin ulcer development in systemic sclerosis patients. Arthritis Rheum. 2009;61(5):688–94.
9. Sebastiani M, Manfredi A, Vukatana G, Moscatelli S, Riato L, Bocci M, et al. Predictive role of capillaroscopic skin ulcer risk index in systemic sclerosis: a multicentre validation study. Ann Rheum Dis. 2012;71(1):67–70.
10. Smith V, De Keyser F, Pizzorni C, Van Praet JT, Decuman S, Sulli A, et al. Nailfold capillaroscopy for day-to-day clinical use: construction of a simple scoring modality as a clinical prognostic index for digital trophic lesions. Ann Rheum Dis. 2011;70(1):180–3.
11. Smith V, Riccieri V, Pizzorni C, Decuman S, Deschepper E, Bonroy C, et al. Nailfold capillaroscopy for prediction of novel future severe organ involvement in systemic sclerosis. J Rheumatol. 2013;40(12):2023–8.
12. Manfredi A, Sebastiani M, Carraro V, Iudici M, Bocci M, Vukatana G, et al. Prediction risk chart for scleroderma digital ulcers: a composite predictive model based on capillaroscopic, demographic and clinico-serological parameters. Clin Hemorheol Microcirc. 2015;59(2):133–43.
13. Cutolo M, Herrick A, Distler O, Becker M, Beltran E, Carpentier P, et al. Nailfold videocapillaroscopy and clinical characteristics to predict digital ulcer risk in systemic sclerosis: a multicenter, prospective cohort study. Arthritis Rheumatol. 2016;68(10):2527–39.
14. Sebastiani M, Manfredi A, Cestelli V, Praino E, Cannarile D, Giuggioli M, et al. Validation study of predictive value of capillaroscopic skin ulcer risk index (CSURI) in scleroderma patients treated with bosentan. Clin Exp Rheumatol. 2015;33(Suppl 91(4)):196.
15. Smith V, Cutolo M. When and how to perform capillaroscopy. In: Cutolo M, editor. Atlas of capillaroscopy in rheumatic diseases, vol. 1. Milano: Elsevier Srl; 2010. p. 33–42.
16. Cutolo M, Sulli A, Pizzorni C, Accardo S. Nailfold videocapillaroscopy assessment of microvascular damage in systemic sclerosis. J Rheumatol. 2000;27(1):155–60.

17. Maricq HR, Leroy EC, D'angelo WA, Medsger TA, Rodnan GP, Sharp GC, et al. Diagnostic potential of invivo microscopy in scleroderma and related disorders. Arthritis Rheum. 1980;23(2):183–9.

18. Maricq HR, Weinberger AB, LeRoy EC. Early detection of scleroderma-spectrum disorders by in vivo capillary microscopy: a prospective study of patients with Raynaud's phenomenon. J Rheumatol. 1982;9(2):289–91.

19. Grassi W, De Angelis R. Capillaroscopy: questions and answers. Clin Rheumatol. 2007;26(12):2009–16.

20. Hofstee HMA, Noordegraaf AV, Voskuyl AE, Dijkmans BAC, Postmus PE, Smulders YM, et al. Nailfold capillary density is associated with the presence and severity of pulmonary arterial hypertension in systemic sclerosis. Ann Rheum Dis. 2009;68(2):191–5.

21. Sulli A, Secchi ME, Pizzorni C, Cutolo M. Scoring the nailfold microvascular changes during the capillaroscopic analysis in systemic sclerosis patients. Ann Rheum Dis. 2008;67(6):885–7.

22. Smith V, Pizzorni C, De Keyser F, Decuman S, Van Praet JT, Deschepper E, et al. Reliability of the qualitative and semiquantitative nailfold videocapillaroscopy assessment in a systemic sclerosis cohort: a two-centre study. Ann Rheum Dis. 2010;69(6):1092–6.

23. Sekiyama J, Camargo C, Eduardo L, Andrade C, Kayser C. Reliability of widefield nailfold capillaroscopy and videocapillaroscopy in the assessment of patients with Raynaud's phenomenon. Arthritis Care Res. 2013;65(11):1853–61.

24. Moore TL, Roberts C, Murray AK, Helbling I, Herrick AL. Reliability of dermoscopy in the assessment of patients with Raynaud's phenomenon. Rheumatology (Oxford). 2010;49(3):542–7.

25. Berks M, Tresadern P, Dinsdale G, Murray A, Moore T, Herrick A, et al. An automated system for detecting and measuring nailfold capillaries. Med Image Comput Comput Assist Interv. 2014;17(Pt 1):658–65.

26. Koenig M, Joyal F, Fritzler MJ, Roussin A, Abrahamowicz M, Boire G, et al. Autoantibodies and microvascular damage are independent predictive factors for the progression of Raynaud's phenomenon to systemic sclerosis: a twenty-year prospective study of 586 patients, with validation of proposed criteria for early systemic sclerosis. Arthritis Rheum. 2008;58(12):3902–12.

27. LeRoy EC, Medsger TA Jr. Raynaud's phenomenon: a proposal for classification. Clin Exp Rheumatol. 1992;10(5):485–8.

28. Avouac J, Fransen J, Walker UA, Riccieri V, Smith V, Muller C, et al. Preliminary criteria for the very early diagnosis of systemic sclerosis: results of a Delphi Consensus Study from EULAR Scleroderma Trials and Research Group. Ann Rheum Dis. 2011;70(3):476–81.

29. van den Hoogen F, Khanna D, Fransen J, Johnson SR, Baron M, Tyndall A, et al. 2013 classification criteria for systemic sclerosis: an American college of rheumatology/European league against rheumatism collaborative initiative. Ann Rheum Dis. 2013;72(11):1747–55.

30. Pain C, Constantin T, Toplak N, Moll M, Iking-Konert C, Piotto D, et al. Raynaud's syndrome in children: systematic review and development of recommendations for assessment and monitoring. Clin Exp Rheumatol. 2016;34(Suppl 100 (5)):200–6.

31. Piotto D, Sekiyama J, Kayser C, Yamada M, Len C, Terreri M. Nailfold videocapillaroscopy in healthy children and adolescents: description of normal patterns. Clin Exp Rheumatol. 2016;34(Suppl 100 (5)):193–9.

32. Andrade LE, Gabriel Junior A, Assad RL, Ferrari AJ, Atra E. Panoramic nailfold capillaroscopy: a new reading method and normal range. Semin Arthritis Rheum. 1990;20(1):21–31.

33. Smith V, Beeckman S, Herrick A, Decuman S, Deschepper E, De Keyser F, et al. An EULAR study group pilot study on reliability of "simple" capillaroscopic definitions to describe capillary morphology in rheumatic diseases. Rheumatology (Oxford). 2016;55(5):883–90.

34. Houtman PM, Kallenberg CG, Fidler V, Wouda AA. Diagnostic significance of nailfold capillary patterns in patients with Raynaud's phenomenon. An analysis of patterns discriminating patients with and without connective tissue disease. J Rheumatol. 1986;13(3):556–63.

35. Preliminary criteria for the classification of systemic-sclerosis (scleroderma). Subcommittee for scleroderma criteria of the American rheumatism association diagnostic and therapeutic criteria committee. Arthritis Rheum. 1980;23(5):581–90.

36. LeRoy EC, Black C, Fleischmajer R, Jablonska S, Krieg T, Medsger TA, et al. Scleroderma (systemic-sclerosis) - classification, subsets and pathogenesis. J Rheumatol. 1988;15(2):202–5.

37. Matucci-Cerenic M, Allanore Y, Czirják L, Tyndall A, Müller-Ladner U, Denton C, et al. The challenge of early systemic sclerosis for the EULAR Scleroderma Trial and Research group (EUSTAR) community. It is time to cut the Gordian knot and develop a prevention or rescue strategy. Ann Rheum Dis. 2009;68(9):1377–80.

38. LeRoy EC, Medsger TA Jr. Criteria for the classification of early systemic sclerosis. J Rheumatol. 2001;28(7):1573–6.

39. Maricq HR. Widefield capillary microscopy. Technique and rating scale for abnormalities seen in scleroderma and related disorders. Arthritis Rheum. 1981;24(9):1159–65.

40. Cutolo M, Sulli A, Smith V. Assessing microvascular changes in systemic sclerosis diagnosis and management. Nat Rev Rheumatol. 2010;6(10):578–87.

41. De Angelis R. The most important capillaroscopic parameters in normal and pathological conditions. In: Cutolo M, editor. Atlas of capillaroscopy in rheumatic diseases. Milano: Elsevier Srl; 2010. p. 61–9.

42. Trombetta A, Smith V, Pizzorni C, Meroni M, Paolino S, Cariti C, et al. Quantitative alterations of capillary diameter have a predictive value for development of the capillaroscopic scleroderma pattern. J Rheumatol. 2016;43(3):599–606.

43. Statham B, Rowell N. Quantification of the nail fold capillary abnormalities in systemic sclerosis and Raynaud's syndrome. Acta Derm Venereol. 1986;66(2):139–43.

44. Ohtsuka T. Quantitative analysis of nailfold capillary abnormalities in patients with connective tissue diseases. Int J Dermatol. 1999;38(10):757–64.

45. Cutolo M, Sulli A, Pizzorni C, Smith V. Capillaroscopy as an outcome measure for clinical trials on the peripheral vasculopathy in SSc-is it useful? Int J Rheumatol. 2010;2010:1. https://doi.org/10.1155/2010/784947.

46. Cutolo M, Smith V. State of art on nailfold capillaroscopy: a reliable diagnostic tool and putative biomarker in rheumatology? Rheumatology (Oxford). 2013;52:1933–40.

47. Avouac J, Vallucci M, Smith V, Senet P, Ruiz B, Sulli A, et al. Correlations between angiogenic factors and capillaroscopic patterns in systemic sclerosis. Arthritis Res Ther. 2013;15(2):R55.

48. Cutolo M, Zampogna G, Vremis L, Smith V, Pizzorni C, Sulli A. Longterm effects of endothelin receptor antagonism on microvascular damage evaluated by nailfold capillaroscopic analysis in systemic sclerosis. J Rheumatol. 2013;40(1):40–5.

49. Sulli A. Reporting and scoring capillaroscopic pictures. In: Cutolo M, editor. Atlas of capillaroscopy in rheumatic diseases. Milano: Elsevier Srl; 2010. p. 77–87.

50. Avouac J, Lepri G, Smith V, Toniolo E, Hurabielle C, Vallet A, et al. Sequential nailfold videocapillaroscopy examinations have responsiveness to detect organ progression in systemic sclerosis. Semin Arthritis Rheum. 2017; [Epub ahead of print].

51. Bruni C, Guiducci S, Bellando-Randone S, Lepri G, Braschi F, Fiori G, et al. Digital ulcers as a sentinel sign for early internal organ involvement in very early systemic sclerosis. Rheumatology (Oxford). 2015;54(1):72–6.

52. Sulli A, Pizzorni C, Smith V, Zampogna G, Ravera F, Cutolo M. Timing of transition between capillaroscopic patterns in systemic sclerosis. Arthritis Rheum. 2012;64(3):821–5.
53. Cutolo M, Sulli A, Smith V. Assessment tools of microvasculopathy. In: 11th EULAR on-line course on systemic sclerosis [Internet]: European League Against Rheumatism; 2015.
54. Cutolo M, Smith V. Nailfold capillaroscopy and other methods to assess the microvasculopathy in systemic sclerosis. In: Hachulla E, Czirjak L, editors. EULAR textbook on systemic sclerosis. London: BMJ; 2013. p. 129–38.
55. Sulli A, Ruaro B, Cutolo M. Evaluation of blood perfusion by laser speckle contrast analysis in different areas of hands and face in patients with systemic sclerosis. Ann Rheum Dis. 2014;73(11):2059–61.
56. Meijs J, Voskuyl A, Bloemsaat-Minekus J, Vonk M. Blood flow in the hands of a predefined homogeneous systemic sclerosis population: the presence of digital ulcers and the improvement with bosentan. Rheumatology (Oxford). 2015;54(2):262–9.
57. Cutolo M, Ferrone C, Pizzorni C, Soldano S, Seriolo B, Sulli A. Peripheral blood perfusion correlates with microvascular abnormalities in systemic sclerosis: a laser-Doppler and nailfold videocapillaroscopy study. J Rheumatol. 2010;37(6):1174–80.
58. Ruaro B, Sulli A, Alessandri E, Pizzorni C, Ferrari G, Cutolo M. Laser speckle contrast analysis: a new method to evaluate peripheral blood perfusion in systemic sclerosis patients. Ann Rheum Dis. 2014;73(6):1181–5.
59. Cutolo M, Ruaro B, Ravera F, Pizzorni C, Smith V, Zampogna G, et al. Long-term treatment with endothelin receptor antagonist bosentan and iloprost improves fingertip blood perfusion in systemic sclerosis. J Rheumatol. 2014;41(5):881–6.
60. Hummers L, Dugowson C, Dechow F, Wise R, Gregory J, Michalek J, et al. A multi-centre, blinded, randomised, placebo-controlled, laboratory-based study of MQX-503, a novel topical gel formulation of nitroglycerine, in patients with Raynaud phenomenon. Ann Rheum Dis. 2013;72(12):1962–7.
61. Cutolo M, Sulli A. Therapy: optimized treatment algorithms for digital vasculopathy in SSc. Nat Rev Rheumatol. 2015;11(10):569–71.
62. Lambrecht V, Cutolo M, De Keyser F, Decuman S, Ruaro B, Sulli A, et al. Reliability of the quantitative assessment of peripheral blood perfusion by laser speckle contract analysis in a systemic sclerosis cohort. Ann Rheum Dis. 2016;75(6):1263–4.
63. Trombetta A, Pizzorni C, Ruaro B, Paolino S, Sulli A, Smith V, et al. Effects of longterm treatment with bosentan and iloprost on nailfold absolute capillary number, fingertip blood perfusion, and clinical status in systemic sclerosis. J Rheumatol. 2016;43(11):2033–41.
64. Ruaro B, Sulli A, Smith V, Paolino S, Pizzorni C, Cutolo M. Short-term follow-up of digital ulcers by laser speckle contrast analysis in systemic sclerosis patients. Microvasc Res. 2015;101:82–5.

Digital Ulcers, Vasculopathy and Internal Organ Involvement

8

Yannick Allanore

Introduction

Systemic sclerosis (SSc) is an autoimmune connective tissue disorder that is characterized by a complex interplay of vascular abnormalities, immune system activation and an uncontrolled fibrotic response. Vascular component is often referred to as vasculopathy and is seen as having a key role in the early pathogenesis of SSc. Furthermore, generalized peripheral microvascular and cardiovascular alterations contribute to some later complications of the disease with converging data supporting that the SSc outcomes depend on the extent and severity of vascular lesions [1].

Patients with SSc develop a broad spectrum of vascular manifestations including the almost universal Raynaud's phenomenon (distal vasospasm), commonly digital ulceration and more rarely critical digital ischaemia. In parallel, within this very heterogeneous disease, some patients will develop some vascular-related organ damages leading to heart or kidney failure. It is still unclear whether there is a continuum between peripheral vasculopathy promoting digital ulceration (DU) or critical ischemia and some other vascular-related complications [2, 3]. The objective of this chapter is to address this question by analysing whether severe digital vasculopathy could be a surrogate for some more severe damages.

Generalized Microvascular Damages

SSc vasculopathy depends on the complex interaction of various pathological processes including autoimmunity, impaired compensatory vasculogenesis, angiogenesis, endothelio-mesenchymal transition, endothelial dysfunction and impaired coagulation/fibrinolysis system. SSc vasculopathy is characterized by a variety of such changes that affect primarily the microcirculation and small arterioles.

The hallmark of functional abnormalities related to SSc vasculopathy is Raynaud's phenomenon. It is characterized by exaggerated but reversible vasospasm in response to cold exposure, stress or emotional upset. It must be pointed out that although it is mainly recognized at the digital level, it is well established that all microcirculatory systems can be affected (heart, nose, etc.) [2]. By example, cardiac imaging showed abnormal perfusion related to small coronary artery disturbances after cold stress [4].

With the progression of structural vascular changes, functional alteration of vascular cells includes endothelial apoptosis, endothelial dysfunction, impaired coagulation/fibrinolysis system, aberrant expression of soluble factors and cell adhesion molecules leading to the pathological inflammation. The next steps include altered neovascularization and vascular remodelling due to the impairment of compensatory vasculogenesis and exaggerated angiogenesis [5–10]. Circulating levels of various angiogenic/angiostatic factors are largely altered, and, so far, most of studies have revealed that pro-angiogenic factors are increased throughout the disease course, especially in the active stage of the disease [5–10]. Regarding the capillaries, structural vascular disease is characterized by distorted and irregular capillary loops in all the involved organs, including in particular the kidneys, lungs and heart. This reflects the systemic nature of the microvascular disorder, even in sites not affected by fibrosis.

Y. Allanore
Service de Rheumatologie A, Hôpital Cochin, Paris, France
e-mail: yannick.allanore@aphp.fr

© Springer Nature Switzerland AG 2019
M. Matucci-Cerinic, C. P. Denton (eds.), *Atlas of Ulcers in Systemic Sclerosis*, https://doi.org/10.1007/978-3-319-98477-3_8

Therefore, destructive vasculopathy characterized by progressive loss of capillaries, leading to tissue hypoxia and dermal fibroblast activation, can co-exist or progress to proliferative obliterative vasculopathy featured by proliferation of vascular cells (endothelial cells, pericytes and vascular smooth muscle cells) [3]. The damages then lead to the occlusion of arterioles and small arteries with fibro-proliferative change and permanent hypoxia which might further promote surrounding fibrosis [11]. Another hallmark of functional abnormalities related to SSc vasculopathy is impaired endothelial function. The vasodilatory response to blood flow-associated shear stress is a useful parameter to quantify endothelial function. In SSc patients, several studies have demonstrated the reduction of flow-mediated dilation (FMD) values supporting impaired nitric oxide production [12].

Altogether, these findings support a generalized microvascular impairment in SSc. One may ask whether the digits might be primarily affected and the exposure to cold of this body area supports some more important or earlier damages that could explain the high risk for digital ulceration. Nevertheless, the pathogenesis of vasculopathy and the findings of abnormal circulating markers as previously highlighted, such as the inverse correlation of FMD values with pulmonary arterial pressure and the association of decreased FMD values with the presence of pulmonary arterial hypertension and digital ulcers, all show some generalized abnormalities [13, 14]. Therefore, it is needed to evaluate in depth the natural course of the disease to see whether proliferative obliterative vasculopathy may gradually and sometimes subclinically progress along with disease duration and eventually become clinically evident with variable degrees of severity leading to recurrent DU, pulmonary arterial hypertension (PAH) and heart failure of renal crisis.

Cross-Sectional Analyses of SSc Patients Having Digital Ulcerations

In order to investigate the clinical manifestations occurring in patients with digital ulceration (DU), the characteristics of SSc-DU patients versus the non-affected patients have been analysed in the report including large series.

A study looking at the natural history of SSc-DU was based on 103 patients among whom 46 had a history of DU. The mean duration of follow-up from the first non-Raynaud SSc symptoms was about 12 years. In 43% of cases, the first DU occurred within 1 year following the first non-Raynaud SSc symptoms and within 5 years in 73% of cases. In multivariable analysis, younger patients at occurrence of first non-Raynaud SSc symptoms and with higher skin score (such has being classified with a diffuse cutaneous subset) experienced earlier DU occurrences. It must also be pointed out that DU was delayed when vasodilator therapy was offered (mainly calcium channel blockers or ACE inhibitors). Pulmonary arterial hypertension (PAH) occurred in 11 patients (11%) during the course of the disease, and its prevalence was comparable between the subgroups (14% PAH in the DU subgroup and 9% PAH in the no DU subgroup; $p = 0.53$) [15].

In a French multicentre study, a cross-sectional analysis of 599 patients with SSc found that 53% had prior or current DU. Looking at associated variables, DU appeared to occur more frequently among males, patients with a higher Rodnan skin score, patients with early onset of disease, patients with carbon monoxide lung diffusion capacity (DLCO) < 60% predicted and patients with anti-topo I antibodies. It must be highlighted that sex and skin disease were the strongest associated variables. The frequency of PAH was not higher in patients with prior or current DU than in those never affected [16].

DLCO measures gas exchanges through the alveolar membrane and can be influenced by the thickness of the alveolar membrane and lung capillary volume. Therefore, a reduced DLCO in the absence of impairment in pulmonary function may represent a surrogate marker of vasculopathy. The association of DLCO impairment and current digital ulcers may indicate the pathophysiological link between vasculopathy and digital ulcers. However, no relationship between prior or current DU and PAH was observed. One of the main studies that highlighted the link between DLCO and vasculopathy was based on the large Pittsburgh Scleroderma Databank from which 106 patients who had the diagnosis of PAH were matched with 106 controls by SSc skin subtype, age, sex, race, disease duration and the mean time to the diagnosis of PAH after the initial Pittsburgh visit. If a decline in DLCO pre-empted PAH, PAH patients and controls had a similar frequency of Raynaud's phenomenon, digital tip ulcers and digital gangrene. However, visual analogue scales for Raynaud's phenomenon showed that cases had significantly higher values for both the severity of Raynaud's phenomenon and the severity of digital tip ulcers [17].

The German network has provided some data derived from 1880 patients from whom 1690 were evaluable for DU. Out of these, 408 (24%) had active DU at the time of entering the registry. In multivariate analysis, datasets from 1164 patients were used and revealed that male sex was the most powerful independent predictor for the presence of DU and that PAH, anti-Scl70 antibodies (but not ACA), involvement of the mouth or oesophagus, elevated erythrocyte sedimentation rate or onset of Raynaud's phenomenon at a young age were all risk factors for the presence of DU. Diffuse skin sclerosis in combination with PAH was the most powerful predictor for the occurrence of DU [18].

In another national project, a total of 19 Spanish centres participated in the recruitment of 1326 SSc patients; out of these, 552 SSc patients had prior or current DU. Multivariate analysis identified that history of prior/current DU in patients with SSc was independently associated to younger age at SSc diagnosis, diffuse cutaneous SSc and peripheral vascular manifestations such as Raynaud's phenomenon, telangiectasia and acro-osteolysis [19]. However, history of DU was not associated with any visceral vasculopathy such as PAH or scleroderma renal crisis.

The Canadian registry was used to determine features associated with DU and their complications and to determine if there were associations of digital ulcers with other evidence of vasculopathy such as PAH and scleroderma renal crisis (SRC). Among 938 SSc patients, 8% had a digital ulcer currently, 44% had a digital ulcer ever, and 53% had digital pitting scars. In the multivariate analysis, the most important variables to predict DU were younger age of onset, ILD, higher hand and finger skin score and higher HAQ score [20]. There was no significant association between the history of digital ulcers and any definition of PAH (prevalence measured at 9%) and neither with renal crisis (prevalence of 5%).

If microcirculation impairment is fundamental in SSc vasculopathy, large vessel disease may contribute although there are still debates about the potential role of atherosclerosis in SSc vascular damages. A Japanese cross-sectional study looked at 254 patients among whom 48 SSc patients had prior or current DU (19%). There were no multivariable analyses performed, but it is of interest to point out that carotid atherosclerosis was not more common in patients with DU as compared to SSc patients without DU. Regarding SSc characteristics, DU were more common in males; in DcSSs, mRSS was higher in patients with a history of DU confirming previous findings coming from other geographical populations [21]. A focus was then done on heart disease, showing no more PAH in DU-SSc patients (9% vs 10% in DU-SSc versus non-DU-SSc). After exclusion of the PAH patients, those with DU had more commonly elevated natriuretic peptide or more mild cardiac abnormalities such as EKG changes or coronary artery disease [21].

The carotid-femoral pulse wave velocity (PWV) is a marker of aortic stiffness that holds prognostic significance in various vascular conditions, including systemic hypertension, renal failure and heart failure. The augmentation index (Aix_75), defined as the amplitude of the reflected wave from the periphery to the heart, can be measured by applanation tonometry and depends on several factors including large artery but also medium and small arteries stiffness. Radial applanation tonometry has been investigated in a group of 63 SSc patients to look at potential association of PWV or Aix_75 with active DU that was observed in 10 SSc patients. No differences existed in baseline characteristics between SSc-DU versus SSc non-DU patients, regarding cutaneous subset of the disease and disease duration, renal and pulmonary function, cardiovascular risk factors, heart function and pulmonary artery pressure [22]. SSc patients with DU versus those without had increased Aix_75, while there was no difference in PWV. The results of the multivariate logistic regression revealed that age, sex, erythrocyte sedimentation rate, aortic pulse pressure and DU were independently associated with Aix_75 [22]. Collectively these results suggest the existence of increased small and medium arteries stiffness in SSc patients with DU without significant aortic increased stiffness, when compared to SSc patients without DU.

Cutaneous telangiectasia is common in SSc and part of the classification criteria. A cross-sectional study aimed at determining whether the number and size of cutaneous telangiectasia were associated with the pattern of microvascular lesions assessed by nailfold videocapillaroscopy (NVC) and markers reflecting the severity of SSc-related vasculopathy.

Among the total of 87 patients, profuse and pseudotumoral cutaneous telangiectasias were both associated with capillary loss and severe neoangiogenesis on NVC [23]. In multivariate analysis, profuse pseudotumoral cutaneous telangiectasias were independently associated with past or current digital ulcers, whereas pseudotumoral cutaneous telangiectasias were independently associated with the late NVC pattern and PAH [23].

Regarding another vascular organ complication, there are few studies about the risk factors of renal crisis; however, none did suggest so far that DU or PAH may be risk factors for such event [24].

The main results of the above studies are summarized in Table 8.1 where associations observed in multivariable analyses are highlighted.

Table 8.1 Digital ulcer associations through multivariable analyses in large multicentre series of SSc patients

Variable	ItinerAIR-SSc (2009) ($n = 599$ patients)	German network (2009) ($n = 1690$)	Canadian network (2011) ($n = 938$)	Spanish registry (2016) ($n = 1326$)
Definition of DU (and prevalence)	Prior or current DU (53%)	Active DU at inclusion (24%)	Past or present DU (44%)	Prior or current DU (42%)
Age	+	−	+	+
Male sex	+	++	−	−
Smoking	−	Not studied	−	−
Disease duration	+	−	−	−
Severe skin involvement	+	NA	+ (finger mRSS)	−
DcSSc	−	−	−	+
Anti-topoisomerase	−	+	−	−
Erythrocyte sedimentation rate	Not studied	+	−	Not studied
Esophageal involvement	Not studied	+	+/−	Not studied
DLCO	+ (<60%)	NA	−	−
Interstitial lung disease	(Severe ILD and exclusion criteria)	−	+	+
Pulmonary hypertension	(Exclusion criteria)	+	−	−
Renal crisis	−	−	−	−
HAQ score	Not studied	Not studied	+	Not studied

Longitudinal and Prospective Studies

Another way to explore if DU may be a surrogate for generalized vasculopathy is to look at prospective data to see whether SSc patients with DU at baseline develop more organ vasculopathy than non-affected patients.

In EULAR Scleroderma Trials and Research (EUSTAR) cohort, it was showed that at presentation, 1092/3196 patients had a history of DU (34.1%). Follow-up at 3 years was the cut-off time to look at the occurrence of complications [25]. In multivariable analyses adjusting for age, gender and other parameters considered potentially significant, a history of DU was strongly predictive for the presence of active DUs at prospective visits but also for an elevated systolic pulmonary arterial pressure on heart ultrasound, for any cardiovascular event (new DUs, elevated US-PAPs or left ventricular failure and for death). Overt PAH could not be analysed and there was no prediction for renal crisis [25].

The German network has also looked at prospective data regarding DU and showed various progressions according to SSc characteristics. Unfortunately, no details are provided about other outcomes unless a statement that the weak or lack of association of DUs with pulmonary hypertension or heart and renal involvement indicates that the vasculopathy in digital arteries and the renal and pulmonary vasculature seem to be affected by different pathophysiological pathways [26].

In the Australian PAH registry, among 1636 patients with SSc, 194 (11.9%) had PAH proven by right heart catheter including 160 who were detected prospectively by screening. The study primarily looked at the outcomes of patients according to the screening programmes, but the characteristics of SSc-PAH are detailed and analysed using univariate analyses. The data show that SSc patients with PAH were older, had longer disease duration from the first non-Raynaud clinical manifestation and were more likely to be anti-centromere positive and to have telangiectasia, calcinosis and joint contractures [27]. Furthermore, digital ulcers were more frequent (53% in PAH-SSc patients and 42% in SSc non-PAH patients), but the strength of association is not very strong, and multivariable analyses would be required to determine independency in prediction.

Biomarker Studies

Many studies investigated in these recent years candidate biomarkers. If some were mainly descriptive using cross-sectional design, some others were based on longitudinal data allowing prediction of vascular risk [28].

The pentraxins are a very conserved family of proteins with a unique architecture. In humans, the two main members of this family are C-reactive protein and serum amyloid

P. Pentraxin 3 (PTX3) is expressed predominantly in atherosclerotic lesions that involve various cells such as macrophages, neutrophils, dendritic cells or smooth muscle cells. Interestingly, PTX3 has been examined, as a novel biomarker for inflammatory cardiovascular disease. In SSc, circulating PTX3 but also fibroblast growth factor 2 (FGF-2) levels has been found to be significantly higher in SSc patients than in healthy control subjects [29]. Of the most interest, PTX3 was elevated in SSc patients who had digital ulcers or PAH, while FGF-2 was reduced in SSc patients with PAH. Multivariate analysis identified elevated PTX3 as an independent parameter associated with the presence of digital ulcers and PAH. Furthermore, PTX3 levels were a useful predictor of future occurrences of digital ulcers, and reduced FGF-2 was independently associated with the presence of PAH. Chemokine CXCL4 levels have been found to be correlated with skin and lung fibrosis and also with pulmonary arterial hypertension. No data were provided regarding DU. But among chemokines, only CXCL4 predicted the risk and progression of systemic sclerosis [30]. Using a cohort of 100 patients and a follow-up of 3 years, vascular biomarkers of new events were investigated, primarily to predict the development of new DU that occurred in 17 SSc patients. Both angiogenic and vasculogenic markers were measured. Using various multivariable models, first the history of previous DU but also placenta growth factor (PlGF) levels and endothelial progenitor cell count were independent predictors of the development of DU [31]. The prediction of other cardiovascular end points were studied suggesting stimulating clues with these markers, but the number of events was low not providing a high statistical power. Interestingly, another study confirmed the interest in regulators of angiogenesis, confirming the promise of PlGF and also of Flit1 as measures of pulmonary hypertension in SSc patients [32].

Angiotensin II type 1 receptor (AT1R) and endothelin 1 type A receptor (ETAR) are functional autoantibodies directed against vascular receptors. A majority of SSc patients have increased levels of anti-AT_1R and anti-ET_AR antibodies compared to healthy donors. Moreover, in SSc patients, the autoantibodies are associated with various vascular symptoms of the disease such as PAH, digital ulcers and renal crisis. Nevertheless, the antibodies are also associated with the diffuse cutaneous subtype as well as with lung fibrosis. Altogether, these data suggest a possible role of the antibodies in disease mechanisms, but their use in clinical practice for predicting damages remains to be established although in the context of DU, it has been shown that anti-ETAR autoantibodies can be used together with the presence of current or past DU to identify patients with SSc who are at risk for the development of subsequent DU [33, 34].

Imaging may also provide some tools to predict DU and vascular outcomes. Few studies have been performed so far, but capillaroscopy was found to be an interesting candidate, and a prospective study of 6 months identified that the mean number of capillaries per millimetre in the middle finger of the dominant hand, the number of DU at enrolment and the presence of critical digital ischemia at enrolment were risk factors for the development of new DUs. Other cardiovascular outcomes were not measured on that duration [35].

Conclusion

Vascular injury and subsequent vascular dysfunction are among the earliest alterations in SSc and are considered to act within the initiating steps in SSc pathogenesis. Microcirculation impairment is the hallmark of the disease, but larger vessels may be affected even if the reality of increased prevalence of atherosclerosis in SSc remains controversial. The process is undoubtedly generalized and all vascular territories are affected. This is strongly supported by autopsy studies that showed lung and kidney vessels involvement despite the lack of any evidence of organ involvement [36]. Nevertheless, DU is the most common clinical expression of advanced vasculopathy. It remains unclear why this area is mostly affected although the permanent exposure to external stress might contribute to its severity. Some have thought that DU could be a marker of damage (vascular and fibrotic changes), but the epidemiological studies do not clearly and reproducibly demonstrate a strong link between DU and other vascular complications. Indeed, cross-sectional studies show that SSc-DU patients have a more severe disease, but there is no demonstration of higher frequency of PAH or renal crisis. The longitudinal studies further support poorer outcomes of SSc-DU patients but do not explicitly found definite higher risk. The main results suggest a potential link between DU and subsequent DU, but several methodological issues preclude firm conclusion. Indeed, the definition of the events differs between the studies; the time of observation is usually not very long for PAH which is usually a mate complication; and because of the scarcity of major cardiovascular events, the sample size may be an issue.

Biomarker studies highlight the systemic component of vasculopathy and suggest some links between DU and PAH, but it seems that additional further and potential regional factors might contribute to more severe remodelling in the fingers or in the lung or in the kidney. Autoantibodies might contribute to these specificities, and it is of interest to see that DU is more common in DcSSc and probably anti-topoisomerase-positive patients, whereas anti-centromere antibodies are reproducibly found in SSc-PAH patients and that anti-RNA polymerase 3 antibodies are strong markers of renal crisis. The role of others and functional antibodies are interesting clues in this context.

One might also add that the natural course of vasculopathy and its complications are moving in the recent years and the recent findings about DU recurrence showing faster healing and less relapse should stimulate further studies to reshape current patients' outcomes and management [37, 38]. Therefore, SSc-DU patients have worse outcomes than non-affected patients, and they should be managed as patients having a severe form of the disease [39]. However, the reason why vasculopathy may be mainly expressed in digital arteries in some patients and in pulmonary or kidney arteries in others remains unclear. Improving the knowledge in the field would distress this part of the disease that is a huge contributor to excessive morbidity and mortality.

References

1. Elhai M, Avouac J, Kahan A, Allanore Y. Systemic sclerosis: recent insights. Joint Bone Spine. 2015;82(3):148–53.
2. Matucci-Cerinic M, Kahaleh B, Wigley FM. Review: evidence that systemic sclerosis is a vascular disease. Arthritis Rheum. 2013;65(8):1953–62.
3. Asano Y, Sato S. Vasculopathy in scleroderma. Semin Immunopathol. 2015;37(5):489–500.
4. Allanore Y, Meune C. Primary myocardial involvement in systemic sclerosis: evidence for a microvascular origin. Clin Exp Rheumatol. 2010;28(5 Suppl 62):S48–53.
5. Manetti M, Romano E, Rosa I, Guiducci S, Bellando-Randone S, De Paulis A, Ibba-Manneschi L, Matucci-Cerinic M. Endothelial-to-mesenchymal transition contributes to endothelial dysfunction and dermal fibrosis in systemic sclerosis. Ann Rheum Dis. 2017;76(5):924–34.
6. Avouac J, Vallucci M, Smith V, Senet P, Ruiz B, Sulli A, Pizzorni C, Frances C, Chiocchia G, Cutolo M, Allanore Y. Correlations between angiogenic factors and capillaroscopic patterns in systemic sclerosis. Arthritis Res Ther. 2013;15(2):R55.
7. Manetti M, Guiducci S, Romano E, Avouac J, Rosa I, Ruiz B, Lepri G, Bellando-Randone S, Ibba-Manneschi L, Allanore Y, Matucci-Cerinic M. Decreased expression of the endothelial cell-derived factor EGFL7 in systemic sclerosis: potential contribution to impaired angiogenesis and vasculogenesis. Arthritis Res Ther. 2013;15(5):R165.
8. Maurer B, Distler A, Suliman YA, Gay RE, Michel BA, Gay S, Distler JH, Distler O. Vascular endothelial growth factor aggravates fibrosis and vasculopathy in experimental models of systemic sclerosis. Ann Rheum Dis. 2014;73(10):1880–7.
9. Derrett-Smith EC, Dooley A, Gilbane AJ, Trinder SL, Khan K, Baliga R, Holmes AM, Hobbs AJ, Abraham D, Denton CP. Endothelial injury in a transforming growth factor β-dependent mouse model of scleroderma induces pulmonary arterial hypertension. Arthritis Rheum. 2013;65(11):2928–39.
10. Avouac J, Wipff J, Goldman O, Ruiz B, Couraud PO, Chiocchia G, Kahan A, Boileau C, Uzan G, Allanore Y. Angiogenesis in systemic sclerosis: impaired expression of vascular endothelial growth factor receptor 1 in endothelial progenitor-derived cells under hypoxic conditions. Arthritis Rheum. 2008;58(11):3550–61.
11. Suliman YA, Distler O. Novel aspects in the pathophysiology of peripheral vasculopathy in systemic sclerosis. Curr Rheumatol Rev. 2013;9(4):237–44.
12. Silva I, Loureiro T, Teixeira A, Almeida I, Mansilha A, Vasconcelos C, Almeida R. Digital ulcers in systemic sclerosis: role of flow-mediated dilatation and capillaroscopy as risk assessment tools. Eur J Dermatol. 2015;25(5):444–51.
13. Hofstee HM, Voskuyl AE, Vonk Noordegraaf A, Smulders YM, Postmus PE, Dijkmans BA, Serné EH. Pulmonary arterial hypertension in systemic sclerosis is associated with profound impairment of microvascular endothelium-dependent vasodilatation. J Rheumatol. 2012;39(1):100–5.
14. Takahashi T, Asano Y, Amiya E, Hatano M, Tamaki Z, Takata M, Ozeki A, Watanabe A, Kawarasaki S, Taniguchi T, Ichimura Y, Toyama T, Watanabe M, Hirata Y, Nagai R, Komuro I, Sato S. Clinical correlation of brachial artery flow-mediated dilation in patients with systemic sclerosis. Mod Rheumatol. 2014;24(1):106–11.
15. Hachulla E, Clerson P, Launay D, Lambert M, Morell-Dubois S, Queyrel V, Hatron PY. Natural history of ischemic digital ulcers in systemic sclerosis: single-center retrospective longitudinal study. J Rheumatol. 2007;34(12):2423–30.
16. Tiev KP, Diot E, Clerson P, Dupuis-Siméon F, Hachulla E, Hatron PY, Constans J, Cirstéa D, Farge-Bancel D, Carpentier PH. Clinical features of scleroderma patients with or without prior or current ischemic digital ulcers: post-hoc analysis of a nationwide multicenter cohort (ItinérAIR-Sclérodermie). J Rheumatol. 2009;36(7):1470–6.
17. Steen V, Medsger TA Jr. Predictors of isolated pulmonary hypertension in patients with systemic sclerosis and limited cutaneous involvement. Arthritis Rheum. 2003;48(2):516–22.
18. Sunderkötter C, Herrgott I, Brückner C, Moinzadeh P, Pfeiffer C, Gerss J, Hunzelmann N, Böhm M, Krieg T, Müller-Ladner U, Genth E, Schulze-Lohoff E, Meurer M, Melchers I, Riemekasten G, DNSS Centers. Comparison of patients with and without digital ulcers in systemic sclerosis: detection of possible risk factors. Br J Dermatol. 2009;160(4):835–43.
19. Tolosa-Vilella C, Morera-Morales ML, Simeón-Aznar CP, Marí-Alfonso B, Colunga-Arguelles D, Callejas Rubio JL, et al. Digital ulcers and cutaneous subsets of systemic sclerosis: clinical, immunological, nailfold capillaroscopy, and survival differences in the Spanish RESCLE registry. Semin Arthritis Rheum. 2016;46(2):200–8.
20. Khimdas S, Harding S, Bonner A, Zummer B, Baron M, Pope J, Canadian Scleroderma Research Group. Associations with digital ulcers in a large cohort of systemic sclerosis: results from the Canadian Scleroderma Research Group registry. Arthritis Care Res (Hoboken). 2011;63(1):142–9.
21. Motegi S, Toki S, Hattori T, Yamada K, Uchiyama A, Ishikawa O. No association of atherosclerosis with digital ulcers in Japanese patients with systemic sclerosis: evaluation of carotid intima-media thickness and plaque characteristics. J Dermatol. 2014;41(7):604–8.
22. Aïssou L, Meune C, Avouac J, Meunier M, Elhaï M, Sorbets E, Kahan A, Allanore Y. Small, medium but not large arteries are involved in digital ulcers associated with systemic sclerosis. Joint Bone Spine. 2016;83(4):444–7.
23. Hurabielle C, Avouac J, Lepri G, de Risi T, Kahan A, Allanore Y. Skin telangiectasia identify a subset of systemic sclerosis patients with severe vascular disease. Arthritis Care Res (Hoboken). 2016;68(7):1021–7.
24. Woodworth TG, Suliman YA, Furst DE, Clements P. Scleroderma renal crisis and renal involvement in systemic sclerosis. Nat Rev Nephrol. 2016;12(11):678–91.
25. Mihai C, Landewé R, van der Heijde D, Walker UA, Constantin PI, Gherghe AM, EUSTAR co-authors, et al. Digital ulcers predict a worse disease course in patients with systemic sclerosis. Ann Rheum Dis. 2016;75(4):681–6.
26. Hunzelmann N, Riemekasten G, Becker MO, Moinzadeh P, Kreuter A, Melchers I, Mueller-Ladner U, Meier F, Worm M, Lee H, Herrgott I, Pfeiffer C, Fierlbeck G, Henes J, Juche A, Zeidler G, Mensing H, Günther C, Sárdy M, Burkhardt H, Koehm M, Kuhr K, Krieg T, Sunderkötter C. The predict study: low risk for digital ulcer development in patients with systemic sclerosis with increas-

ing disease duration and lack of topoisomerase-1 antibodies. Br J Dermatol. 2016;174(6):1384–7.

27. Morrisroe K, Stevens W, Sahhar J, Rabusa C, Nikpour M, Proudman S, Australian Scleroderma Interest Group (ASIG). Epidemiology and disease characteristics of systemic sclerosis-related pulmonary arterial hypertension: results from a real-life screening programme. Arthritis Res Ther. 2017;19(1):42.

28. Chora I, Guiducci S, Manetti M, Romano E, Mazzotta C, Bellando-Randone S, Ibba-Manneschi L, Matucci-Cerinic M, Soares R. Vascular biomarkers and correlation with peripheral vasculopathy in systemic sclerosis. Autoimmun Rev. 2015;14(4):314–22.

29. Shirai Y, Okazaki Y, Inoue Y, Tamura Y, Yasuoka H, Takeuchi T, Kuwana M. Elevated levels of pentraxin 3 in systemic sclerosis: associations with vascular manifestations and defective vasculogenesis. Arthritis Rheumatol. 2015;67(2):498–507. https://doi.org/10.1002/art.38953.

30. van Bon L, Affandi AJ, Broen J, Christmann RB, Marijnissen RJ, Stawski L, Farina GA, et al. Proteome-wide analysis and CXCL4 as a biomarker in systemic sclerosis. N Engl J Med. 2014;370(5):433–43.

31. Avouac J, Meune C, Ruiz B, Couraud PO, Uzan G, Boileau C, Kahan A, Chiocchia G, Allanore Y. Angiogenic biomarkers predict the occurrence of digital ulcers in systemic sclerosis. Ann Rheum Dis. 2012;71(3):394–9.

32. McMahan Z, Schoenhoff F, Van Eyk JE, Wigley FM, Hummers LK. Biomarkers of pulmonary hypertension in patients with scleroderma: a case-control study. Arthritis Res Ther. 2015;17:201.

33. Cabral-Marques O, Riemekasten G. Vascular hypothesis revisited: role of stimulating antibodies against angiotensin and endothelin receptors in the pathogenesis of systemic sclerosis. Autoimmun Rev. 2016;15(7):690–4.

34. Avouac J, Riemekasten G, Meune C, Ruiz B, Kahan A, Allanore Y. Autoantibodies against endothelin 1 type a receptor are strong predictors of digital ulcers in systemic sclerosis. J Rheumatol. 2015;42(10):1801–7.

35. Cutolo M, Herrick AL, Distler O, Becker MO, Beltran E, Carpentier P, Ferri C, Inanç M, Vlachoyiannopoulos P, Chadha-Boreham H, Cottreel E, Pfister T, Rosenberg D, Torres JV, Smith V, CAP Study Investigators. Nailfold videocapillaroscopic features and other clinical risk factors for digital ulcers in systemic sclerosis: a multicenter, prospective cohort study. Arthritis Rheumatol. 2016;68(10):2527–39.

36. D'Angelo WA, Fries JF, Masi AT, Shulman LE. Pathologic observations in systemic sclerosis (scleroderma). A study of fifty-eight autopsy cases and fifty-eight matched controls. Am J Med. 1969;46(3):428–40.

37. Khanna D, Denton CP, Merkel PA, Krieg T, Le Brun FO, Marr A, Papadakis K, Pope J, Matucci-Cerinic M, Furst DE, DUAL-1 Investigators.; DUAL-2 Investigators. Effect of Macitentan on the development of new ischemic digital ulcers in patients with systemic sclerosis: DUAL-1 and DUAL-2 randomized clinical trials. JAMA. 2016;315(18):1975–88.

38. Hachulla E, Hatron PY, Carpentier P, Agard C, Chatelus E, Jego P, Mouthon L, Queyrel V, Fauchais AL, Michon-Pasturel U, Jaussaud R, Mathian A, Granel B, Diot E, Farge-Bancel D, Mekinian A, Avouac J, Desmurs-Clavel H, Clerson P, SEDUCE study group. Efficacy of sildenafil on ischaemic digital ulcer healing in systemic sclerosis: the placebo-controlled SEDUCE study. Ann Rheum Dis. 2016;75(6):1009–15.

39. Hughes M, Ong VH, Anderson ME, Hall F, Moinzadeh P, Griffiths B, et al. Consensus best practice pathway of the UK Scleroderma Study Group: digital vasculopathy in systemic sclerosis. Rheumatology (Oxford). 2015;54(11):2015–24.

Guya Piemonte, Francesca Braschi, and Laura Rasero

Introduction

In patients with systemic sclerosis (SSc), the presence of fistulas, skin lesions, and gangrene is a complication associated with vascular involvement which requires prolonged treatment (over 1 year), sometimes evolving to amputation of the phalanx, finger, or limbs [1].

The common definition of "fistulas" is the "abnormal communication most commonly seen between two internal organs or between an internal organ and the surface of the body" [2]. In the skin, fistula is defined a fistulous tract communicating between an ulcer and an adjacent area or between an injury and the deeper layers of the skin. In these cases, the risk of an increase of the length and depth of the lesion is amplified due to the difficulty to assess the extent and to place a local antiseptic device. This may lead to complications such as the progressive infections of tissue that can affect the tendons, joints, and bones.

Two SSc patients with fistulas have been successfully treated with the association of negative topical pressure (NTP) and split-thickness skin grafting [1]. In both cases, the combination of the two therapies represented the last attempt before proceeding to amputation, while they were treated for

Table 9.1 Negative topical pressure (NTP) uses

Indications	Contraindications	Use with caution
Burns	Blood vessels exposed	Impaired hemostasis
Chronic wounds of the lower extremities	Organs exposed	Anticoagulant therapy in progress
Diabetic ulcers	Tendons exposed	
Wounds on the abdomen opened with fistulas	Malignancy wound	
Trauma with extensive tissue loss	Unexplored fistulas	
Skin grafts		
Sternal wounds infected		

a month of intravenous prostacyclins, oral antibiotics, and povidone-iodine ointment [1]. Table 9.1 shows the different uses of NTP.

The placement of a silk thread (seton stitch) for fistulas in skin lesions associated with lymphedema of the legs and complicated by comorbidity and associated with compression bandaging was proposed. This procedure facilitates the drainage of cavities and promotes healing, avoiding the surgical incision that has little benefit [3].

Prevention

A correct approach to prevent this complication should include close monitoring of the wound and planning a follow-up of the patient at least twice weekly by experienced staff. The main purpose is to promptly identify wound signs and symptoms that indicate a potential evolution to a fistula. The main changes of the characteristics of the lesion can be specific and nonspecific.

G. Piemonte
Department of Health Science, University of Florence, Florence, Italy

F. Braschi (✉)
Health Professions Department, Azienda Ospedaliera Universitaria Careggi, Florence, Italy
e-mail: braschif@aou-careggi.toscana.it

L. Rasero
Department of Health Sciences, University of Florence – Careggi of Hospital, Florence, Tuscany, Italy

© Springer Nature Switzerland AG 2019
M. Matucci-Cerinic, C. P. Denton (eds.), *Atlas of Ulcers in Systemic Sclerosis*, https://doi.org/10.1007/978-3-319-98477-3_9

Specific Signs

1. Appearance of satellite lesions and/or detachment of the surrounding tissue (Fig. 9.1)
2. Depression and/or endowment of the wound edges (Fig. 9.2)
3. Undermining margins assessed by the placement of a cannula or a surgical tool as an ideal environment for microbial growth (Figs. 9.3 and 9.4)

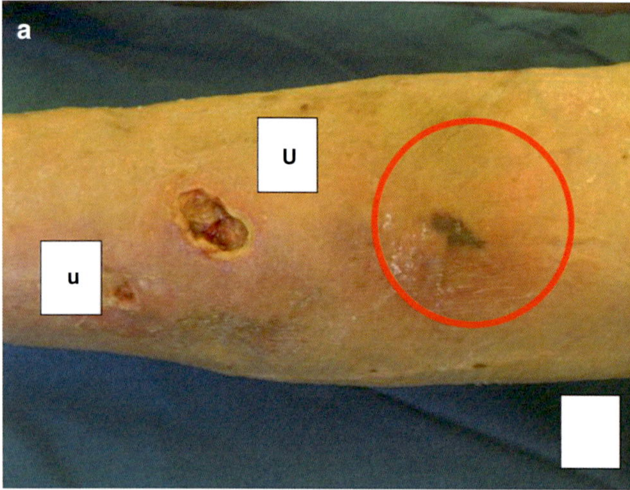

Fig. 9.1 The lesion indicated by the letter "U" is the lesion appeared as first; the lesion indicated by the letter "u" appeared after, and it is correlated to the first. The presence of a darker area (circled in red) above the lesion "U" constitutes a potential signal of expansion of the infectious process (**a**). Systemic antibiotic therapy targeted, silver dressings, and close monitoring of the patient have averted this possibility (**b**)

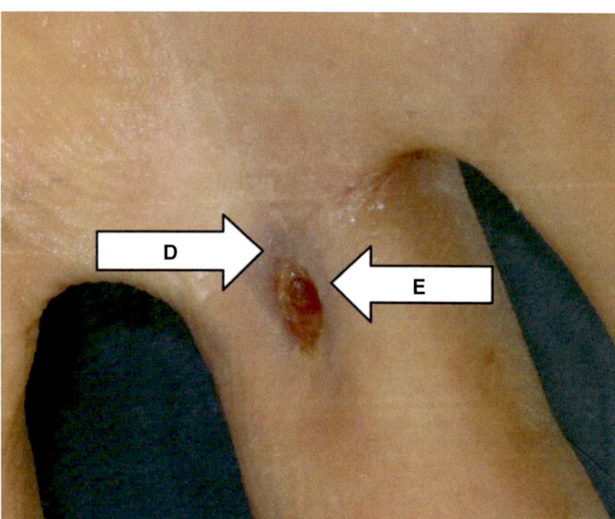

Fig. 9.2 Depression of the wound (D) and endowment (E) of the wound edges

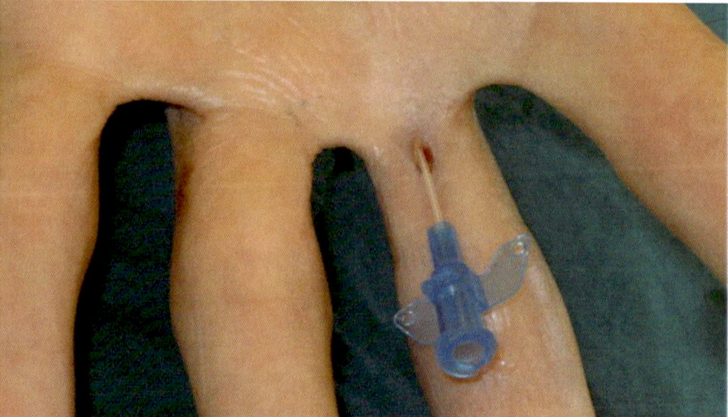

Fig. 9.3 Evaluation of the fistulas depth by a cannula

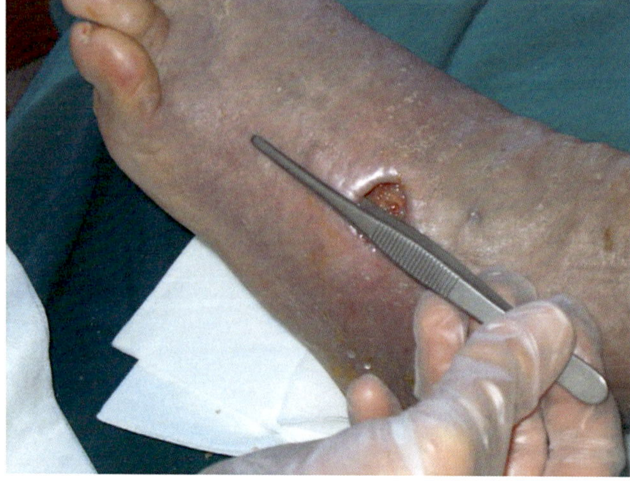

Fig. 9.4 Evaluation of the depth of the fistula through a surgical instrument

Nonspecific Signs

1. Spread in the local and/or spread in the surrounding tissue (Fig. 9.5)
2. Marked redness around the wound (Fig. 9.5)
3. Increase of necrotic tissue and/or occurrence of slough (Fig. 9.5)
4. Increase in the size of the wound
5. Purulent material
6. Bad smell

One or more than one of these signs may be present but not yet determine the presence of a fistula and thus be only prognostic signs. However it is essential to monitor the evolution in association or not to the appearance of other symptoms reported by the patient:

- Increase in pain that can become pulsating
- Feeling of tension around the lesion
- Impaired quality of life

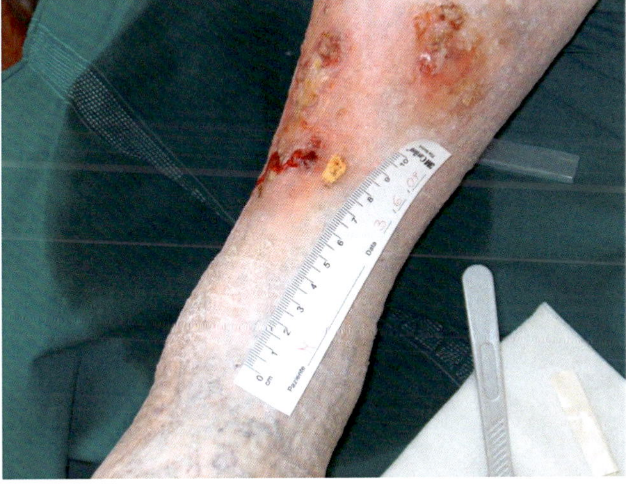

Fig. 9.5 Presence of local edema, redness surrounding the skin, and slough

Local Treatment

In the presence of a fistula, the presence of purulent material is always needed to verify, and drainage must be performed to collect a sample for analysis. Abscesses originating from deep tissue are frequent in the course of immunosuppressive therapies and comorbidity such as diabetes. In this case a broad-spectrum antibiotic therapy is mandatory to prevent deeper skin layer infection, and continue it as a preventive measure even if antibiogram is negative.

Local treatment can be summarized in seven steps:

1. Wash the wound with saline solution using a 10 ml syringe for digital ulcers and a 20/30 ml syringe for the injuries to the lower limbs. Use a cannula 14Fr to ensure cleansing within the fistula. Be careful not to touch the bottom of the wound to avoid pain. The evaluation of the depth of the fistula may be performed later only after the application of local anesthetic.
2. Disinfect the wound with non-cytotoxic products.
3. Repeat the cleansing.
4. Aspirate the abscess material and provide the laboratory a sample for analysis to start a specific antibiotic therapy [4].
5. Proceed with the application of a local anesthetic.
6. Evaluation of the fistula and of the edges of the wound with a cannula or by a surgical tool (Fig. 9.6). In case of undermining dead end, sterile saline can be injected within the fistula by measuring the amount in ml injected and removing it again immediately after. This allows, even if in a very empirical mode, to obtain a comparison parameter for the subsequent follow-up. Sometimes the fistula is extremely low, in the order of a few millimeters, so it is more suitable to assess the fistula through a cannula, with a marker to indicate the depth along the lumen and subsequently measuring with a ruler. In the presence of two adjacent lesions, inject the liquid into a wound using a syringe and cannula allows to confirm the presence of a communication between the two.
7. Apply of a hydrofiber device with antiseptic properties. Medications containing silver ensure a slow and prolonged antiseptic action. These kinds of products are

required when containment of exudate and protection of the perilesional skin is needed, thanks to its vertical absorption capacity [5]. In the present case, it is essential to employ devices able to absorb exudate and/or purulent materials and fill the fistula. Care should be taken not to overfill the fistula with the device to avoid pressure on the walls of the cavity and interactions between the dressing and the purulent material with transformation of the medication that acquires occluding characteristics. The placement of the dressing into the wound should be performed to ensure an easy removal, thus preventing residue deposit of dressings on the bottom of the lesion. For this reason, the products that have a structure that prevents it from flaking and loss within the fistula are largely preferred.

It is necessary to evaluate with a Doppler ultrasonography of the vessels of the lower limbs and an x-ray examination to document any possible involvement of the bone. When silver devices are used, x-ray should not be performed because they may interfere with the radiographic imaging.

Lesions due to calcinosis, according to the classification and staging of Amanzi [6], represent a threatening condition that predisposes the patient to fistula formation as through between the deposits of calcium formed in the deeper layers of skin surface. Alternatively they may determine the formation of skin lesions very close and often adjoining or potentially likely to become (Fig. 9.7). These kinds of ulcers require very long treatment times that can establish phenomena of self-maintenance with consequent chronicity of the lesion.

An x-ray examination can be a great help to know size, placement, and depth of the calcium deposits in the soft tissue in order to identify the areas most at risk of infectious processes with onset of abscesses and fistulas (Fig. 9.8).

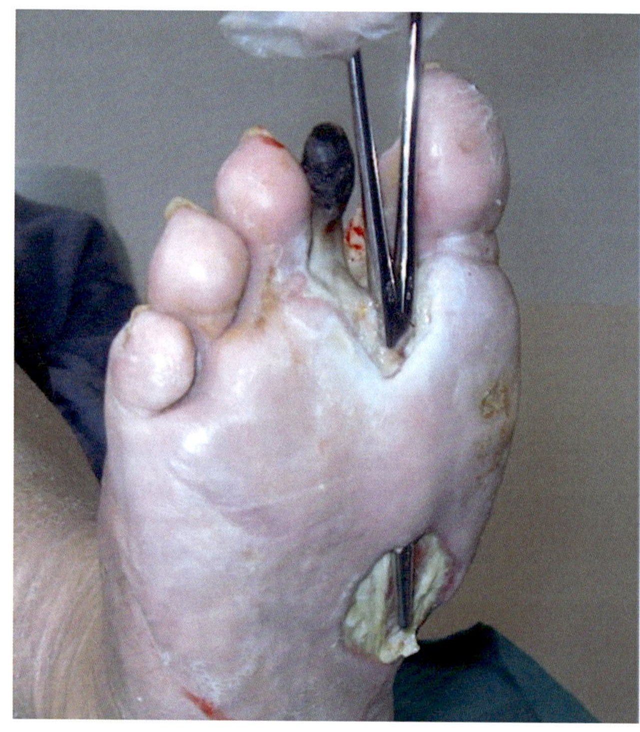

Fig. 9.6 Evaluation of the depth of the fistula through surgical instrument

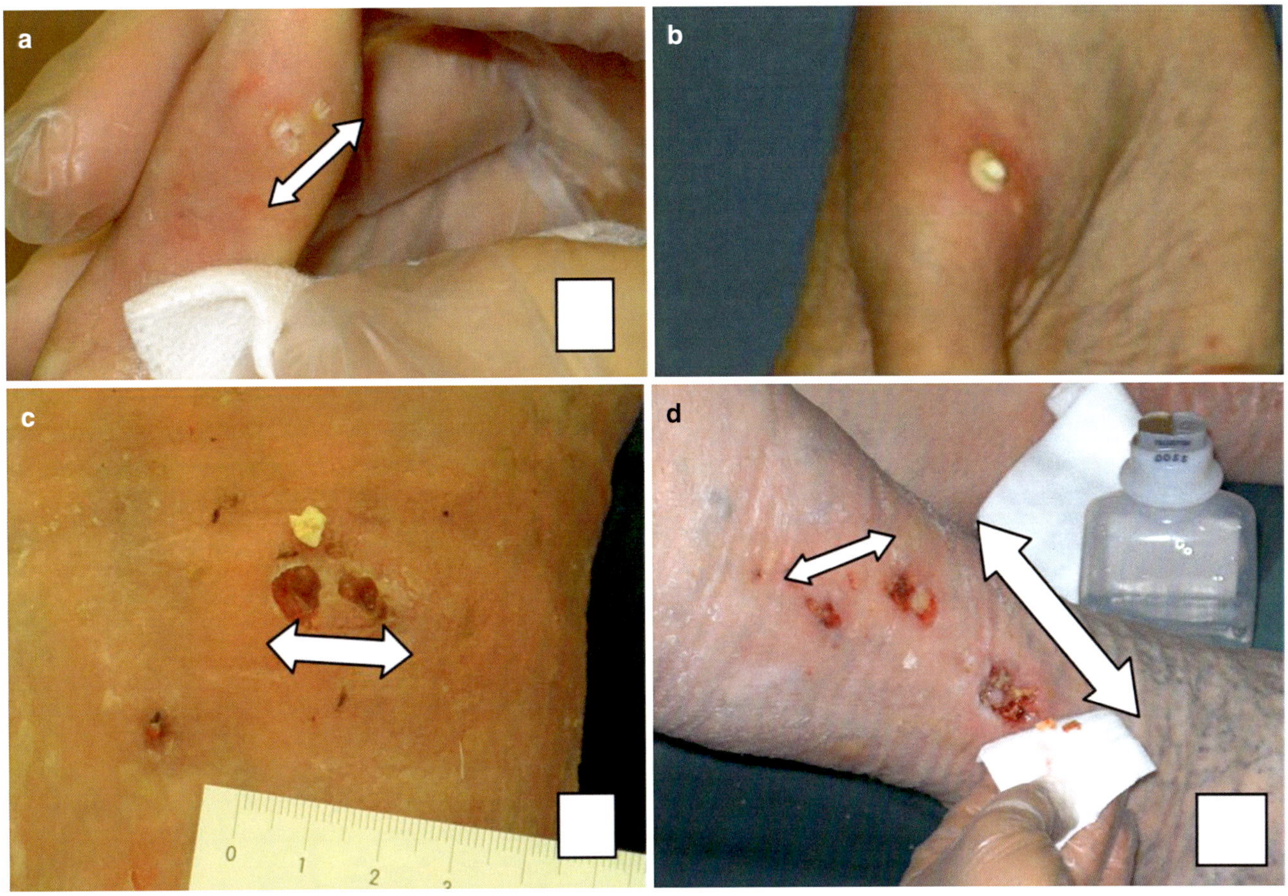

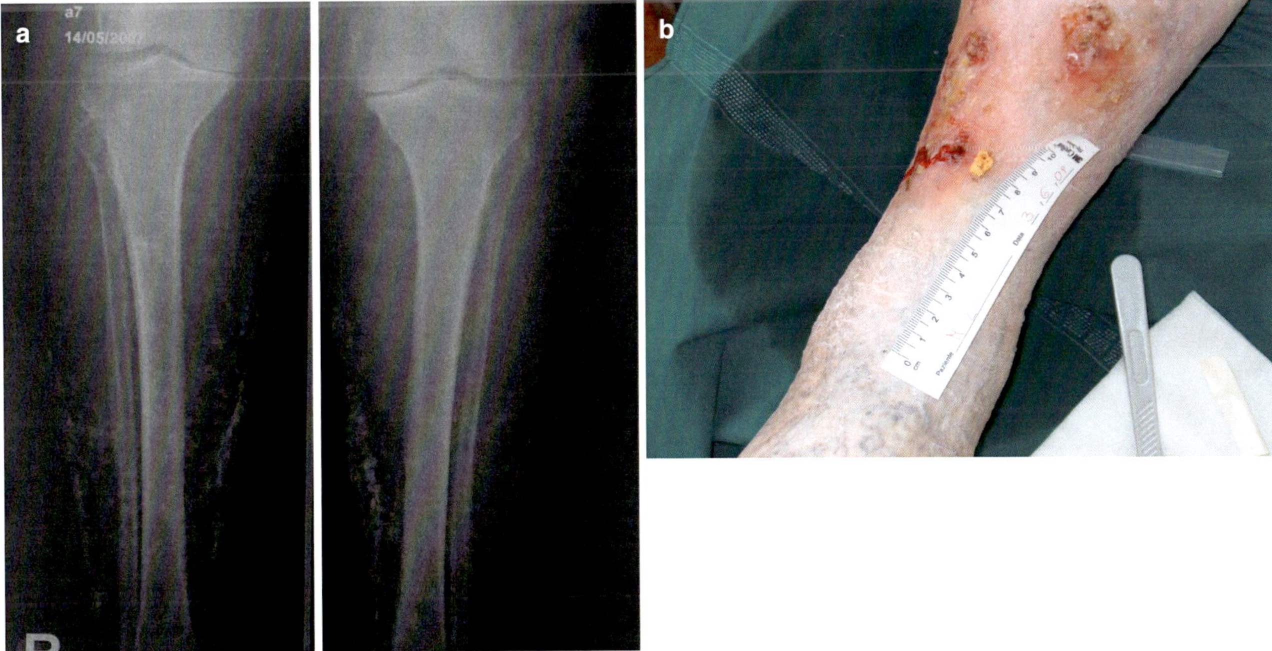

Fig. 9.7 Lesions due to digital calcinosis of the hands (**a, b**) and lower limbs (**c, d**) potentially communicating

Fig. 9.8 X-ray of the lower limbs with evident extensive deposits of calcium linked together (**a**). In the same patient, the appearance of close skin lesions incurred by phenomena of calcinosis radiologically confirmed and predisposes to a high risk of fistulas (**b**)

Conclusions

Fistulas are complications that must be avoided, because it exposes the patient to a higher risk of bacterial infection. It can result in sepsis and interventions that may require amputation of the affected district. In SSc patients, ischemia and immunosuppressive therapies may contribute to facilitate the formation of fistulas.

References

1. Kajihara I, Jinnin M, Yamada S, Ichihara A, Makino T, Igata T, Masuguchi S, Fukushima S, Ihn H. Successful treatment of skin fistulas in systemic sclerosis patients with the combination of topical negative pressure therapy and split-thickness skin grafting. Mod Rheumatol. 2014;24(2):374–6. https://doi.org/10.3109/14397495.2 013.854065.
2. European Wound Management Association (EWMA). Position document Topical negative pressure in wound management. London: MEP Ltd; 2007.
3. Lane TA, Shalhoub J, Franklin OJ. Seton sutures for leg ulcers associated fistulous tracts. Ann R Coll Surg Engl. 2010;92(6):533.
4. Dutronc H, Gobet A, Daucgy FA, Klotz R, Cazave C, Garcia C, Lafarie-Castet S, Fabre T, Dupon M. Stump infection after major lower-limb amputation: a 10-years retrospective. Med Mal Infect. 2013;43(12–12):456–60. study. https://doi.org/10.1016/j.medmal.2013.09.00.
5. Walker M, Metcalf D, Parsons D, Bowler P. A real-life clinical evaluation of a next-generation antimicrobial dressing on acute and chronic wounds. J Wound Care. 2015;24(1):11–22. https://doi.org/10.12968/jowc.2015.24.1.11.
6. Amanzi L, Fiori G, Galluccio F, Miniati I, Guiducci S, Conforti ML, Kaloudi O, Nacci F, Sacu O, Candelieri A, Moggi Pignone A, Rasero L, Conforti D, Matucci-Cerinic M. Digital ulcers in scleroderma: staging, characteristics and subsetting through observation of 1614 digital lesions. Rheumatology (Oxford). 2010;49(7):1374–82.

Silvia Bellando-Randone and Gemma Lepri

In systemic sclerosis (SSc), it is well known that infection of digital ulcers (DU) may provoke pain and disability, affecting patients' quality of life and prognosis, thus representing a high socioeconomic cost. In fact, DU may evolve to complications as infection of soft tissue, cellulitis and osteomyelitis, and gangrene, often requiring amputation [1, 2].

In SSc-DU, infection is a very common complication slowing significantly wound healing. In infected DU, some clinical signs are important (pain, heat, redness, and swelling) (Figs. 10.1, 10.2, 10.3, and 10.4) in order to raise the suspicion and adopt a careful approach to identify the nature of the infection. Usually, the development of an infection is favored either by SSc microangiopathy and defective immune system, with the possible contribution of immunosuppressive treatments. The reduction of tissue blood perfusion and the response to systemic antibiotics may further contribute to deteriorate the infected tissues. These factors may represent the most favorable conditions for ulcer infection by different agents (S. *aureus*, E. *coli* P. *aeruginosa*, E. *faecalis*, S. *agalactiae*, S. *marcescens*, S. *epidermidis*, E. *aerogenes*, S. *maltophilia*, P. *mirabilis*). Moreover, during the wound care procedures, patients can be exposed to microorganisms. Therefore, the prevention and treatment of preexisting local or systemic infections is of crucial importance.

The most common sources of infectious agents are the patient himself, the contact with other patients and the health care personnel, and also the hospital environment where contaminated medical equipment and/or medications are the most frequent cause of infection [3]. An important reservoir of infective agents is the patient's endogenous flora, in particular bacteria present on the skin, mucous membranes, and gastrointestinal tract. Besides the most common agents such as S. *aureus* and P. *aeruginosa*, the frequent detection of fecal pathogens strongly emphasizes the importance of patient's education to optimize the methodology of home self-medications. In fact, a high incidence (in one-quarter of cases) of fecal pathogens in infected SSc-DU has been shown [4]. For these reasons, a rigorous asepsis is mandatory during all therapeutic procedures. It must include hand hygiene of doctors, nurses, and patients and a careful surveillance of the hospital environment and cross-transmission of infection among patients. Regular sterilization of the rooms where wounds are usually managed is absolutely mandatory [5].

A further complication of a DU is monomicrobial or polymicrobial osteomyelitis (OM) [6], which is an infection and inflammation of the bone or bone marrow. In general, microorganisms may reach the bone via the bloodstream, contiguously from infected areas (as in cellulitis and in DU) or following a penetrating trauma. Although DU occurs very frequently in SSc [7], at the moment, the prevalence of OM in SSc patients is not clearly defined. Only one study on 248 SSc patients has shown a 7.7% (19/248 patients) prevalence of OM [8]. OM was associated with infected DU highlighting the importance of DUs' infection as a main predisposing condition [8]. In addition, patients with DU complicated by OM showed a significantly higher percentage of serum anti-Scl70 autoantibodies and a lower mean age compared to those without OM [8]. These correlations suggest that OM may complicate DU in patients with more severe SSc clinical variants, characterized by more pronounced immune-system depression and marked deterioration of the patient's general conditions, including nutritional status [4]. Moreover, the prevention strategies and treatment of OM complicating SSc-DU are still largely empiric. For the management of OM, a multidisciplinary team is required including infectivologist, orthopedic surgeon, radiologist, and nuclear medicine physician [9]. OM usually manifests with symptoms and signs of acute infection like pain, swelling, and fever [6]. In chronic OM, the presence of fistulas with purulent secre-

S. Bellando-Randone (✉) · G. Lepri
Department of Clinical and Experimental Medicine,
University of Florence, Florence, Italy

Department of Geriatric Medicine, Division of Rheumatology
AOUC, Florence, Italy

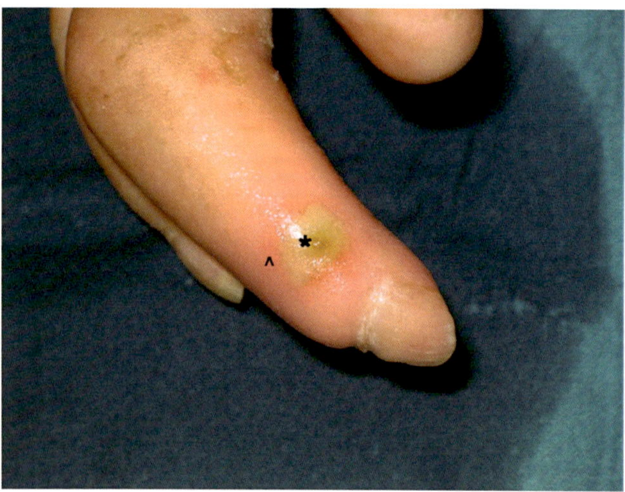

Fig. 10.1 Presence of infection with purulent material (*) and redness (^)

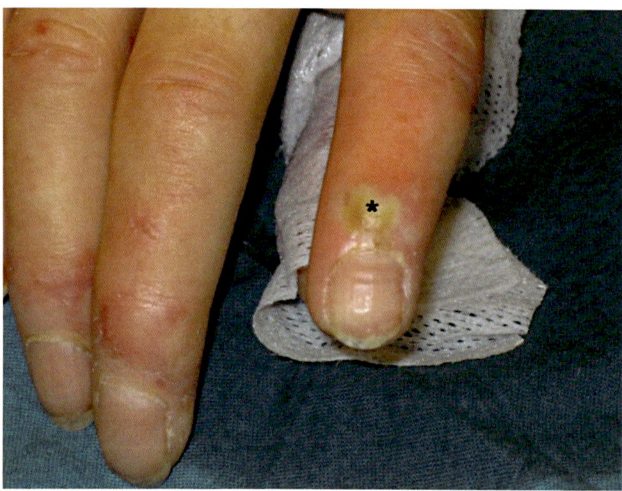

Fig. 10.2 Fibrin (*)

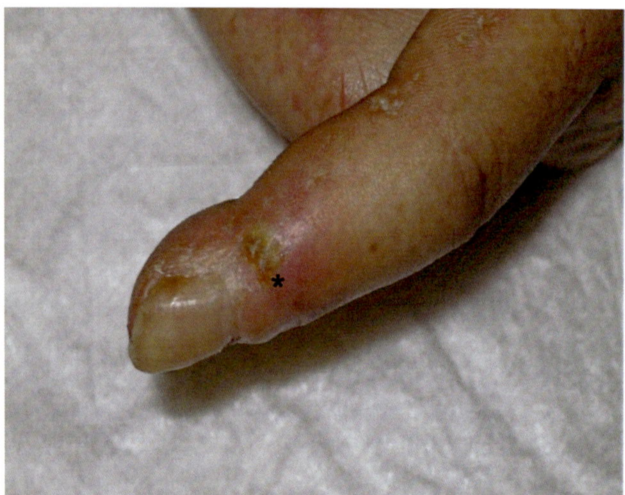

Fig. 10.3 Presence of redness and swelling (*)

tion, skin discoloration and dystrophy, occasional or chronic pain, and fever are observed. These symptoms may alternate with asymptomatic phases. Few data are reported about SSc OM related to complicated DU. In the literature, most of the knowledge about the diagnosis and treatment of OM complicating DU derive from data on diabetic ulcers. Despite the different etiology and pathogenesis of DU, the algorithm to suspect and diagnose OM may be substantially similar. The aspecific laboratory findings (leukocytosis, C-reactive protein (CRP), and erythrocyte sedimentation rate (ESR) elevation) [6], together with clinical history, are the main signs to suspect an OM in the case of DU. However in chronic OM, leukocyte levels greater than $15.000/mm^3$ are rarely found [10]. For this reason, the pathogen identification is crucial for the diagnosis and the choice of the most effective therapy. Surgical sampling or the biopsy of the infected tissue is an efficacious procedure to identify the microbial agent [10]. The culture examination of bone allowed identification of the microorganism in 94% of cases of OM [10, 11]. Often in clinical practice, a DU swab may help in detecting the microorganism and start as soon as possible the best antibiotic therapy. At histopathological examination, OM is characterized by "bone fragmentation or necrosis", with cells' infiltration (inflammatory cells). With Gram staining, the presence of the etiologic agent may be also detected [10]. X-rays may be considered the first instrumental examination in the suspect of OM even if its sensitivity is poor in the first phases of OM as it allows to detect bone alterations after several days (at least 2 weeks) only [6, 10]. Osteopenia, often considered the first sign of OM, and soft tissue's swelling, periostea reaction, and thickening with sclerosis are the x-ray modifications most frequently seen [10, 12] (Fig. 10.5). Magnetic resonance imaging (MRI) is a sensitive tool, in particular in the early phase of bone infection (approximately in the first 5 days), and it provides more information about the extent of the infective process, the soft tissue involvement [12], and marrow edema. In addition, inflammation and alterations of soft tissue (including abscesses, cellulitis, and ulcers) are detected by MRI [6, 12]. Also ultrasound (US) could be useful in the detection of abscesses and fluid collections of soft tissue involved in OM. In fact, US is the first examination when cellulitis, frequently found in OM, is suspected. This complication, as well as OM, often requires patient's hospitalization and a rapid control with intravenous antibiotic therapy to avoid evolution to sepsis [13, 14]. X-rays are not a useful in detecting cellulitis. However, CT is an accurate imaging tool to show the cortical bone and of the soft tissue involvement [14]. Scintigraphy (technetium-99-m-labeled diphosphonates) may be helpful in the early identification of bone infection, usually starting from 2 days after the onset of infectious symptoms and signs. This technique shows not only the infectious process but also the rate of new bone formation. Scintigraphy is helpful to investigate OM when "bone is not affected by underlying conditions" [10]. Gallium

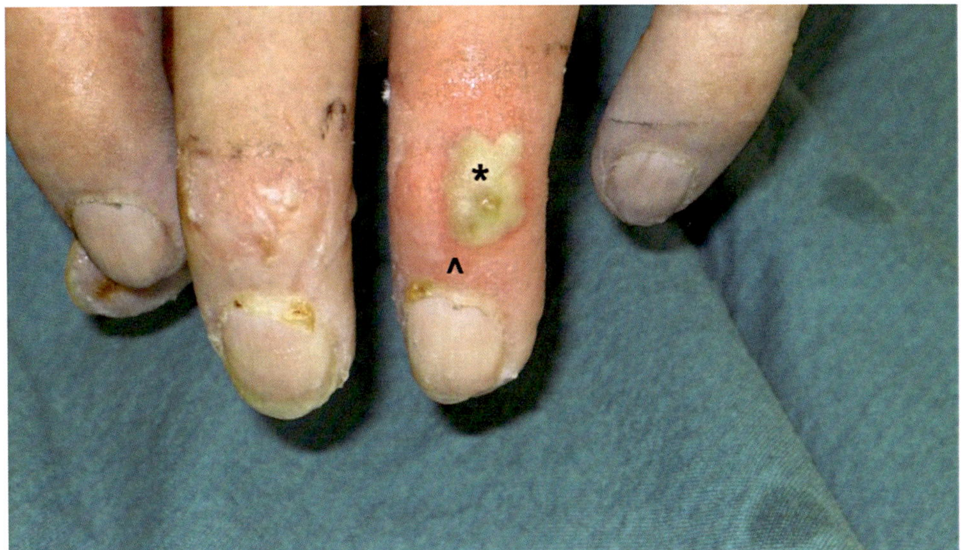

Fig. 10.4 Presence of fibrin (*) and redness (^)

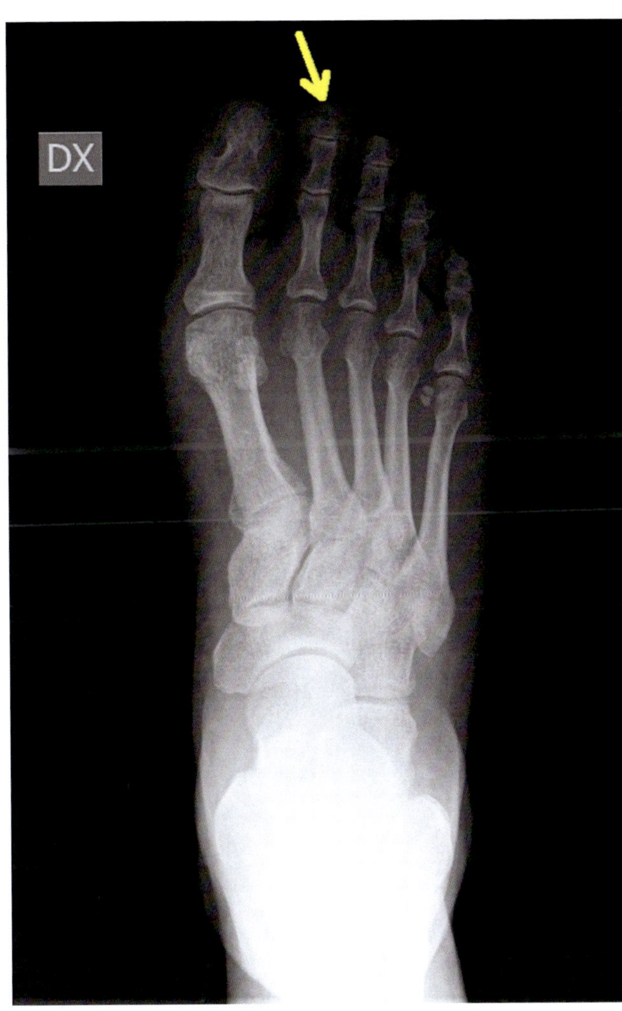

Fig. 10.5 Millimetric area of bone resorption

scan exploits the fact that radiolabeled isotopes attach to phase reactant proteins present in the bone and in the soft tissue. However, in many other conditions (such as malignancy and inflammatory diseases), gallium scans may be positive. It should be also considered that scintigraphy may also provide false-negative results in SSc because vasculopathy may significantly decrease blood perfusion. Recently, FDG-PET has been shown to have a promising role in the detection of bone infection [10, 12].

Conclusions

In SSc, DU may evolve to complications involving soft tissue (cellulitis) and/or the bone (osteomyelitis) representing a great socioeconomic cost. Therefore, an early diagnosis and a prompt treatment are mandatory also to limit the patient's disability and the worsening of quality of life. A crucial element is the self-care education of patients to limit the possibility of contamination and infection. Clinical signs of DU, bone, soft tissue, or systemic infection together with an appropriate use of imaging are most important factors useful to plan a correct management of SSc DUs and of their complications.

References

1. Steen V, Denton CP, Pope JE, Matucci-Cerinic M. Digitalulcers: overt vascular disease in systemic sclerosis. Rheumatology. 2009;48(Suppl 3):iii19–24.
2. Schiopu E, Impens AJ, Philips K. Digital ischemia in scleroderma spectrum of diseases. Int J Rheumatol. 2010, 2010; https.//doi.org/10.1155/2010/923743.

3. Gastmeier P, Stamm-Balderjahn S, Hansen S, Nitzschke-Tiemann F, Zuschneid I, Groneberg K, et al. How outbreaks can contribute to prevention of nosocomial infection: analysis of 1,022 outbreaks. Infect Control Hosp Epidemiol. 2005;26:357–61.

4. Giuggioli D, Manfredi A, Colaci M, Lumetti F, Ferri C. Scleroderma digital ulcers complicated by infection with fecal pathogens. Arthritis Care Res. 2012;64(2):295–7.

5. Longtin Y, Sax H, Allegranzi B, Schneider F, Pittet D. Handhygiene. N Engl J Med. 2011;364:e24.

6. Jeffcoate WJ, Lipsky BA. Controversies in diagnosis and managing osteomyelitis of the foot in diabetes. Clin Infect Dis. 2004;39:S115–22.

7. Ferri C, Valentini G, Cozzi F, Sebastiani M, Michelassi C, LaMontagna G, et al. Systemic sclerosis: demographic, clinical and serologic features and survival in 1,012 Italian patients. Medicine. 2002;81:139–53.

8. Giuggioli D, Manfredi A, Colaci M, Lumetti F, Ferri C. Osteomyelitis complicating scleroderma digital ulcers. Clin Rheumatol. 2013;32(5):623–7.

9. Concia E, Prandini N, Massari L, Ghisellini F, Consoli V, Menichetti F, et al. Osteomyelitis: clinical update for practical guidelines. Nucl Med Commun. 2006;27(8):645–60.

10. Esposito S, Leone S, Bassetti M, Borrè S, Leoncini F, Meani E, et al. Italian guidelines for the diagnosis and infectious disease management of osteomyelitis and prosthetic joint infections in adults. Infection. 2009;37(6):378–496.

11. Zuluaga AF, Galvis W, Saldarriaga JG, Agudel M, Salazar BE, Vesga O. Etiologic diagnosis of chronic osteomyelitis: a prospective study. Arch Intern Med. 2006;166:95–100.

12. Pineda C, Vargas A, Rodríguez AV. Imaging of osteomyelitis: current concepts. Infect Dis Clin N Am. 2006;20(4):789–825.

13. Cranendonk DR, Opmeer BC, Prins JM, Wiersinga WJ. Comparing short to standard duration of antibiotic therapy for patients hospitalized with cellulitis (DANCE): study protocol for a randomized controlled trial. BMC Infect Dis. 2014;14:235.

14. Swartz MN. Cellulitis. N Engl J Med. 2004;350:904–12.

Jelena Blagojevic

Introduction

Digital loss is the most serious and fearful complication of SSc-related peripheral vasculopathy. It may occur as a consequence of gangrene leading to an autoamputation or to surgical amputation or as a result of amputation performed for other reasons, as severe osteomyelitis. Patients which experience gangrene and amputation usually have a history of recurrent ischemic DUs. Digital necrosis requiring amputation is preceded by critical ischemia that manifests with persistent finger discoloration (blue or white), increasing severe pain, extreme tenderness, and digital ulceration. Critical digit-threatening ischemia must be considered a medical emergency and should require rapid and aggressive treatment in order to prevent digital loss.

Gangrene

Gangrene is the most severe clinical manifestation of peripheral vasculopathy in SSc and is the most frequent cause of digital loss in SSc. It consists in necrosis of soft tissues, occurring when the arterial blood supply falls below minimal metabolic requirements. It may occur in DU setting as a consequence of persistent severe ischemia and/or as a result of severe infection.

Gangrene can be classified in a dry and a wet form.

1. Dry gangrene is far more common type of gangrene in SSc and it is caused by chronic ischemia leading slowly to tissue death, dehydration, and eventually mummification of the tissues. The color of the area interested by gangrene is at the beginning dark brown and then switches to black and becomes dry, horny, and shriveled (Fig. 11.1). At the beginning, gangrene may be associated with severe pain, but later the affected area becomes numb and finally anesthetized. If not treated surgically, dead tissue will gradually separate from the healthy tissue and fall off; this process is called autoamputation.

2. Wet gangrene is a liquefactive necrosis with bacterial putrefaction. It is usually an acute process, due to the sudden interruption of the blood flow, the dead part retaining its fluids, furnishing a favorable soil for the bacterial growth. Furthermore, it may develop as an infection of dry gangrene or be a consequence of a severe bacterial infection that contributes to critical tissue ischemia. The area affected by this kind of gangrene becomes moist, edematous, and macerated containing dark-colored fluids and emanates a characteristic odor. The tissues become violaceous or greenish-black, progressing to a bronze, brown, or black color. In the affected tissues, pain is intense with a sense of tension. Systemic symptoms (as fever, malaise etc.) are usually present. This type of gangrene is rare in SSc, usually occurring as a complication of severely infected DU or as a result of dry gangrene infection (Fig. 11.2).

Areas of gangrene are initially characterized by a red line on the skin that marks the border of the affected tissues, called the line of demarcation. This line represents an inflammatory reaction triggered by the dead tissue. Subsequently, granulation tissue forms between the dead and the living parts, in order to cause their separation. This granulation tissue penetrates into the dead tissue until is unable to get adequate nourishment. Ulceration follows and thus a final line of demarcation forms separating the gangrene from healthy parts.

In the case of dry gangrene, the demarcation line forms rapidly and it is sharp, if the blood supply of the proximal tissues is adequate, separating neatly the dead from the viable tissue. As regards wet gangrene, the spread of tissue damage is rapid and the demarcation line is not clear. The infection and suppuration extend into the neighboring living

J. Blagojevic
Department of Experimental and Clinical Medicine,
Division of Rheumatology, University of Florence, Florence, Italy

© Springer Nature Switzerland AG 2019
M. Matucci-Cerinic, C. P. Denton (eds.), *Atlas of Ulcers in Systemic Sclerosis*, https://doi.org/10.1007/978-3-319-98477-3_11

tissue, thereby causing the final line of demarcation to be more proximal than in dry gangrene.

In SSc patients with gangrene, it is of paramount importance to assess the patency of the large vessels, in order to verify the blood supply to the healthy tissues and to rule out the stenosis of large vessels as a contributory cause of gangrene. As the macrovascular arterial involvement may be observed in the upper limbs of SSc patients, especially involving the ulnar artery [1], the assessment of peripheral pulses and Allen's test should be performed in all patients with DU and gangrene. Doppler ultrasound is mandatory if the involvement of large vessels is suspected. Digital subtraction angiography should be performed in case of significant stenosis of large vessels detected by Doppler ultrasound, especially if amenable to angioplasty or surgical revascularization. Angiography computed tomography and magnetic resonance angiography may be done if conventional angiography is contraindicated or in selected cases before surgical revascularization. In the case of ischemia of sudden onset, other causes of gangrene as thromboembolism, hematological disorders, and overlap syndromes should be ruled out.

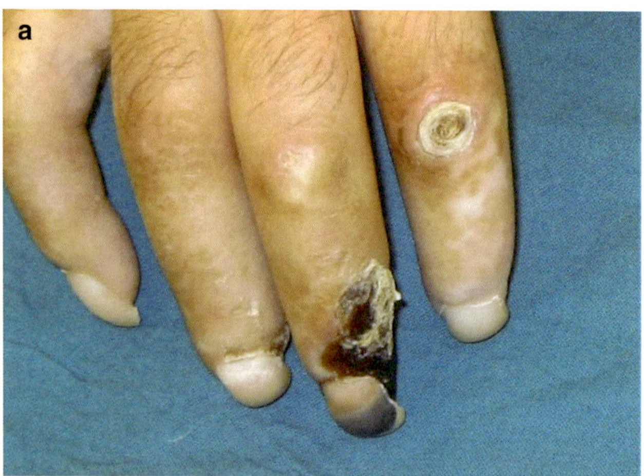
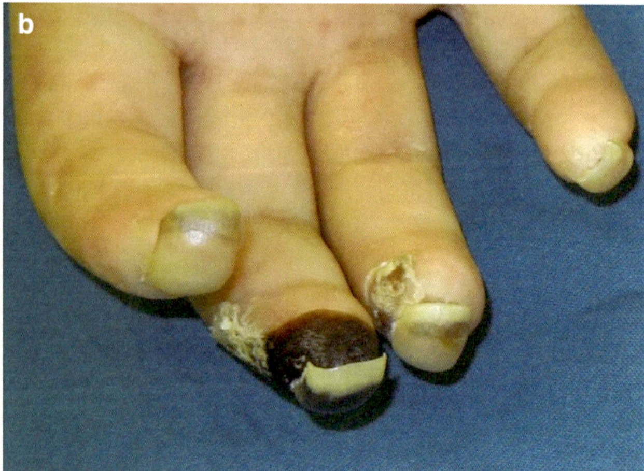

Fig. 11.1 (**a**, **b**) Dry gangrene

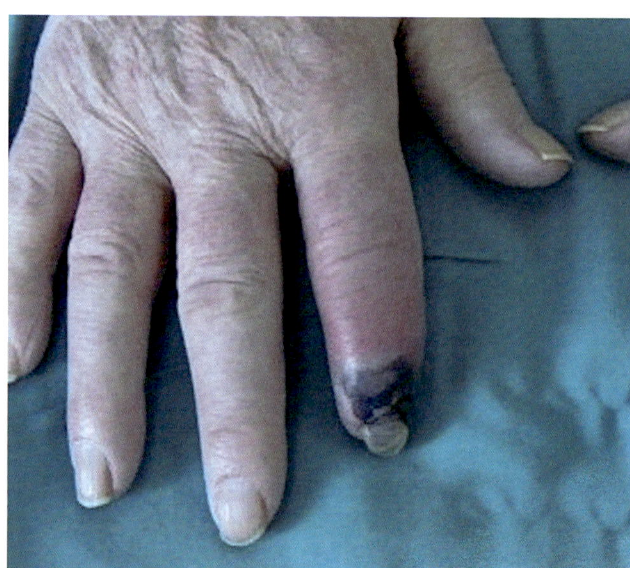

Fig. 11.2 Wet gangrene

Amputation and Autoamputation

The final treatment of gangrene is surgical, by amputation of the necrotic tissues. Wet gangrene requires a prompt surgical approach in order to prevent spreading of the infection to the adjacent healthy tissues and in the circulation, causing life-threatening sepsis. The surgical treatment of dry gangrene can be postponed to the formation of definite demarcation line. In SSc, this process may be long-lasting and disturbing. The line of demarcation usually develops slowly and irregularly or does not develop because of the impairment of the blood supply in the tissues adjacent to gangrene. These patients are also at high risk of infection.

As regards the medical treatment, the maximal vasodilating therapy is mandatory, in order to improve the blood supply, to help the demarcation of dry gangrene, and to promote wound healing. Infection must be also prevented and readily treated if it occurs. In selected cases, hyperbaric oxygen treatment may be applied to combat the infection and to accelerate the demarcation [2]. The maintenance of adequate nutritional status is also needed, as well as the achievement of prompt analgesia.

When planning the amputation, the first step is to determine the precise level of the amputation. For this reason, local treatment of dry gangrene before amputation is very important: surgical debridement of desiccated skin and necrotic tissue will assist in identifying the demarcation.

In selected cases with very small and well-limited areas of dry gangrene, gangrene may be treated only by the surgical debridement in order to maximize the amount of residual viable tissue.

Dry gangrene must be kept as aseptic as possible in order to avoid its transformation into wet form, as the line of demarcation with granulation tissue represents the site of the infection entrance. If it occurs anyway, drainage of the area by incision and removal of any dead tissue is required, together with systemic antibiotic treatment.

Other indications for surgical amputation in patients with DUs are infected DUs complicated by refractory osteomyelitis and severe nonhealing DUs. Nevertheless surgical amputation should be the last resort for the treatment of DUs in SSc.

Potential risks of the surgical amputation are represented by bleeding, infection, thrombosis, and adverse effects of anesthesia, while common complications consist in infection and in impaired wound healing. SSc patients who undergo surgery for DU or gangrene are at high risk of impaired healing, due to the disease-related vasculopathy [3]. Wound dehiscence occurs frequently and healing usually takes place by the second intention (Fig. 11.3).

Autoamputation is the spontaneous separation of nonviable from viable tissues usually associated with dry gangrene, as described above. Ulceration follows the formation of the granulation tissue which allows gradual separation of two parts; eventually the gangrenous part falls off. The ulcer that has been created between living and gangrenous tissue is now on the top of the part that was previously covered by gangrene. This type of ulcer can be defined as ulcer secondary to or derived from gangrene. The phenomenon of autoamputation of fingers and toes may be seen in non-treated scleroderma patients with dry gangrene. It is usually associated with risk of infection and poor healing; thus, it has to be avoided.

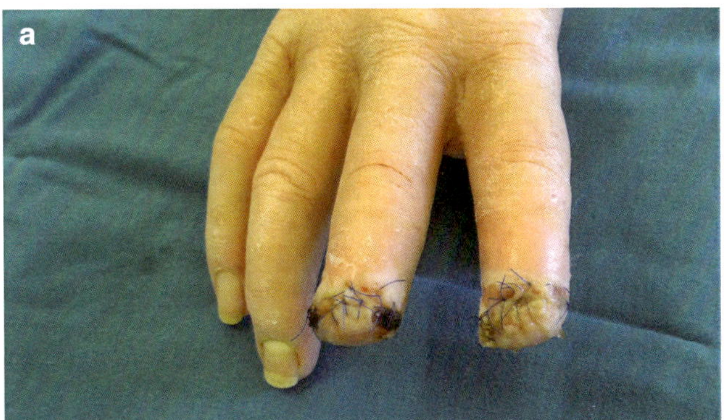

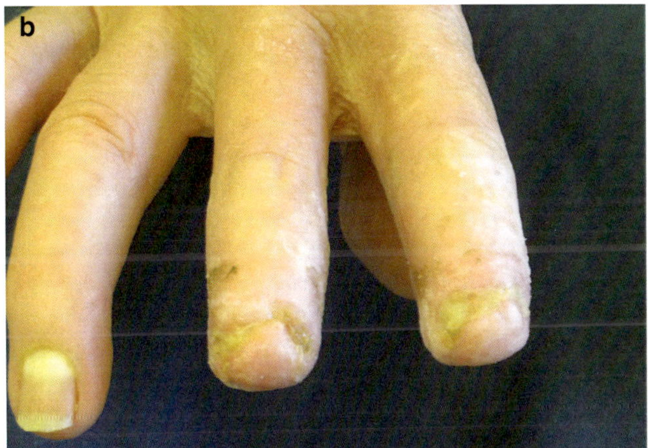

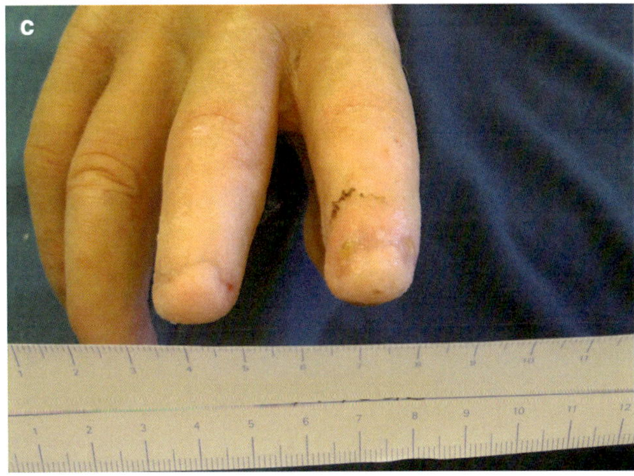

Fig. 11.3 The second intention wound healing. (**a**) Wound dehiscence. (**b**) Healing by the second intention. (**c**) Resolution

Clinical Burden of Digital Loss in SSc

Data on prevalence of gangrene and amputation in large cohorts of SSc patients vary between the registries and differ between patients with previous history of DUs and gangrene and in those without.

It has been estimated that 5–10% of SSc patients develops gangrene or undergo amputation [4–6]. The risk of gangrene and amputation increases to 20% in patients with DUs [7–9], while the incidence of amputation ranges from 1% to 2% of patients/year [7, 8].

Data from the Pittsburgh database refer to 2080 patients with SSc, identified between 1972 and 1995 and prospectively followed for a mean of 10 years. Fifty-eight percent of subjects enrolled in this cohort experienced DU during the course of disease. Eleven percent all patients underwent amputation or had gangrene over the observational period, while in patients with persistent DUs, the probability of losing a part of finger was 20% [4].The incidence of gangrene increased with time since the development of DUs, particularly after 4 years [4].

A retrospective study performed on 1168 SSc patients in the Royal Free Hospital in London, in 2008, showed that 16.6% of the subjects had at least one recorded episode of DU and that 1.4% of them developed digital gangrene, over the observational period of 18 months. Sixty-eight percent of patients with gangrene experienced autoamputation or required surgical amputation [10].

The analysis of 1043 patients included in the Canadian scleroderma research registry from August 2004 to April 2010 showed that digital necrosis/gangrene was observed in 1.1% and digital loss/amputation in 5.9% of patients, while DU occurred in 8.8% of patients [6].

The analysis of DUO registry, the European multicenter observational registry of SSc patients with DUs, performed on 2439 subjects enrolled from April 2008 to November 2010, showed that 22.6% of patients experienced gangrene, 9.5%surgical amputation and 8.6% autoamputation [7].

A retrospective study conducted in 2006 on 103 SSc patients with and without history of DU, included into the French screening program for pulmonary arterial hypertension (PAH) by a single center, showed that 18% of patients with DU had gangrene and that the incidence of finger amputation was 1.2% per patient-year in patients with history of DU [8].

In our large prospective study on more than 1600 digital cutaneous lesions in 100 SSc patients, performed from January 2004 to January 2008, less than 1% of patients experienced gangrene. Autoamputation occurred in 14% of cases of gangrene [11].

Reported potential risk factors for digital loss and amputation in SSc patients are diffuse cutaneous subtype [10], current smoking [12], older age [13], long history of RP, and long disease duration [13]. Other possible risk factors for the occurrence of digital loss are anti-centromere antibodies [13, 14] and anti-beta2-glycoprotein I antibodies [15].

Allanore et al. have recently evaluated features of SSc patients enrolled into DUO registry which presented history of gangrene or which experienced gangrene within the observational period going from April 2008 to June 2014 [9]. Eight hundred eight patients (8% percent of 4534 patients enrolled in the registry by June 2014) had gangrene at the time of enrollment and/or had a history of gangrene. There were no differences regarding Raynaud's phenomenon or disease duration, cutaneous subset, autoantibodies, major organ involvement, or smoking between patients with current and/or previous gangrene and those without. The preliminary analysis showed that the only risk factor for the occurrence of new gangrene during the follow-up was represented by a history of previous gangrene. Moreover, 34% of patients with previous and/or current gangrene at the inclusion visit and only 2.4% of patients without history of gangrene underwent surgical amputation during the follow-up period.

Conclusion

Prevalence of gangrene, amputation, and autoamputation seems to be still too high in SSc, despite novel vasodilating and vasoactive therapies, now available in the clinical practice.

SSc patients who undergo digital loss have a significant disability, functional impairment, and psychological repercussions, usually worsening previous damage. Since the amputation and the autoamputation represent the severe and debilitating consequence of DU, every effort has to be made in order to avoid their occurrence.

References

1. Taylor MH, McFadden JA, Bolster MB, Silver RM. Ulnar artery involvement in systemic sclerosis (scleroderma). J Rheumatol. 2002;29:102–6.

2. Kaide CG, Khandelwal S. Hyperbaric oxygen: applications in infectious disease. Emerg Med Clin North Am. 2008;26(2):571–95.

3. Tagil M, Dieterich J, Kopylov P. Wound healing after hand surgery in patients with systemic sclerosis--a retrospective analysis of 41 operations in 19 patients. J Hand Surg Eur. 2007;32(3):316–9.

4. Steen V, Denton CP, Pope JE, Matucci-Cerinic M. Digital ulcers: overt vascular disease in systemic sclerosis. Rheumatology (Oxford). 2009;48(Suppl 3):S19–24.

5. Poormoghim H, Moghadam AS, Moradi-Lakeh M, Jafarzadeh M, Asadifar B, Ghelman M, Andalib E. Systemic sclerosis: demographic, clinical and serological features in 100 Iranian patients. Rheumatol Int. 2013;33(8):1943–50.

6. Muangchan C, Canadian Scleroderma Research Group, Baron M, Pope J. The 15% rule in scleroderma: the frequency of severe organ complications in systemic sclerosis: a systematic review. J Rheumatol. 2013;40(9):1545–56.

7. Denton CP, Krieg T, Guillevin L, Schwierin B, Rosenberg D, Silkey M, Zultak M, Matucci-Cerinic M, DUO Registry investigators. Demographic, clinical and antibody characteristics of patients with digital ulcers in systemic sclerosis: data from the DUO registry. Ann Rheum Dis. 2012;71(5):718–21.

8. Hachulla E, Clerson P, Launay D, et al. Natural history of ischemic digital ulcers in systemic sclerosis: single-center retrospective longitudinal study. J Rheumatol. 2007;34:2423–30.

9. Allanore Y, Denton CP, Krieg T, Cornelisse P, Rosenberg D, Schwierin B, Matucci-Cerinic M. Clinical characteristics of systemic sclerosis patients with digital ulcer disease who developed gangrene: data from DUO registry. Ann Rheum Dis. 2015;74(Suppl2):818.

10. Nihtyanova SI, Brough GM, Black CM, Denton CP. Clinical burden of digital vasculopathy in limited and diffuse cutaneous systemic sclerosis. Ann Rheum Dis. 2008;67:120–3.

11. Amanzi L, Braschi F, Fiori G, Galluccio F, Miniati I, Guiducci S, Conforti ML, Kaloudi O, Nacci F, Sacu O, Candelieri A, Pignone A, Rasero L, Conforti D, Matucci-Cerinic M. Digital ulcers in scleroderma: staging, characteristics and sub-setting through observation of 1614 digital lesions. Rheumatology (Oxford). 2010;49:1374–82.

12. Harrison BJ, Silman AJ, Hider SJ, Herrick AL. Cigarette smoking as a significant risk factor for digital vascular disease in patients with systemic sclerosis. Arthritis Rheum. 2002;46(12):3312–6.

13. Caramaschi P, Biasi D, Caimmi C, Barausse G, Sabbagh D, Tinazzi I, LA Verde V, Tonetta S, Adami S. Digital amputation in systemic sclerosis: prevalence and clinical associations: a retrospective longitudinal study. J Rheumatol. 2012;39(8):1648–53.

14. Wigley FM, Wise RA, Miller R, Needleman BW, Spence RJ. Anticentromere antibodies as a predictor of digit ischemic loss in patients with systemic sclerosis. Arthritis Rheum. 1992;35:688–93.

15. Boin F, Franchini S, Colantuoni E, Rosen A, Wigley FM, Casciola-Rosen L. Independent association of anti-β2-glycoprotein I antibodies with macrovascular disease and mortality in scleroderma patients. Arthritis Rheum. 2009;60(8):2480–9.

Pain

Felice Galluccio

Background

In systemic sclerosis (SSc), skin ulcers are persistent and often recurrent complications, difficult to manage, slow to heal, and can cause tissue loss [1]. Moreover, these are frequently infected and may lead to osteomyelitis, gangrene, autoamputation, and in some cases septicemia [2, 3].

General principles of ulcer management include the establishment of a clean and healthy wound base, often through surgical debridement, treatment of infection, coverage with an appropriate dressing and maintenance of a moist environment [4].

In SSc, ulcers cause considerable pain with a disabling effect on patients, limiting hand function and daily activities, such as feeding, dressing, and hygiene [5], heavily impairing quality of life [6]. Indeed, the progressive scarring and tissue loss that patients experience daily can lead to some degree of depression and anxiety [7] that has been shown to be a significant predictor of the intensity of pain [8]. Ongoing inflammation and infection may amplify pain experience [8, 9]. Evidence suggests that stress significantly slows wound healing and multiple cellular and biochemical mechanisms have been identified that link to stress and healing [10, 11]. Additionally, pain activates the sympathetic branch of the autonomic nervous system, triggering a physiological response that slows wound healing [12]. Moreover, pain interferes with treatment protocols because patients are unwilling or unable to comply with necessary regimens and protocols. Treatments, like debridement or bandaging, may cause extreme discomfort and noncompliance that significantly delays healing.

Understanding the different types and the neurobiology of pain pathways is a critical step in pain management for SSc patients with skin ulcers.

F. Galluccio
Division of Rheumatology, Department of Clinical and Experimental Medicine, University of Firenze – Aou Careggi, Firenze, Italy

Neurobiology of Ulcer-Related Pain

Ulcer-related pain may occur as one or both nociceptive and neuropathic. Nociceptors are the free nerve endings that respond to tissue injury. These nerve endings are either small myelinated A-δ fibers, which conduct pain quickly and produce sharp localized discomfort, or larger unmyelinated C fibers, which conduct pain slowly and are responsible for dull or throbbing pain.

Generally, once damaged tissue has healed, nociceptive pain subsides. If nociceptive pain continues for a prolonged period and the nerve fibers are in a constant inflammatory state – such as with repeated ulcer debridement or dressing changes – sensitization of the nerve fibers may lead to hyperalgesia (amplified pain) [13] or allodynia (pain from a benign stimulus, such as light touch). Allodynia, which is more characteristic of neuropathic pain [14] may confound evaluation and treatment [10].

Neuropathic pain is caused by insult to the actual nerve fibers or central nervous system. It often occurs after prolonged nociceptive pain from an injury, although it may also be caused by inflammation or compression of a nerve by a lesion or scar tissue. Usually it is chronic and described as burning, tingling, or shooting. Unlike nociceptive pain, neuropathic pain often continues even after the tissue has healed because the damaged nerve fibers continue to misfire [10, 14].

The complex neural connections involved in the processing of pain are difficult to understand. The "gate control" theory asserts that a pain stimulus is first regulated in the peripheral nervous system and spine. The dorsal horn of the spinal cord receives nociceptive or pain stimuli from A-δ and C nerve fibers as well as non-nociceptive or sensory stimuli from large A-β fibers. A-β fibers transmit sensory input faster than both A-δ and C fibers. When A-β nerve fibers are simultaneously stimulated with the smaller pain fibers, signals race ahead of the pain transmissions and, by synapsing with inhibitory and projection neurons, "close the

© Springer Nature Switzerland AG 2019
M. Matucci-Cerinic, C. P. Denton (eds.), *Atlas of Ulcers in Systemic Sclerosis*, https://doi.org/10.1007/978-3-319-98477-3_12

gate" for transmission of pain stimuli to the brain. This theory would explain why pain is lessened when an injured area is massaged. If only the smaller A-δ and C nerve fibers are stimulated or if an abundance of smaller fibers are stimulated, they inactivate the inhibitory and projection neurons and "open the gate" to the brain [15]. Once nerve fibers have been stimulated, electrical signals are transmitted through the opening and closing of sodium and other ionic channels through the peripheral nerves and ascending pathways and through the spinal cord to the thalamus, hypothalamus, limbic system, and cerebral cortex. Pain transmission of a small A-δ nerve fiber is quickly relayed to the thalamus and cerebral cortex for an immediate response, withdrawal, and pain relief, which occurs through descending pathways. The C nerve fiber travels the same ascending pathway through the spinal cord, only more slowly. In the brain, the signal takes a path through the hypothalamus, which releases certain hormones including those for stress, and the limbic system, which affects emotions. This might explain why chronic pain often is associated with depression and anxiety. Descending pathways originating in the cortex inhibit the ascending pathways in the midbrain and spinal cord, "closing the gate" and diminishing pain perception. Natural opioid neurotransmitters endorphins, dynorphins, and enkephalins are released from the hypothalamus and work to alter pain perception [16].

The pain experience may be changed by anxiety, stress, emotions, and cognition [16]. High levels of anxiety and the release of stress hormones may inhibit descending pathways and "open the gate" causing pain perception to intensify. This explains why individuals experience pain differently and why an individual may respond to the same type of pain differently each time it occurs [12]. Moreover, pain thresholds are largely influenced by previous pain experiences.

Management of Ulcer-Related Pain

Management of skin ulcers requires a multifaceted approach that includes pain control and emotional support at the very outset of treatment. It is necessary to determine the underlying pathology causing the pain. Worsening or change in the type or intensity of pain may indicate a deteriorating condition or impending infection [2].

First, we must differentiate pain by subtypes:

- *Background or chronic pain*: continuous pain stemming from the ulcer itself. This includes pain associated with an infection. Pain levels may fluctuate for background pain over the course of the day due to changes in the wound or whether or not the patient is able to distract themselves.
- *Incident pain*: caused by movement of some kind whether from friction and shear when the patient moves or the movement of the dressing.
- *Procedural cycling pain*: experienced during repetitive procedures like dressing change.
- *Operative non-cycling pain*: operative pain is severe enough to require anesthesia for a procedure like occasional debridement.

It is therefore evident that each of these should be managed at every level of treatment.

Type, intensity, location, and cause of pain must be assessed, as well as the patient physical and emotional status. It is crucial to remember that pain is a complex, subjective, and perceptual phenomenon and pain experience is never in the same way or with the same intensity and responses to treatment modalities vary as well. For this reason, pain management must be individualized.

Non-pharmacological approach is the first line of treatment. Standard topical care treatment includes the maintenance of a warm and humid environment and the application of various medications such as hydrogel, hydrocolloid, paraffin gauze, and antiseptic dressings like silver-coated medications. Healthcare professionals must openly discuss their fears and expectations with patients and encourage them to participate in treatment, such as cleaning or dressing changes. Communication is not only crucial for assessing the state and characteristics of pain but is a way to distract and relax the patient during medications. It is proven that establishing a relationship with the patient helps reduce the level of anxiety and the fear of experiencing procedural or operative pain, thereby allowing to naturally readjust pain perception and raising tolerance to future treatment.

Pharmacological treatment must be targeted according to the subtype of pain. Pain triggers, like infections, ischemia, edema, etc., should be promptly identified and treated.

Local anesthetics must be used for procedural and operative pain; nonsteroidal fast-acting anti-inflammatory drugs can be used for incident or breakthrough pain, while analgesics like paracetamol, NSAIDs or COX-2 inhibitors, cannabinoids, and weak or strong opioids can be used in the control of chronic background pain. Adjunctive therapies, like anticonvulsants, sodium and calcium channel blockers, botulinum toxin injection, or surgical treatments, should be considered if appropriate conservative measures fail.

Take-Home Messages

- Controlling pain at every level of treatment.
- Patients should be encouraged to actively participate in their treatment.
- The primary etiology, size, depth, and extent of skin ulcers help guide treatment.
- All contributing factors should be identified and treated (e.g., ischemia, edema, infections, etc.).

References

1. Galluccio F, Matucci-Cerinic M. Registry evaluation of digital ulcers in systemic sclerosis. Int J Rheumatol. 2010;2010. pii: 363679
2. Amanzi L, Braschi F, Fiori G, Galluccio F, Miniati I, Guiducci S, et al. Digital ulcers in scleroderma: staging, characteristics and subsetting through observation of 1614 digital lesions. Rheumatology (Oxford). 2010;49(7):1374–82.
3. Korn JH. Scleroderma: a treatable disease. Cleve Clin J Med. 2003;70(11):954, 956, 958 passim.
4. Barbul A. Wound healing. In: Bruncardi CF, Anderson DK, Billiar TR, Dunn DL, Pollack RE, editors. Schwartz's principles of surgery. 8th ed. New York: McGraw-Hill; 2005.
5. Merkel PA, Herlyn K, Martin RW, Anderson JJ, et al. Measuring disease activity and functional status in patients with scleroderma and Raynaud's phenomenon. Arthritis Rheum. 2002;46(9):2410–20.
6. Mouthon L, Mestre-Stanislas C, Bérezné A, Rannou F, et al. Impact of digital ulcers on disability and health-related quality of life in systemic sclerosis. Ann Rheum Dis. 2010;69(1):214–7.
7. Newland PK, Wipke-Tevis DD, Williams DA, et al. Impact of pain on outcomes in long-term care residents with and without multiple sclerosis. J Am Geriatr Soc. 2005;53:1490–6.
8. Aaron LA, Patterson DR, Finch CP, et al. The utility of a burn specific measure of pain anxiety to prospectively predict pain and function: a comparative analysis. Burns. 2001;27:329–34.
9. Pediani R. What has pain relief to do with acute surgical wound healing? World Wide Wounds. http://www.worldwidewounds.com/2001/march/Pediani/Pain relief-surgical wounds.html. Accessed 01 April 2010.
10. Popescu A, Salcido RS. Wound pain: a challenge for the patient and wound care specialist. Adv Skin Wound Care. 2004;17(1):14–20.
11. Vileikyte L. Stress and wound healing. Clin Dermatol. 2007;25(1):49–55.
12. Fleck CA. Managing wound pain: today and in the future. Adv Skin Wound Care. 2007;20(3):138–45.
13. Sussman C, Bates-Jenson C. Wound care. In: A collaborative practice manual for health professionals. 3rd ed. Philadelphia: Lippincott Williams & Wilkins; 2006. p. 278–81.
14. Richeimer S. The Richeimer pain update (Richeimer Pain Medical Group), www.helpforpain.com/arch2000dec.htm.
15. Melzak R, Wall PD. Pain mechanisms: a new theory. Science. 1965;150:971–9.
16. Hunt S, Koltzenburg M. The neurobiology of pain: (molecular and cellular neurobiology). Oxford: Oxford University Press; 2005.

Paul Legendre and Luc Mouthon

Introduction

Digital ulcers (DUs), defined as well-localized loss of dermis, distal to the metacarpophalangeal (MCP) joints, occur in up to 50% of patients with systemic sclerosis (SSc) [1]. In a recent study conducted in a cohort of SSc patients, DUs were episodic in 9.4%, recurrent in 46.2%, and chronic in 11.2% of the patients [2]. Recurrent DUs on the fingertips and over the interphalangeal joints lead to scars and digital resorption.

Complications may occur such as superinfection that may lead to osteitis and progression to gangrene requiring amputation. Beyond pain and superinfection, recurrent DUs lead to major hand disability with clinical, social, and psychological impact and poor quality of life (QoL) in patients with SSc [3, 4].

Clinical Assessment in Global and Hand Disability

As for many chronic diseases, several tools could be used to evaluate patient's disability from a self-assessment (by the patient himself) or from medical evaluation.

Quality of Life Assessment

SF 36

QoL could be self-assessed using the Medical Outcomes Study 36-item Short-Form Health Survey (SF-36) that investigates 8 scales related to QoL. Scale scores are normalized to a mean of 50 and standard deviation of 10 based on the normal US population [5].

Patient-Reported Outcomes Measurement Information System

Patient-Reported Outcomes Measurement Information System (PROMIS) is also a valid instrument of self-evaluation to measure the health status of SSc patients [6, 7]. PROMIS includes four items each for seven domains (physical function, anxiety, depression, fatigue, sleep disturbance, pain interference, ability to perform social roles), plus a single pain intensity item.

Global Disability Assessment

The Health Assessment Questionnaire (HAQ) is a global self-assessment evaluation of disability. In SSc patients experiencing DUs, HAQ could be a good reflect of hand disability as it is still a major instrument to assess disability in many musculoskeletal disorders [8]. HAQ was validated in SSc patients [9]. In SSc, a more specific version of HAQ was proposed with five patient-generated visual analog scales added to the original HAQ, assessing Raynaud's phenomenon, DUs, gastrointestinal and lung symptoms, and overall disease severity from the patient's perspective [10]. HAQ evaluates 20 items related to daily activities divided into 8 domains scored between 0 (no disability) and 3 (maximal disability) [11]. The disability index (HAQ-DI) is also measured on a scale of 0–3 units, representing an average score across the domains.

P. Legendre · L. Mouthon (✉)
Internal Medicine Department, Reference Center for Rare Systemic Autoimmune Diseases of Ile de France,
Hospital Cochin, Paris, France
e-mail: luc.mouthon@aphp.fr

© Springer Nature Switzerland AG 2019
M. Matucci-Cerinic, C. P. Denton (eds.), *Atlas of Ulcers in Systemic Sclerosis*, https://doi.org/10.1007/978-3-319-98477-3_13

Hand Disability Assessment

Cochin Hand Function Scale (CHFS)

In patients with SSc, hand disability can be assessed by the patient himself using the Cochin hand function scale (CHFS) (Fig. 13.1). This self-assessment questionnaire has been first set up for patients with rheumatoid arthritis [12] and secondary validated in patients with SSc [13, 14]. CHFS is based on 18 items related to daily activities, each scored on a scale of 0 (performed without difficulty) to 5 (impossible to do). The total score is obtained by adding individual scores (range 0–90) [14]. More recently, a 6-item short form of the CHFS (CHFS-6) was validated in SSc patients [15].

Other Tools

Hand Mobility in Scleroderma index (HAMIS) has also been proposed to specifically assess hand global mobility in patients with SSc [16]. However, this hetero-assessment index does not evaluate hand disability for activities of daily living.

Global hand and wrist mobility could be evaluated by physician using the hand functional index (HFI) from Keitel [17] ranges from 4 (best mobility) to 42 (worst mobility). The Kapandji index is assessed by the physician to evaluate hand disability, testing the opposition and the counter-opposition of the thumb. Kapandji scores range from 0 (worst mobility) to 100 (best mobility) [18].

Michigan Hand Outcome Questionnaire (MHOQ) has been widely used for nearly 20 years to assess patients with a variety of hand and upper extremity conditions and allowed a self-assessment of esthetic consideration [19]. MHOQ has a good internal consistency and adequate convergent validity in SSc [20].

Without the help of adapted instruments, in the past two weeks, did you:	0	1	2	3	4	5
Section 1: In the kitchen, can you						
Hold a bowl?						
Seize a fill bottle and raise it?						
Hold a full plate of food?						
Pour liquid for a bottle into a glass?						
Unscrew the lid from a jar opened before?						
Cut meat with a knife?						
Prick things well with a fork?						
Peel fruit?						
Section 2: Dressing, can you						
Button your shirt?						
Open and close a zipper?						
Section 3: Hygiene, can you						
Squeeze a new tube of toothpaste?						
Hold a toothbrush efficiently?						
Section 4: In the office						
Write a short sentence with a pencil or ordinary pen?						
Write a letter with a pencil or ordinary pen?						
Section 5: Other, can you						
Turn a round door knob?						
Cut a piece of paper with scissors?						
Pick up coins from a table top?						
Turn a key in a lock?						

Fig. 13.1 Cochin hand function scale (CHFS)

0 = Yes, without difficulty; 1 = Yes, with a little difficulty; 2 = Yes with some difficulty; 3 = Yes, with much difficulty; 4 = Nearly impossible to do; 5 = Impossible

Patients Categorization

In order to better describe the impact of DUs on QoL, several authors proposed to study specifically SSc patients experiencing digital lesions in homogenous groups [2, 21]. In a first study, digital lesions were classified in four groups: digital pitting scars, DU, calcinosis, or gangrene [21]. Then, in a large prospective study based on 4534 patients, included in the "Digital Ulcers Outcome" (DUO) Registry, four groups of SSc patients were individualized: non-DU, episodic DUs, recurrent DUs, and chronic DUs [2].

Clinical Impact

In fact, observations made in a large prospective cohort of SSc patients show that concomitant DUs could occur on several fingers of the dominant hand and both hands in one-third of cases (Fig. 13.2) [4].

Furthermore, SSc patients with active DUs have reduced wrist and hand mobility (assessed by Kapandji scale) and increased global (HAQ) and hand disabilities (CHFS) compared to those without active DUs [4, 22]. Hand disability may occur as soon as the patient develops one DU [4]. In EUSTAR cohort, DU-related complications were reported in 23% of patients, and 27% of patients required ≥1 DU procedure during follow-up [23]. Then, as stated before, recurrent DUs lead to sequelae such as auto or surgical amputations, arthrodesis, or scars that alter hand ability [4].

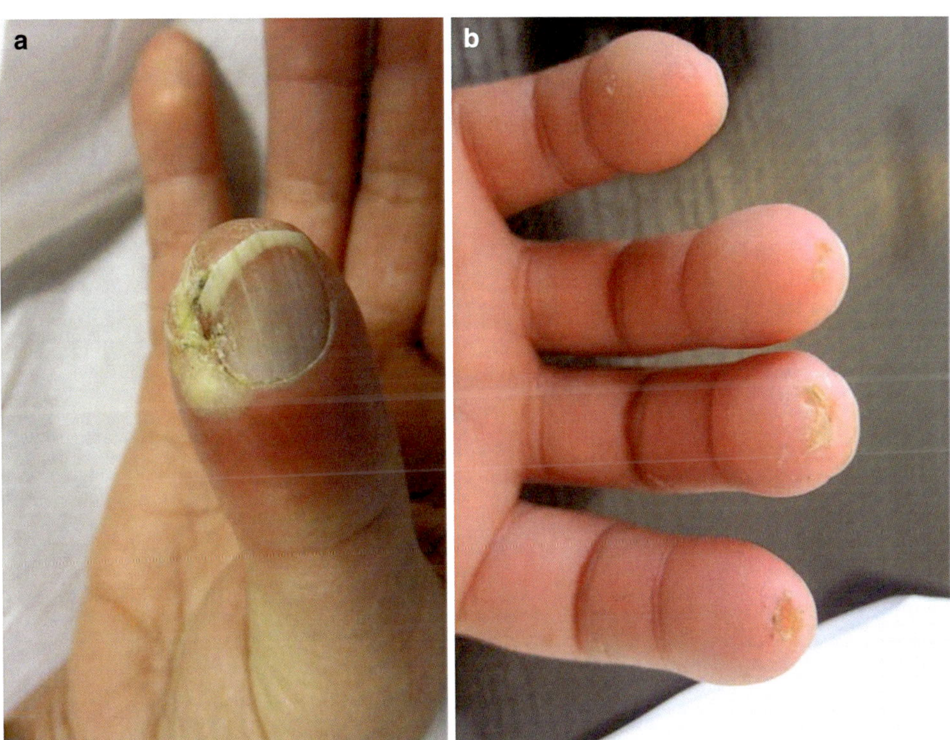

Fig. 13.2 Systemic sclerosis: digital ulcers (**a**) superinfection of a digital ulceration of the right thumb. (**b**) Digital ulcers scars of the pulp of 2nd, 3rd and 4th fingers of the left hand

Quality of Life

The social impact of DUs in SSc patients has to be integrated in the global impact of the disease in professional and activities of daily living. In fact, DU consequences, together with asthenia, pain dyspnea, and discomfort linked to sclerosis, are major complaints of patients with SSc [24]. Furthermore, recurrent hospitalizations due to DUs or complications impact both daily living and professional activities [23].

Patients needing help from their family may negatively impact both the familial balance and their own well-being, explaining why SSc patients with DUs had significantly poorer QOL compared to non-DUs patients [22]. Moreover, patients with active DUs had significantly poorer QoL and mental health subscale of SF-36 compare to patients with non-active DUs [4]. One study suggested that anxiety was significantly higher in patients with DUs than in others using HAQ, CHFS, and Hospital Anxiety and Depression Scale [25]. In case of DUs, PROMIS-29 is also altered in patients with hand disability [26].

Ulcerations and their sequelae induce also esthetic prejudice leading to limited social activities.

Professional Impact

Fitness to work is a multifactorial phenomenon and depends on individual factors such as physical capacity and psychological characteristics, as well as the requirements of work [27]. Patients suffering SSc commonly have to change jobs and go on full-time sick leave [27, 28]. According to different series, 23.9–60.9% of SSc patients were on full-time sick leave, 35.6% were receiving a disability pension, and 31–34.5% experienced occupational changes [25, 27]. Factors associated with employment status were general health status: global, hand and mouth disability, and depression [27]. Although DUs were not significantly associated with full-time sick leave or professional changes in these studies, hand disability was significantly increased in patients on sick leave [17].

Focusing on DUs, data extracted from EUSTAR cohort reported an overall work impairment of 35% [23]. In the DUO registry, category of patients that experienced a new DU at every follow-up visit (chronic category) had the highest rate of incident complications, highest work impairment, and greatest need for help compared with the other categories [2]. Moreover, patients experiencing chronic DUs were younger at disease onset, with implications for their working life. When younger patients develop chronic DUs, they are affected with a burdensome disease at time period of their life where they need and/or want to maintain employment [2].

Overall, SSc has a significant impact on activities of daily living (ADL) and work disability. The decision to stop work is likely influenced by the patient's health. Disability and the need for external home help are increased in SSc patients with DUs.

Economic Impact

Economic burden of DUs is difficult to quantify in SSc patients. However, some considerations could help us to understand that DUs could represent an important global healthcare problem.

First, patients experiencing DUs underwent one or repeated hospitalizations. Hachulla et al. reported in a study conducted in France that the number of days of hospitalization related to the care of DU was estimated of 1.43 days per patient-year. Considering the cost of hospitalization and cost of treatments such as Iloprost, the authors estimated a cost of 1,542 € per patient-year for national assurance healthcare [1]. Additional costs could be added such as antibiotic prescription or surgical procedures.

We have reported that SSc patients with DUs needed more external home help and more paid and nonpaid household help than SSc patients without DUs [25]. Most patients reported a limitation in daily activities related to SSc, as assessed by a daily activity limitation scale and an increased need for home help [25, 27]. In the DUO registry, median daily activity impairment increased from 10% in the non-DU category to 40% in the recurrent and 60% in the chronic categories. The chronic category also recorded the highest proportion of patients who needed help and the highest number of hours needed for unpaid help [2]. Similar conclusions were made in Brand et al. and Bérezne et al. studies [23, 27]. In a retrospective study, conducted in Italy, the treatment of 20 SSc patients experiencing DUs represented a cost of 535,117€ per patient per year for the society [29]. These data highlighted the elevated direct costs of treatments for public assurance healthcare. Then, prevention of the occurrence of DUs in SSc patients is a major issue to prevent disability.

Conclusion

In SSc patients, DUs contribute to hand disability. Hand disability related to DU negatively impacts social, professional, and daily living activities of SSc patients but has also a significant economic impact. Several tools could be used to assess the consequences of DU and better define the patient's needs. As a consequence, prevention of DUs recurrences must be a major goal for physicians in order to diminish disability and improve patient's global burdens.

References

1. Hachulla E, Clerson P, Launay D, Lambert M, Morell-Dubois S, Queyrel V, et al. Natural history of ischemic digital ulcers in systemic sclerosis: single-center retrospective longitudinal study. J Rheumatol. 2007;34(12):2423–30.
2. Matucci-Cerinic M, Krieg T, Guillevin L, Schwierin B, Rosenberg D, Cornelisse P, et al. Elucidating the burden of recurrent and chronic digital ulcers in systemic sclerosis: long-term results from the DUO Registry. Ann Rheum Dis. 2016;75(10):1770–6.
3. Lok C, Mouthon L, Ségard M, Richard M-A, Guillevin L. Les ulcères digitaux de la sclérodermie systémique. /data/revues/01519638/v138i11/S0151963811003620/ [Internet]. 2011 Nov 10 [cited 2017 Sep 7]; Available from: http://www.em-consulte.com/en/article/669717.
4. Mouthon L, Carpentier PH, Lok C, Clerson P, Gressin V, Hachulla E, et al. Ischemic digital ulcers affect hand disability and pain in systemic sclerosis. J Rheumatol. 2014;41(7):1317–23.
5. Ware JE, Gandek B, Kosinski M, Aaronson NK, Apolone G, Brazier J, et al. The equivalence of SF-36 summary health scores estimated using standard and country-specific algorithms in 10 countries: results from the IQOLA Project. International Quality of Life Assessment. J Clin Epidemiol. 1998;51(11):1167–70.
6. Hinchcliff ME, Beaumont JL, Carns MA, Podlusky S, Thavarajah K, Varga J, et al. Longitudinal evaluation of PROMIS-29 and FACIT-dyspnea short forms in systemic sclerosis. J Rheumatol. 2015;42(1):64–72.
7. Hinchcliff M, Beaumont JL, Thavarajah K, Varga J, Chung A, Podlusky S, et al. Validity of two new patient-reported outcome measures in systemic sclerosis: patient-reported outcomes measurement information system 29-item health profile and functional assessment of chronic illness therapy-dyspnea short form. Arthritis Care Res. 2011;63(11):1620–8.
8. Ramey DR, Raynauld JP, Fries JF. The health assessment questionnaire 1992: status and review. Arthritis Care Res. 1992;5(3):119–29.
9. Poole JL, Steen VD. The use of the health assessment questionnaire (HAQ) to determine physical disability in systemic sclerosis. Arthritis Care Res. 1991;4(1):27–31.
10. Steen VD, Medsger TA. The value of the health assessment questionnaire and special patient-generated scales to demonstrate change in systemic sclerosis patients over time. Arthritis Rheum. 1997;40(11):1984–91.
11. Georges C, Chassany O, Mouthon L, Tiev K, Toledano C, Meyer O, et al. Validation of French version of the scleroderma health assessment questionnaire (SSc HAQ). Clin Rheumatol. 2005;24(1):3–10.
12. Duruöz MT, Poiraudeau S, Fermanian J, Menkes CJ, Amor B, Dougados M, et al. Development and validation of a rheumatoid hand functional disability scale that assesses functional handicap. J Rheumatol. 1996;23(7):1167–72.
13. Brower LM, Poole JL. Reliability and validity of the Duruoz Hand Index in persons with systemic sclerosis (scleroderma). Arthritis Rheum. 2004;51(5):805–9.
14. Rannou F, Poiraudeau S, Berezné A, Baubet T, Le-Guern V, Cabane J, et al. Assessing disability and quality of life in systemic sclerosis: construct validities of the Cochin hand function scale, health assessment questionnaire (HAQ), systemic sclerosis HAQ, and medical outcomes study 36-item short form health survey. Arthritis Rheum. 2007;57(1):94–102.
15. Levis AW, Harel D, Kwakkenbos L, Carrier M-E, Mouthon L, Poiraudeau S, et al. Using optimal test assembly methods for shortening patient-reported outcome measures: development and validation of the Cochin hand function scale-6: a Scleroderma Patient-Centered Intervention Network Cohort Study. Arthritis Care Res. 2016;68(11):1704–13.
16. Sandqvist G, Eklund M. Validity of HAMIS: a test of hand mobility in scleroderma. Arthritis Care Res. 2000;13(6):382–7.
17. Keitel W, Hoffmann H, Weber G, Krieger U. Evaluation of the percentage of functional decrease of the joints using a motor function test in rheumatology. Dtsch Gesundheitsw. 1971;26(40):1901–3.
18. Kapandji A. Clinical test of apposition and counter-apposition of the thumb. Ann Chir Main. 1986;5(1):67–73.
19. Chung KC, Pillsbury MS, Walters MR, Hayward RA. Reliability and validity testing of the michigan hand outcomes questionnaire. J Hand Surg Am. 1998;23(4):575–87.
20. Schouffoer AA, van der Giesen FJ, Beaart-van de Voorde LJ, Wolterbeek R, Huizinga TW, Vliet Vlieland TP. Validity and responsiveness of the Michigan Hand Questionnaire in patients with systemic sclerosis. Rheumatology. 2016;55(8):1386–93.
21. Amanzi L, Braschi F, Fiori G, Galluccio F, Miniati I, Guiducci S, et al. Digital ulcers in scleroderma: staging, characteristics and subsetting through observation of 1614 digital lesions. Rheumatology (Oxford). 2010;49(7):1374–82.
22. Mouthon L, Mestre-Stanislas C, Bérezné A, Rannou F, Guilpain P, Revel M, et al. Impact of digital ulcers on disability and health-related quality of life in systemic sclerosis. Ann Rheum Dis. 2010;69(1):214–7.
23. Brand M, Hollaender R, Rosenberg D, Scott M, Hunsche E, Tyndall A, et al. An observational cohort study of patients with newly diagnosed digital ulcer disease secondary to systemic sclerosis registered in the EUSTAR database. Clin Exp Rheumatol. 2015;33(4 Suppl 91):S47–54.
24. Morell-Dubois S, Condette-Wojtasik G, Clerson P, Berezné A, Launay D, Lambert M, et al. Plaintes et besoins des patients atteints de sclérodermie systémique: une meilleure connaissance afin d'améliorer le suivi. /data/revues/02488663/v32i9/S0248866311000683/ [Internet]. 2011 Aug 31 [cited 2017 Sep 10]; Available from: http://www.em-consulte.com/en/article/536624.
25. Bérezné A, Seror R, Morell-Dubois S, de Menthon M, Fois E, Dzeing-Ella A, et al. Impact of systemic sclerosis on occupational and professional activity with attention to patients with digital ulcers. Arthritis Care Res. 2011;63(2):277–85.
26. Kwakkenbos L, Thombs BD, Khanna D, Carrier M-E, Baron M, Furst DE, et al. Performance of the patient-reported outcomes measurement information system-29 in scleroderma: a Scleroderma Patient-centered Intervention Network Cohort Study. Rheumatology. 2017;56(8):1302–11.
27. Nguyen C, Poiraudeau S, Mestre-Stanislas C, Rannou F, Bérezné A, Papelard A, et al. Employment status and socio-economic burden in systemic sclerosis: a cross-sectional survey. Rheumatology (Oxford). 2010;49(5):982–9.
28. Sandqvist G, Scheja A, Eklund M. Working ability in relation to disease severity, everyday occupations and well-being in women with limited systemic sclerosis. Rheumatology (Oxford). 2008;47(11):1708–11.
29. Cozzi F, Tiso F, Lopatriello S, Ciprian L, Sfriso P, Berto P, et al. The social costs of digital ulcer management in scledoma patients: an observational Italian pilot study. Joint Bone Spine. 2010;77(1):83–4.

Calcinosis

14

Francesca Bartoli, Laura Cometi,
and Marco Matucci-Cerinic

Definition

Calcinosis is a disorder characterized by deposition of calcium in the skin and subcutaneous tissues [1].

It is one of the typical manifestations of systemic sclerosis (SSc), especially in the limited cutaneous SSc (lcSSc) subtype, identified in 40% of patients and having a substantial impact on quality of life. Calcinosis is frequently associated with Raynaud's phenomenon, esophageal alterations, sclerodactyly, and telangiectasia configuring the CREST syndrome.

It most commonly involves the hands, particularly the fingers, and it is often associated with pain, recurrent episodes of local inflammation, and functional impairment [1].

Etiopathogenesis and Classification

Two general mechanisms of calcification in soft tissues have been described: metastatic calcification (deposition of calcium in normal cutaneous or subcutaneous tissue in the presence of elevated levels of serum calcium and/or phosphate) and dystrophic calcification (deposition of calcified material in diseased tissues, associated with normal serum calcium and phosphate levels). Calcinosis occurring in SSc can be considered a subtype of dystrophic calcification [1, 2].

The pathophysiology of calcinosis remains poorly understood; preliminary data suggest that digital vasculopathy, leading to insufficient blood flow and tissue hypoxia up to ischemia, may have a central role [3–6].

The alterations of some biomarkers such as osteonectin, parathyroid hormone, vitamin D, and calcitonin have been implicated in the pathophysiology of calcinosis. In fact, it was found a relationship between bone metabolism alteration and calcinosis [2]; two case reports showed successful use of bisphosphonates for the treatment of calcinosis in SSc patients, suggesting that impaired bone metabolism may play a role in the pathogenesis of calcinosis [7, 8]. Further research is needed to confirm the association between calcinosis and osteoporosis and to determine its implication in the development of targeted therapies.

To date, a universally used and broadly accepted classification of calcinosis is not available. A classification based on clinical (shape and consistency) features allows identification of two kinds of calcinosis: mousse (soft consistency and white, cream-like material) (Fig. 14.1) and stone (calcium deposits forming small, round, hard aggregates) (Figs. 14.2, 14.3 and 14.4). For these two types, X-ray is not needed for their identification. On the other hand, using X-ray, three kinds of calcinosis may be recognized: net (calcium deposits forming a network), plate (large uniform and flat agglomerate), and stone (calcium deposits forming small, round, hard aggregates) [8].

F. Bartoli (✉) · L. Cometi
Rheumatology Department, Azienda Ospedaliero – Universitaria Careggi, Florence, Italy

M. Matucci-Cerinic
Department of Experimental and Clinical Medicine, University of Florence, Florence, Italy

Department of Geriatric Medicine, Division of Rheumatology, AOUC, Florence, Italy

© Springer Nature Switzerland AG 2019
M. Matucci-Cerinic, C. P. Denton (eds.), *Atlas of Ulcers in Systemic Sclerosis*, https://doi.org/10.1007/978-3-319-98477-3_14

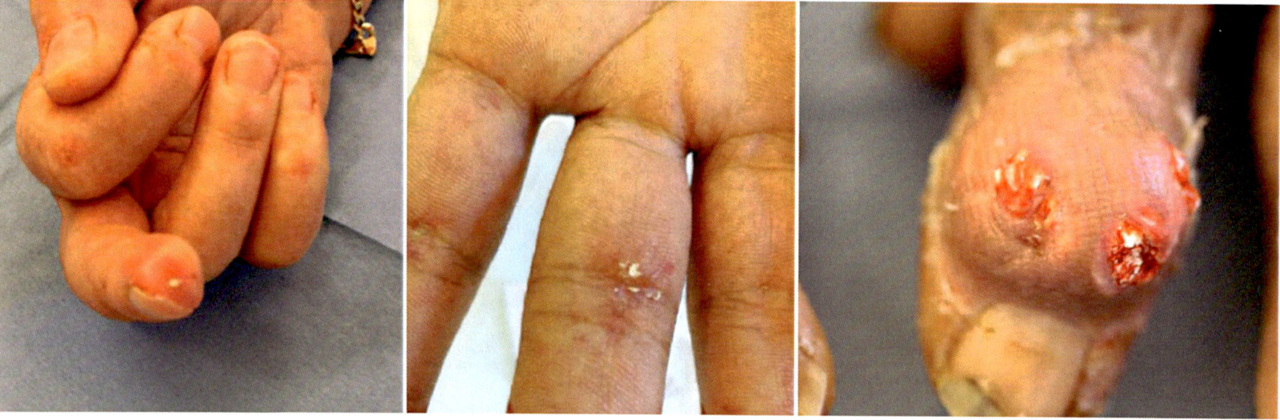

Fig. 14.1 Visible and palpable calcinosis on clinical examination: stone calcinosis of the finger

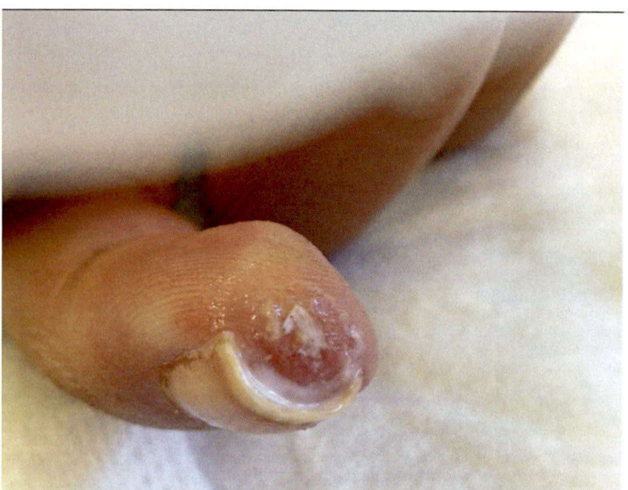

Fig. 14.2 Visible and palpable calcinosis on clinical examination: mousse calcinosis on the finger provoking an ulcer

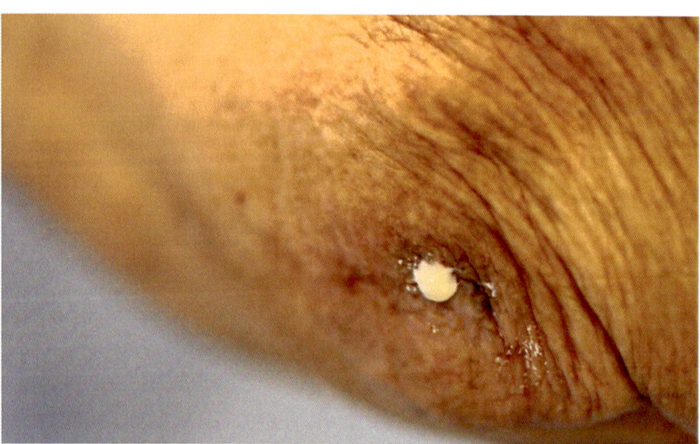

Fig. 14.3 Visible and palpable calcinosis on clinical examination: mousse calcinosis of the elbow

In collaboration with the Scleroderma Clinical Trials Consortium, Valenzuela et al. recently developed a novel radiographic scoring system for potential use in clinical trials.

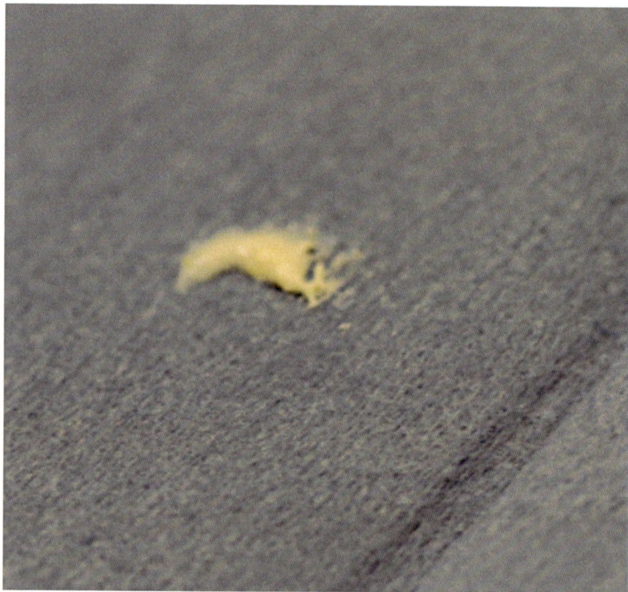

Fig. 14.4 Mousse calcinosis material

This scoring system provides an estimate of the calcinosis burden affecting the hands in patients with SSc, taking into account the area coverage, density, number, and anatomic location of calcinosis lesions, with excellent reliability [1].

Clinical and Laboratory Features

Calcinosis in patients with SSc is a late manifestation, most often occurring more than 7.5 years after the diagnosis. It typically involves the extremities such as hands and feet, particularly the fingers. It can be typically found on parts that have suffered micro-traumatisms, repetitive stress, or pressure such as the extension surfaces of elbows and buttocks. Calcinosis can inflame, infect, ulcerate, and drain white chalky material. When infected, calcium deposits become more painful and debilitating and require the use of antibiotics and surgical removal.

The study conducted by Valenzuela et al. demonstrated an association between calcinosis and digital ulcers, as well as other ischemic manifestations of SSc, as digital tip pitting scars, loss of digital pulp, nailfold capillary changes, and acro-osteolysis [1]. These findings were also confirmed in many other subsequent publications [6, 9–11].

Moreover, Morardet et al. suggested an association between calcinosis and late capillaroscopic pattern, demonstrating a significant reduction of the mean number of capillaries in patients with calcinosis [5].

Calcinosis in SSc has also been associated with male gender [3], long disease duration, anticentromere antibody (ACA) [12], anti-PM/Scl antibody [13], and anticardiolipin. The study of Baron et al. showed also an association with anti-RNA polymerase III and dcSSc, in contradistinction to the commonly held belief [9].

Cases of scleroderma patients suffering from calcinosis in uncommon parts, sometimes associated with exuberant symptomology, have been reported. In this case, the term of "tumoral calcinosis" has been used, despite this name does not refer the presence of neoplasm process [14–16].

Ulcers as Complication of Calcinosis

A frequent complication of calcinosis in SSc patients are skin ulcers, defined as lesions on the skin surface, produced by the sloughing of inflammatory necrotic tissue. The most common sites are the hands, followed by the knee, hip, upper arm, pretibial region, elbow, foot, wrist, and abdomen. It has been shown that ulcers develop mostly in 48.7% of the calcinotic areas [17] and that the time to healing is longer (93.64 days +/− 59.22 days) than in ischemic ulcers (76.2 +/−64 days) [18]. Usually the surrounding skin becomes edematous, with signs of inflammation and with jagged edges. Fibrin is usually absent, differently from the granulation tissue that is always present. Skin ulcers could be complicated by infection and fistulas, mainly on the hip, pretibial area, knees, and elbows [17]. A history of digital ulcers seems to be a significant independent predictor for radiographic progression of calcinosis [3].

Diagnosis

As yet reported, hand X-ray may be useful to detect subcutaneous calcinosis and to follow the progression [6, 19], while ultrasound seems not very sensitive. In fact, calcinosis is one of the most common findings observed on hand radiographs from SSc patients (23–33%).

To follow-up the progression of hand calcinosis, some scoring systems have been proposed. In the radiographic scoring system of Chung et al., the severity of calcinosis is assessed evaluating the area coverage, density, and anatomic location. This complex scoring system was feasible in a mean time of 4 min with excellent inter- and intra-rater reliability and performed better than a more simple scoring system [19].

CT scanning produces three-dimensional images which have the potential of measuring calcinosis "volume" and give a very visual demonstration of the extent of calcinosis [6].

Dual-energy computed tomography (DECT) imaging can be useful in the evaluation of scleroderma-related calcinosis of the hands [20].

Treatment

General measures to improve blood flow to the extremities, such as avoiding trauma, smoking, stress, and cold exposure, are of crucial importance. For the same reason, medical treatment of Raynaud's phenomenon and digital ulcers may play a role in prevention of calcinosis.

Supportive therapies such as antibiotics for infections, pain medications, and wound care are also a key [1].

Calcium channel blockers, diltiazem in particular, have been used most frequently for the medical treatment of calcinosis. By reducing the intracellular calcium influx in the affected tissues and local macrophages, diltiazem alters the formation and crystallization of calcium [1, 21]. Bisphosphonates may be useful in reversing the calcification process by inhibiting macrophage proinflammatory cytokine production and reducing bone resorption [1].

Although several studies suggest that low-dose warfarin may be effective for small calcinosis, evidence supporting the use of warfarin in calcinosis is conflicting [1, 21].

The use of intravenous immunoglobulin, due to its anti-inflammatory properties, is limited and has shown mixed results [1]. Regarding biologic therapies, rituximab and anti-TNF agents may be a promising therapy to treat calcinosis in patients with SSc [1, 22], although there are also some studies with conflicting results [23].

Finally colchicine and minocycline seem to be more effective in reducing the inflammation associated with calcinosis than the size of calcium deposits [1, 21].

Favorable results were obtained by local steroid injection at sites of calcinosis, although caution for local infection is needed [21].

Surgical resection and CO2 laser treatment may be useful options to reduce pain, relieve restriction of the range of joint motion, and prevent the occurrence of skin ulcers [21].

Conclusion

The presence of calcinosis, regardless of extension or severity, leads to morbidity and affects the life quality of patients suffering from scleroderma. Means to prevent or delay its occurrence have not yet been identified. The lack of sufficient clinical studies addressing scleroderma calcinosis and medical treatment is a major challenge for the clinician [11].

It is not uncommon that the fortuitous identification of subcutaneous calcium deposits occurs when image exams are requested for other purposes. Despite being difficult to treat and not always with evident results, the physician has to investigate for the presence of calcinosis.

References

1. Valenzuela A, Chung L. Calcinosis: pathophysiology and management. Curr Opin Rheumatol. 2015;27:542–8.
2. Valenzuela A, Baron M, Canadian Scleroderma Research Group, Herrick AL, et al. Calcinosis is associated with digital ulcers and osteoporosis in patients with systemic sclerosis: A Scleroderma Clinical Trials Consortium study. Semin Arthritis Rheum. 2016;46:344–9.
3. Avouac J, Mogavero G, Guerini H, Drapé JL, Mathieu A, Kahan A, Allanore Y. Predictive factors of hand radiographic lesions in systemic sclerosis: a prospective study. Ann Rheum Dis. 2011;70(4):630–3. https://doi.org/10.1136/ard.2010.134304. Epub 2010 Dec 3
4. Avouac J, Guerini H, Wipff J, Assous N, et al. Radiological hand involvement in systemic sclerosis. Ann Rheum Dis. 2006;65:1088–92.
5. Morardet L, Avouac J, Sammour M, Baron M, Kahan A, Feydy A, Allanore Y. Late nailfold videocapillaroscopy pattern associated with hand calcinosis and acro-osteolysis in systemic sclerosis. Arthritis Care Res (Hoboken). 2016;68(3):366–73. https://doi.org/10.1002/acr.22672.
6. Herrick AL, Gallas A. Systemic sclerosis-related calcinosis. J Scleroderma Relat Disord. 2016;1(2):194–203.
7. Rabens SF, Bethune JE. Disodium etidronate therapy for dystrophic cutaneous calcification. Arch Dermatol. 1975;111:357–61.
8. Fujii N, Hamano T, Isaka Y, Ito T, Imai E. Risedronate: a possible treatment for extraosseous calcification. Clin Calcium. 2005;15(Suppl.1):75–8.
9. Baron M, Pope J, Robinson D, Jones N, et al. Calcinosis is associated with digital ischaemia in systemic sclerosis—a longitudinal study. Rheumatology. 2016;55:2148–55.
10. Koutaissoff S, Vanthuyne M, Smith V, De Langhe E, Depresseux G, Westhovens R, De Keyser F, Malghem J, Houssiau FA. Hand radiological damage in systemic sclerosis: comparison with a control group and clinical and functional correlations. 2011; Elsevier Inc. Semin Arthritis Rheum 40:455–60.
11. Johnstone EM, Hutchinson CE, Vail A, Chevance A, Herrick AL. Acro-osteolysis in systemic sclerosis is associated with digital ischaemia and severe calcinosis. Rheumatology (Oxford). 2012;51(12):2234–8. https://doi.org/10.1093/rheumatology/kes214. Epub 2012 Aug 25
12. Steen VD, Ziegler GL, Rodnan GP, Medsger TA Jr. Clinical and laboratory associations of anticentromere antibody in patients with progressive systemic sclerosis. Arthritis Rheum. 1984;27(2):125–31.
13. D'Aoust J, Hudson M, Tatibouet S, Wick J, Canadian Scleroderma Research Group, Mahler M, Baron M, Fritzler MJ. Clinical and serologic correlates of anti-PM/Scl antibodies in systemic sclerosis: a multicenter study of 763 patients. Arthritis Rheumatol. 2014;66(6):1608–15. https://doi.org/10.1002/art.38428.
14. Daumas A, Rossi P, Ariey-Bonet D, Bernard F, Dussol B, Berbis P, Granel B. Generalized calcinosis in systemic sclerosis. Q J Med. 2014;107:219–21.
15. Onishi S, Homma Y, Hasegawa H, Yasukawa M. Multiple tumoral calcinosis in systemic sclerosis. Intern Med. 2013;52:2689.
16. Audemard A, Silva NM, Boutemy J, Maignè G, Bienvenu B. Tumoral calcinosis during the course of systemic sclerosis. J Rheumatol. 2015;42:348.
17. Bartoli F, Fiori G, Braschi F, Amanzi L, et al. Calcinosis in systemic sclerosis: subsets, distribution and complications. Rheumatology. 2016;55:1610–4.
18. Amanzi L, Braschi F, Fiori G, Galluccio F, et al. Digital ulcers in Scleroderma: staging, characteristics and sub-setting through observation of 1614 digital lesions. Rheumatology (Oxford). 2010;49:1374–82.
19. Chung L, Valenzuela A, Fiorentino D, Stevens K, et al. Validation of a novel radiographic scoring system for calcinosis affecting the hands of patients with systemic sclerosis. Arthritis Care Res (Hoboken). 2015;67(3):425–30.
20. Hsu V, Bramwit M, Schlesinger M. Dual-energy computed tomography for the evaluation of calcinosis in systemic sclerosis. J Rheumatol. 2015;42:2.
21. Fujimoto M, Asano Y, Ishii T, Ogawa F, et al. The wound/burn guidelines – 4: Guidelines for the management of skin ulcers associated with connective tissue disease/vasculitis. J Dermatol. 2016;43:729–57.
22. Tosounidou S, MacDonald H, Situnayake D. Successful treatment of calcinosis with infliximab in a patient with systemic sclerosis/myositis overlap syndrome. Rheumatology (Oxford). 2014;53(5):960–1.
23. Poormoghim H, Andalib E, Almasi AR, Hadibigi E. Systemic sclerosis and calcinosis cutis: response to rituximab. J Clin Pharm Ther. 2016;41:94–6.

Part V

General Approach to Digital Ulceration: Algorithm

Cosimo Bruni, Tiziana Pucci, Laura Rasero,
and Christopher P. Denton

Introduction

Digital ulcers (DU) are considered a major vascular complication in systemic sclerosis (SSc) and represent a clinical, social and economical burden for the patients, the clinicians and nurses and the health system. The field of DU is still matter of basic and clinical research since new vasodilating and vasoactive drugs are available [1, 2].

The Team

The DU management team is structured with a rheumatologist and a specialist nurse. A tight collaboration between these two figures is mandatory to cover all the features related to DUs. The clinician is responsible for identifying, after an overall evaluation of SSc, comorbidities and concomitant medications which might influence the development of DUs and the evolution of current lesions. The specialist nurse can evaluate the needs and priorities of the patient, schedule the frequency of visits to monitor the DU status and illustrate the possibility of social welfare facilities (such as transportation and local dressing services). She can also educate the patient to keep a correct lifestyle (smoking cessation, prevention of cold exposure, moisturizing) and stimulate his active participation in the care process. Using dedicated nutritional scale [3], a dietician can help to implement the quality of food intake to favour DU healing. To complete the team, an occupational therapist can educate the patient on movements and the use of tools to overcome disabilities and the difficulties related to the DU presence and to prevent further DU worsening.

How to Assess

When evaluating a patient with DU, it is mandatory to assess the number, location, pain of DU and the loss of hand function. The DU count mirrors the severity of peripheral vascular damage, providing an indirect and reliable measure of the severity of microvascular involvement. The number of DU may also be a predictor of the disease course [4]. Furthermore, it is important to distinguish between persistent and recurrent/new DU, guiding the clinician towards possible different therapeutic approaches. DU count and healing of the main ("cardinal") DU have been used as main outcomes in randomized clinical trials assessing the drug effect, but also pain, disability and functionality are being used as secondary outcome measures.

Pain

DUs are well known to be extremely painful and disabling, thus limiting the daily social and working life. For this reason, different scores and scales have been used in SSc patients with DU. One of the easiest outcome tool is the Visual Analogue Scale (VAS): it is a 10-cm-long line, with the left extremity meaning the lowest value and the right extremity representing the highest score possible. VAS scale can give a subjective evaluation of the chosen parameter, including pain related to DU, general health assessment, specific organ or symptom evaluation, and it can be patient- or clinician-oriented [5]. As it is a subjective assessment, the assessor should always be the same in the different visits.

C. Bruni (✉)
Department of Experimental and Clinical Medicine, Division of Rheumatology, University of Florence, Florence, Italy

T. Pucci
Department of Geriatric Medicine, Division of Rheumatology, AOUC, Florence, Italy

L. Rasero
Department of Health Sciences, University of Florence Careggi of Hospital, Florence, Tuscany, Italy

C. P. Denton
Division of Medicine, University College London, Centre for Rheumatology, Royal Free Hospital, London, UK

© Springer Nature Switzerland AG 2019
M. Matucci-Cerinic, C. P. Denton (eds.), *Atlas of Ulcers in Systemic Sclerosis*, https://doi.org/10.1007/978-3-319-98477-3_15

Moreover, there can even be a significant discrepancy between the clinician and the patient assessment on the same measurement.

Global Disability Scales

From a patient-oriented perspective, many scales have been developed to assess global and hand-specific disabilities that have been validated for scleroderma patients. The standard Health Assessment Questionnaire Disability Index (HAQ-DI) is a multisystem self-reported questionnaire assessing eight different domains of daily activities: dressing/grooming, arising, eating, walking, hygiene, reaching, gripping and other activities. Each item inside every domain is scored 0–3, with higher values meaning maximal disability. HAQ-DI showed a good performance in evaluating functional status in patients with scleroderma, despite the presence of digital ulcers, in many studies [6]. A non-validated HAQ shortened version (also called Hand Function Index, HFI) also exists, mainly focussed on hand function, which showed improvement in a clinical study on the treatment of digital ulcers, but it was only done as a post hoc analysis [7]. More recently, variation in both the HAQ and HFI showed association with changes in the DU status, when analysed as a post hoc evaluation of two randomized clinical trials [8]. As an evolution of the HAQ score, Steen et al. added patient self-reported VAS on pain, patient general disease assessment, vascular features including Raynaud's, digital ulcers assessment, lung involvement and gastrointestinal involvement evaluation. This may reflect also the major organ involvement which frequently characterize SSc. The implemented HAQ, called Scleroderma HAQ or SHAQ [9], showed reliability and validity in evaluating SSc patients. The UK scleroderma functional score (UKFS) was also previously validated, showing a cross-sectional correlation with HAQ-DI, with the SHAQ and with clinical/laboratory markers of disease severity in SSc [10]. More recently, the UKFS has also been demonstrated to reflect disease worsening or improvement longitudinally, including DU evolution [11].

Hand Disability Scales

Other scales have been developed that are completely focussed on hand function and that have been used to monitor SSc patients with DU:

- Cochin hand function scale (CHFS or Duruoz Hand Index) [12] is an 18-question scale, with each item ranging from 0 to 5 according to maximal disability, with a total score from 0 to 90. The CHFS was initially created for rheumatoid arthritis (RA) and only subsequently validated also for SSc [13]. It reflects higher disability and stronger impact on occupational performance in SSc patients with DU [14].

- The Michigan Hand Questionnaire (MHQ) is centred on hand function investigating six different aspects: overall hand functionality, activities of daily living, pain, performance at work, aesthetics and satisfaction on pain according to hand function. This is another scale previously validated for RA, which showed to be influenced also by DU in SSc patients [15].

- The Hand Disability in SSc-Digital Ulcer (HDISS-DU) is the most recently developed tool to assess DU in SSc. It represents a reviewed version of the CHFS including 26 items administered to patients and was reported to be comprehensive, therefore suitable of being used for future validation studies [16].

The various clinical outcome measures currently available have shown to correlate one to each other, reflecting the DU-related disability in SSc patients [17]. As a limitation, all these tools are patient-oriented, being influenced by subjectivity. Therefore, the need for objective outcome measure remains still unmet [18]. Two recent publications have proposed new scoring systems to assess DU. Ahrens et al. published a severity score based on depth and diameter of both hyperkeratosis and ulcers, showing the ability to reflect changes in time [19], while Bruni et al. proposed the DUCAS, a composite clinical score based on DU number and new appearance, taking into consideration all the possible complications related to the presence of DU (from infection to amputation) [20]. Both scores are currently presented with preliminary results, thus further studies will be necessary for their complete and formal validation.

Future Perspectives

From both epidemiological and clinical points of view, the development of a clinical objective DU evaluation scale or assessment method is of pivotal importance. These scales are a useful tool for the clinician in clinical practice, allowing a follow-up focussed on DU burden. At the same time, it could be a fundamental item in randomized clinical trials, especially those built for the evaluation of disease-modifying drugs and for treatments acting directly on DUs.

The Team and the Assessment of DU

1. A multidisciplinary team is needed to evaluate DU, including physicians, nurses, dieticians and physiotherapists
2. DU count, appearance of new DU, together with disability and functionality scales, and pain evaluation are the most frequently used measures to assess DU
3. Composite scores to evaluate evolution in time and severity of DU are needed in future clinical practice and to be used as outcome measures in randomized clinical trial

References

1. Wigley FM, Seibold JR, Wise RA, McCloskey DA, Dole WP. Intravenous iloprost treatment of Raynaud's phenomenon and ischemic ulcers secondary to systemic sclerosis. J Rheumatol. 1992;19(9):1407–14.
2. Matucci-Cerinic M, Denton CP, Furst DE, Mayes MD, Hsu VM, Carpentier P, et al. Bosentan treatment of digital ulcers related to systemic sclerosis: results from the RAPIDS-2 randomised, double-blind, placebo-controlled trial. Ann Rheum Dis. 2011;70(1):32–8.
3. Malnutrition Universal Screening Tool BAPEN, registered no: 1023927. First published May 2004 by the Malnutrition Advisory Group, a Standing Committee of BAPEN. Reviewed and reprinted March 2008 and September 2010. British Dietetic Association, the Royal College of Nursing and the Registered Nursing Home Association. Available on: www.bapen.org.uk.
4. Steen V, Denton CP, Pope JE, Matucci-Cerinic M. Digital ulcers: overt vascular disease in systemic sclerosis. Rheumatology (Oxford). 2009;48(Suppl 3):iii19–24. https://doi.org/10.1093/rheumatology/kep105. Review
5. Pope J. Measures of systemic sclerosis (scleroderma): Health Assessment Questionnaire (HAQ) and Scleroderma HAQ (SHAQ), physician- and patient-rated global assessments, Symptom Burden Index (SBI), University of California, Los Angeles, Scleroderma Clinical Trials Consortium Gastrointestinal Scale (UCLA SCTC GIT) 2.0, Baseline Dyspnea Index (BDI) and Transition Dyspnea Index (TDI) (Mahler's Index), Cambridge Pulmonary Hypertension Outcome Review (CAMPHOR), and Raynaud's Condition Score (RCS). Arthritis Care Res (Hoboken). 2011;63 Suppl 11:S98–111.
6. Merkel PA, Herlyn K, Martin RW, Anderson JJ, Mayes MD, Bell P, et al. Measuring disease activity and functional status in patients with scleroderma and Raynaud's phenomenon. Arthritis Rheum. 2002;46(9):2410–20.
7. Korn JH, Mayes M, Matucci Cerinic M, Rainisio M, Pope J, Hachulla E, et al. Digital ulcers in systemic sclerosis: prevention by treatment with bosentan, an oral endothelin receptor antagonist. Arthritis Rheum. 2004;50(12):3985–93.
8. Zelenietz C, Pope J. Differences in disability as measured by the Health Assessment Questionnaire between patients with and without digital ulcers in systemic sclerosis: a post hoc analysis of pooled data from two randomized controlled trials in digital ulcers using bosentan. Ann Rheum Dis. 2010;69(11):2055–6.
9. Steen VD, Medsger TA Jr. The value of the Health Assessment Questionnaire and special patient-generated scales to demonstrate change in systemic sclerosis patients over time. Arthritis Rheum. 1997;40(11):1984–91.
10. Smyth AE, MacGregor AJ, Mukerjee D, Brough GM, Black CM, Denton CP. A cross- sectional comparison of three self-reported functional indices in scleroderma. Rheumatology. 2003;42:732–8.
11. Serednicka K, Smyth AE, Black CM, Denton CP. Using a self-reported functional score to assess disease progression in systemic sclerosis. Rheumatology (Oxford). 2007;46(7):1107–10.
12. Duruöz MT, Poiraudeau S, Fermanian J, Menkes CJ, Amor B, Dougados M, et al. Development and validation of a rheumatoid hand functional disability scale that assesses functional handicap. J Rheumatol. 1996;23(7):1167–72.
13. Brower LM, Poole JL. Reliability and validity of the Duruoz Hand Index in persons with systemic sclerosis (scleroderma). Arthritis Rheum. 2004;51(5):805–9. Erratum in: Arthritis Rheum. 2005;53(2):303
14. Mouthon L, Mestre-Stanislas C, Bérezné A, Rannou F, Guilpain P, Revel M, et al. Impact of digital ulcers on disability and health-related quality of life in systemic sclerosis. Ann Rheum Dis. 2010;69(1):214–7.
15. Impens AJ, Chung KC, Buck MH, Schiopu E, Kotsis S, Burns P, et al. Influences of clinical features of systemic sclerosis (Ssc) on the Michigan Hand Questionnaire (MHQ). [abstract]. Arthritis Rheum. 2006;54(Suppl,9):S483.
16. Khanna D, Poiraudeau S, Gelhom H, Hunsche E, Papadakis K, Perchenet L, et al. Development and content validity of the Hand Disability in systemic sclerosis Digital ulcers (HDISS-SU) scale. [abstract]. Arthritis Rheum. 2011;63 Suppl 10:1863.
17. Ingegnoli F, Boracchi P, Ambrogi F, Meroni PL. Comparative analysis of different specific indices of hand impairment in systemic sclerosis. J Rheumatol. 2010;37(10):2192–3.
18. Matucci-Cerinic M, Seibold JR. Digital ulcers and outcomes assessment in scleroderma. Rheumatology (Oxford). 2008;47 Suppl 5:v46–7.
19. Ahrens HC, Siegert E, Tomsitz D, Mattat K, March C, Worm M, et al. Digital ulcers score: a scoring system to assess digital ulcers in patients suffering from systemic sclerosis. Clin Exp Rheumatol. 2016;34 Suppl 100(5):142–7.
20. Bruni C, Ngcozana T, Braschi F, Piemonte G, Benelli L, Guiducci S, et al. The Ducas: proposal for a digital ulcer assessment score in scleroderma. [abtract]. Arthritis Rheumatol. 2016;68(suppl 10)

Diagnostic Tools

16

Yannick Allanore

Despite the widespread prevalence of Raynaud's phenomenon, standardized diagnostic criteria have not been thoroughly established [1]. A recent attempt has provided a preliminary set of classification criteria that will need further validation [2]. Raynaud's phenomenon is clinically defined, and there is no tool to use to confirm the vasospastic process. However, when identified, there might be a need for investigations when a secondary Raynaud's is suspected, the main criteria being the late onset (over 40 years), tissular damages (digital ulcer), presence of sign or symptom of an associated disease (mainly connective tissue disease), asymmetrical attacks and abnormality of pulses, and laboratory findings evocative of an etiology (antinuclear antibodies, hematological disorder, or atherosclerosis risk factors).

Prevalence of Severe Peripheral Vasculopathy in SSc

In the EUSTAR cohort, a recent report identified that 36% of the patients ever had DU and 17% had active ongoing ulceration at inclusion [3]. There are less data about critical ischemia and escalation to gangrene. Of the 2080 Pittsburgh SSc patients, 32% ($n = 666$) of all patients with SSc have had persistent DUs, and overall 11% of the SSc patients had undergone amputation or experienced gangrene [4]. In the RAPIDS-2 trial, conducted in 188 patients with active DUs, 11% experienced amputation (1–2% per patient-year of follow-up) [5]. In a retrospective cohort of 1168 British patients with SSc, 12% of the cohort required hospital admissions for treatment with intravenous therapies for severe vasculopathy. Of the 194 patients, 184 had finger ulcers, and 18 had toe ulcers (16% and 1.5% of the SSc cohort, respectively). Furthermore, 19 patients (2%) developed critical digital

ischaemia, and 16 (1.4%) developed digital gangrene [6]. An Italian study has reported that 9 out of 188 patients (5%) underwent partial or total surgical digital amputation because of necrotic process [7]. The DU Outcomes (DUO) Registry is a European, prospective, multicenter, observational cohort of patients with SSc and past and/or current DUs at enrolment. Among the 4944 patients enrolled in the DUO Registry from April 2008 to November 2014, 4642 had information recorded on their gangrene status: 81.6% ($n = 3787$) were categorized as "never gangrene," 18.4% ($n = 855$) as "ever gangrene," and 5.6% ($n = 258$) as "current gangrene" [8].

These data show that critical ischemia leading to gangrene is not common and seems to occur in 1–5% of patients according to the series and that digits are far more frequently affected than the toes.

Risk Factors for Critical Ischemia in SSC-Raynaud

In the Italian study cited above, all patients who required surgery for vasculopathy had concomitant large vessel involvement. Comparison of cases with and without digital amputation showed that this complication was associated with older age, long history of RP, long disease duration, presence of anti-centromere antibody, and coexistence of peripheral artery disease and hypercholesterolemia [7]. This raises the question of SSc-Raynaud's patients having the highest risk of DU and of critical ischemia. The above suggested higher risk for SSc patients with classical cardiovascular risk is supported by few additional studies. Indeed, among patients with SSc, current smokers are three to four times more likely than never smokers to incur digital vascular complications. After adjusting for age, sex, and disease duration, current smokers were significantly more likely than never smokers to have had debridement (OR 4.5, 95% CI 1.1–18.3) or admission for IV vasodilators (OR 3.8, 95% CI 1.1–12.9). Patients smoking at higher intensity were more likely to require admission for

Y. Allanore
Service de Rhumatologie A, Hôpital Cochin, Paris, France
e-mail: yannick.allanore@aphp.fr

© Springer Nature Switzerland AG 2019
M. Matucci-Cerinic, C. P. Denton (eds.), *Atlas of Ulcers in Systemic Sclerosis*, https://doi.org/10.1007/978-3-319-98477-3_16

IV vasodilators [9]. These findings are supported by another report showing that smoking had a strong negative effect on vascular outcomes in SSc, although severe vascular damages such as gangrene were not evaluated [10]. Other potential risk factors for severe vascular damages are the presence of anti-centromere antibodies [11] or the overlap between SSc micro-angiopathy and cryoglobulinemic vasculitis [12].

In the DUO Registry analyses, 3809 patients were eligible for inclusion in the longitudinal part. On multivariate analyses, being a current/former smoker, having ≥3 finger DUs, previous gangrene and previous upper limb sympathectomy were independent risk factors at enrolment for the development of incident gangrene [8].

Although more data are needed before drawing any conclusion, large vessel vasculopathy and classical cardiovascular risk factors seem to increase the risk of critical ischemia and gangrene in SSc-Raynaud suggesting that SSc-Raynaud's patients with these conditions must be followed up more accurately and may need specific examinations.

Work-Up of Raynaud's Phenomenon

As stated above, the diagnosis of Raynaud's phenomenon is clinical and does not require systematic specific tests for the identification of the syndrome. Investigations are required (i) to classify RP in primary versus secondary and (ii) when DUs are severe and recurrent and/or when vessel obstruction is suspected, investigations are indicated.

One of the main clinical finding evocative of vessel obstruction or compression is the *unilateral presentation* of the symptoms. Indeed, unilateral Raynaud's phenomenon or an asymmetric expression must always lead to vascular investigations looking at large vessel obstruction. In some other than SSc systemic disease such as vasculitis, Buerger's disease, Takayasu, or antiphospholipid syndromes, Raynaud's phenomenon can be present and vascular investigations required because of critical ischemia. Unilateral Raynaud's phenomenon first suggests an arterial lesion or compression and can be favored by some occupational injury. Unilateral Raynaud's phenomenon must lead to performed vascular tests to establish the cause in addition to vascular examination (artery pressures, ankle/brachial index) and imaging including first vascular Doppler ultrasound. Arterial damages can be due to mechanical factors or background inflammatory disease (vasculitis). Hypothenar hammer syndrome is related to dysplasia of the ulnar artery anterior to the superficial palmar arch. Vibration injury can occur in workers (jackhammers, chisels, rivet presses, drills, compacters, chain saws, buffers, or sanders). Thoracic outlet syndrome, which manifests chiefly as pain and neurological symptoms, is associated with Raynaud's phenomenon in about half of the cases. When the diagnosis is suspected, cervical spine and clavicle imaging

(X-ray, CT scan) should be performed to look for a cervical rib or elongated transverse process.

In the context of SSc, there is no recommendation for the performance of vascular imaging, but taking into account the above data, it can be suggested that recurrent DU and mainly critical ischemia and gangrene, in particular when classical cardiovascular risks are present, should lead to the evaluation of large vessels first by Doppler ultrasound.

The first vascular investigation is indeed usually Doppler ultrasound because it is simple, not expensive, and noninvasive. Color Doppler produces a picture of the artery that shows different flow rates allowing the identification with good sensitivities and specificities of vessel obstruction. Another advantage of this technique is the possibility to perform dynamic tests. They are of particular importance in the thoracic outlet syndrome resulting from excess pressure placed on a neurovascular bundle passing between the scalene muscles, and that can generate severe arterial consequences. Limitations of Doppler ultrasound include sequential stenosis and difficulty in imaging the inflow arteries.

Beyond the assessment of the whole vascular tree, power Doppler ultrasonography has been recently used to evaluate radial and ulnar artery to compare blood flow velocity, resistive indices, and presence of occlusion in unselected patients. A first study included a total of 79 SSc patients and 40 healthy controls. Overall, radial and ulnar arteries showed altered velocities and high resistive indices higher in SSc patients compared with controls. Seventeen (21.5%) SSc patients had ulnar artery occlusion (11 patients bilateral) compared with none in the control subjects [13]. At baseline, there was no association between ulnar artery occlusion and digital ulcers, but during follow-up, new or recurrent DU occurred more often in patients with ulnar artery occlusion as compared to unaffected SSc patients [14/28 (50%) vs 24/113 (21%); relative risk = 2.4; 95% CI 1.4, 3.7; $P = 0.002$]. Another study included 55 SSc patients and 19 controls. The prevalence of ulnar artery occlusion was 36%. A total of 56% of SSc patients had a pathologic finger pulp blood flow. Both parameters were associated with a history of multiple DU episodes and the occurrence of new DUs during the follow-up [14]. Power Doppler ultrasonography could be used as prognostic factors and considered in further studies evaluating DU treatment strategies. However, some other studies did not identify any association between Doppler ultrasound and digital ulcers in unselected patients [15].

Both in unilateral Raynaud's and in severe bilateral presentation leading to critical ischemia or gangrene, Doppler ultrasound is the first investigation to perform. Thereafter, if it does not provide evidence for a cause, angiography, magnetic resonance imaging, and angio-computed tomography need to be discussed. In unselected patients, preliminary studies have raised some interest in power Doppler ultrasound to identify ulnar artery occlusion and to predict recurrent DU.

Angiography

When a causal lesion is suspected and when vascular damages are severe and might suggest large vessel narrowing, angiography can be required in Raynaud and mainly in SSc-Raynaud. However, different techniques are available.

Arteriography remains the most accurate and informative test and is therefore the criterion standard, although it is an invasive diagnostic method. This examination can be associated with complications such as hematoma at the puncture site or arterial wall rupture, those due to radiation exposure and nephrotoxicity due to the intravenous contrast material. If some old studies have reported in RP magnification hand angiography and cold exposure with pharmacodynamic tests, the diagnostic and predictive value of such examination has never been demonstrated, and this contrasts with the potential serious adverse events [16]. Indeed, in series of 103 patients suffering from bilateral Raynaud's phenomenon without any obvious underlying disease and who were unresponsive to nifedipine and aspirin, standardized angiograms showed vasculopathy compatible with primary vasospasm in 42 patients and atherosclerotic vascular disease in 44 patients, but these data were not correlated with the outcomes of the patients [17]. Therefore, arteriography is not anymore used in Raynaud's assessment but preserved for severe cases and mostly within the context of preoperative evaluation. Indeed, patients with SSc and severe RP characterized by refractory digital ulcerations have been investigated for large artery involvement and related endovascular therapy [18]. In a retrospective series of 15 patients, all having a positive Allen test and ulnar artery occlusive disease documented by angiography 8/15 underwent ulnar artery revascularization combined with digital sympathectomy, and all 8 experienced major improvement in RP and healing of digital ulcers [18]. Although retrospective and uncontrolled, this study suggests that in case of occlusion, ulnar artery revascularization with or without digital sympathectomy can be considered in patients who failed conventional medical therapy. A classification of the damages observed in refractory RP patients has been proposed [19]. It suggested to stratify the patients as follows: Types I and II involve the radial or ulnar arteries (Type I with complete occlusion, while Type II involved partial occlusion); Type IIIa showed tortuous, narrowed, or stenosed common and digital vessels, and Type IIIb is a subset which involved the digital vessel of the index finger related to exposure to prolonged vibration; and Types IV and V showed global involvement from the main to digital vessels (Type IV showed diffused tortuosity, narrowing, and stenosis, and Type V is the most severe, with paucity of vessels and very scant flow) [19].

Several noninvasive techniques for evaluating perfusion of hand and wrist arteries have been introduced into clinical practice. Recently, *magnetic resonance angiography* (MRA) has been used with and without contrast material as a safe, reliable, and accurate technique for evaluation of vascular pathologies of the hand. However, conversely to the data reported for arteriography, all the subsequent studies used angiography in less selected patients and mainly not in the context of critical ischemia. Therefore, angiography conversely to arteriography was not performed as a preoperative test. Indeed, our group utilized MRA of the hand with a phased array wrist coil at 1.5 T with the following protocol (Fig. 16.1): 2mMol/kg gadolinium injected intravenously, and 30 s later four successive coronal 3D gradient echo sequences (TR = 8.4 msec, TE = 3 msec) of 52 s each were acquired. The maximum intensity projection (MIP) reformatting technique was then used to deliver four successive coronal views of the whole volume. The primary second to fifth fingers predefined criteria were [20]:

- Quality of arterial opacification with stop site (metacarpophalangeal joint for the common digital arteries, proximal phalanx, middle phalanx, or distal phalanx for the proper digital arteries) and caliber (normal or reduced)
- Quality of venous flux (same sites as for arteries)
- Presence of tissular blockage and avascular areas on the more delayed sequence

In a series of 38 consecutive and unselected SSc patients, 35 (92%) patients had at least 1 true digital artery which did not reach the first phalanx, as assessed at the initial arterial analysis, and 23 (61%) had 4 or more damaged arteries. Twenty-eight (74%) patients had thin arteries, and 23 (61%) had more than 1 avascular area. Current digital ulcers were substantially more frequent among SSc patients with more than four proper digital arteries which did not reach the first phalanx than other patients (10/23 vs 0/15; $p = 0.003$). All the patients had abnormal venous flux, and general venous blockage was found in 12 patients (32%) [20]. The main findings of this study are the substantial arterial and venous damage detected by MRA in patients with systemic sclerosis, and examples are provided in Fig. 16.1. Our study emphasizes that both the microcirculation and also small caliber vessels are involved in SSc as shown by previous studies using angiography. However, MRA has a major advantage over arteriography in that it is a noninvasive examination and image quality is comparable to that of conventional angiography without risk of induced vasospasm. This technique can be used for repeated examinations allow-

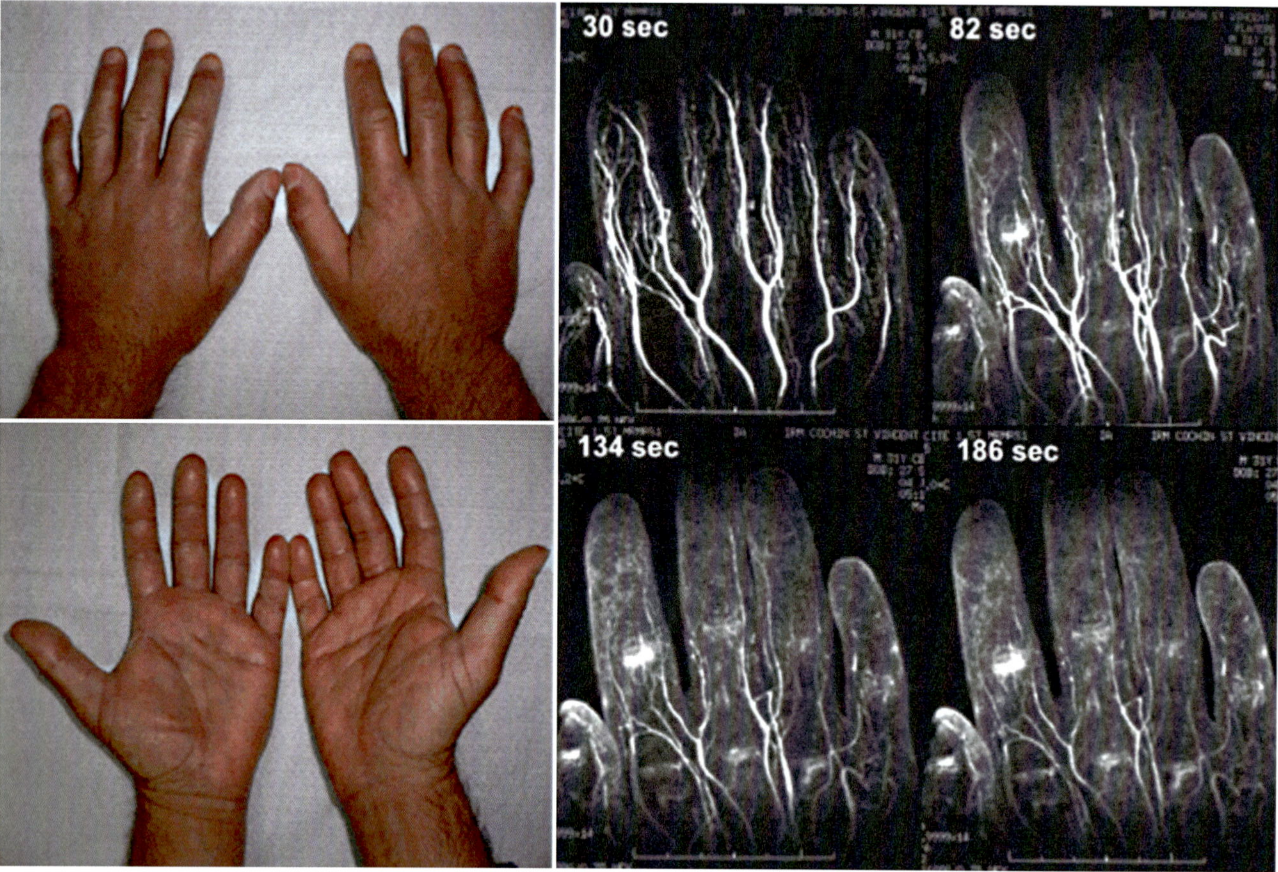

Fig. 16.1 Hand pictures of a patient with early diffuse cutaneous SSc together with successive magnetic resonance angiography images. Representative images of the successive acquisition at 52 s intervals, starting with arterial filling, tissular enhancement, and then venous return

ing comparisons. However, its ability to detect changes in SSc patients should now be tested to determine whether it has value as an outcome measure for vascular therapies and predictive value for clinical outcomes. Non-enhanced magnetic resonance imaging has been investigated in a pilot study of six SSc patients and six controls and showed similar qualitative and semiquantitative findings as compared to the contrast-enhanced MR [21]. However, it must be emphasized that the non-enhanced technique requires long imaging time owing to electrocardiographic triggering and conversely, the contrast-enhanced method offers the ability to acquire time-resolved images that show blood flow dynamics. MRA is noninvasive and does not require the use of ionizing radiation, and the contrast agent used, if any, is relatively non-nephrotoxic. The limitations are as follows: its cost, its availability, the limited depiction of small vessels, MRI contraindications, and the possible overestimation of the degree of stenosis. Furthermore, both techniques were not compared in the context of Raynaud's and SSc to the reference standard digital subtraction angiography limiting the possibility to make firm conclusions. High-resolution

three-dimensional time-of-flight (3D-TOF) MRA at three Tesla has also been used for the visualization of digital arteries in SSc patients. In a controlled series of 33 patients with SSc, some vessel lumen obstruction could be identified, but the technique mainly appeared as feasible with a good presentation rate of all digital arteries [22]. It is a promising method such as the above stated for judging the severity of microvascular involvement in finger vessels of SSc patients. Scoring system and patient prospective follow-up are now required to look for correlation with clinical events.

When damages are very severe according to Doppler ultrasound, arteriography or angiography might be considered mainly when a revascularization is envisaged. The strategy might be to use first MR angiography because it is noninvasive, but when revascularization is confirmed, arteriography might be required and used to perform revascularization. The development of noninvasive methods might lead to the use of this tool to risk-stratify SSc patients in the future and even guide therapy, but more work is indeed expected in this avenue.

Conclusion

Raynaud's phenomenon relates to microcirculation impairment. In the very large majority of cases, vascular imaging is unnecessary, and very often even no test is required in front of Raynaud's phenomenon. However, when Raynaud's phenomenon is unilateral or when it leads to very severe damages, mainly in the context of SSc, some tests might be indicated. Apart from detailed clinical examination, Doppler ultrasound will be the first-line tool to evaluate large vessel compression or endovascular damages. However, more accurate tests like arteriography or MR angiography can be indicated to narrow the lesion and support any decision regarding revascularization. However, these cases are very rare, and if endovascular procedures might be envisaged, very trained multidisciplinary teams should be queried.

References

1. Matucci-Cerinic M, Kahaleh B, Wigley FM. Review: evidence that systemic sclerosis is a vascular disease. Arthritis Rheum. 2013;65(8):1953–62.
2. Maverakis E, Patel F, Kronenberg DG, Chung L, Fiorentino D, Allanore Y, Guiducci S, Hesselstrand R, Hummers LK, Duong C, Kahaleh B, Macgregor A, Matucci-Cerinic M, Wollheim FA, Mayes MD, Gershwin ME. International consensus criteria for the diagnosis of Raynaud's phenomenon. J Autoimmun. 2014;48–49:60–5.
3. Meier FM, Frommer KW, Dinser R, Walker UA, Czirjak L, Denton CP, Allanore Y, Distler O, Riemekasten G, Valentini G, Müller-Ladner U, EUSTAR Co-authors. Update on the profile of the EUSTAR cohort: an analysis of the EULAR Scleroderma Trials and Research group database. Ann Rheum Dis. 2012;71(8):1355–60.
4. Steen V, Denton CP, Pope JE, Matucci-Cerinic M. Digital ulcers: overt vascular disease in systemic sclerosis. Rheumatology (Oxford). 2009;48 Suppl 3:iii19–24.
5. Korn JH, Mayes M, Matucci Cerinic M, Rainisio M, Pope J, Hachulla E, Rich E, Carpentier P, Molitor J, Seibold JR, Hsu V, Guillevin L, Chatterjee S, Peter HH, Coppock J, Herrick A, Merkel PA, Simms R, Denton CP, Furst D, Nguyen N, Gaitonde M, Black C. Digital ulcers in systemic sclerosis: prevention by treatment with bosentan, an oral endothelin receptor antagonist. Arthritis Rheum. 2004;50(12):3985–93.
6. Nihtyanova SI, Brough GM, Black CM, Denton CP. Clinical burden of digital vasculopathy in limited and diffuse cutaneous systemic sclerosis. Ann Rheum Dis. 2008;67:120–3.
7. Caramaschi P, Biasi D, Caimmi C, Barausse G, Sabbagh D, Tinazzi I, LA Verde V, Tonetta S, Adami S. Digital amputation in systemic sclerosis: prevalence and clinical associations. A retrospective longitudinal study. Rheumatology. 2012;39(8):1648–53.
8. Allanore Y, Denton CP, Krieg T, Cornelisse P, Rosenberg D, Schwierin B, Matucci-Cerinic M, DUO Investigators. Clinical characteristics and predictors of gangrene in patients with systemic sclerosis and digital ulcers in the Digital Ulcer Outcome Registry: a prospective, observational cohort. Ann Rheum Dis. 2016;75(9):1736–40.
9. Harrison BJ, Silman AJ, Hider SL, Herrick AL. Cigarette smoking as a significant risk factor for digital vascular disease in patients with systemic sclerosis. Arthritis Rheum. 2002;46(12):3312–6.
10. Hudson M, Lo E, Baron M, Steele R, Canadian Scleroderma Research Group. Modeling smoking in systemic sclerosis: a comparison of different statistical approaches. Arthritis Care Res (Hoboken). 2011;63(4):570–8.
11. Takahashi M, Okada J, Kondo H. Six cases positive for anti-centromere antibodies with ulcer and gangrene in the extremities. Br J Rheumatol. 1997;36(8):889–93.
12. Giuggioli D, Manfredi A, Colaci M, Manzini CU, Antonelli A, Ferri C. Systemic sclerosis and cryoglobulinemia: our experience with overlapping syndrome of scleroderma and severe cryoglobulinemic vasculitis and review of the literature. Autoimmun Rev. 2013;12(11):1058–63.
13. Frerix M, Stegbauer J, Dragun D, Kreuter A, Weiner SM. Ulnar artery occlusion is predictive of digital ulcers in SSc: a duplex sonography study. Rheumatology (Oxford). 2012;51(4):735–42.
14. Lescoat A, Coiffier G, Rouil A, Droitcourt C, Cazalets C, de Carlan M, Perdriger A, Jégo P. Vascular evaluation of the hand by power doppler ultrasonography and new predictive markers of ischemic digital ulcers in systemic sclerosis: results of a prospective pilot study. Arthritis Care Res (Hoboken). 2017;69(4):543–51.
15. Rosato E, Gigante A, Barbano B, Cianci R, Molinaro I, Pisarri S, Salsano F. In systemic sclerosis macrovascular damage of hands digital arteries correlates with microvascular damage. Microvasc Res. 2011 Nov;82(3):410–5.
16. Rösch J, Porter JM. Hand angiography and Raynaud's syndrome. Rofo. 1977;127(1):30–7.
17. van Vugt RM, Kater L, Dijkstra PF, Schardijn GH, Kastelein JJ, Bijlsma JW. The outcome of angiography in patients with Raynaud's phenomenon: an unexpected role for atherosclerosis and hypercholesterolemia. Clin Exp Rheumatol. 2003;21(4):445–50.
18. Taylor MH, McFadden JA, Bolster MB, Silver RM. Ulnar artery involvement in systemic sclerosis (scleroderma). J Rheumatol. 2002;29(1):102–6.
19. Kim YH, Ng SW, Seo HS, Chang AH. Classification of Raynaud's disease based on angiographic features. J Plast Reconstr Aesthet Surg. 2011;64(11):1503–11.
20. Allanore Y, Seror R, Chevrot A, Kahan A, Drapé JL. Hand vascular involvement assessed by magnetic resonance angiography in systemic sclerosis. Arthritis Rheum. 2007;56(8):2747–54.
21. Sheehan JJ, Fan Z, Davarpanah AH, Hodnett PA, Varga J, Carr JC, Li D. Nonenhanced MR angiography of the hand with flow-sensitive dephasing-prepared balanced SSFP sequence: initial experience with systemic sclerosis. Radiology. 2011;259(1):248–56.
22. Zhang W, Xu JR, Lu Q, Ye S, Liu XS. High-resolution magnetic resonance angiography of digital arteries in SSc patients on 3 Tesla: preliminary study. Rheumatology (Oxford). 2011;50(9):1712–9.

Part VI

Differential Diagnosis

Benjamin Chaigne and Loïc Guillevin

Introduction

An ulcer is defined as the cutaneous loss of every part of the epidermis and at least the superficial layer of the dermis. In systemic sclerosis (SSc), digital ulcer (DU) can be simply defined as a digitally located loss of continuity in the epidermidis and adjacent layers, but sometimes, loss of ≥2 mm of palmar dermis reflects an ischemic etiology [1]. Although SSc is the predominant systemic DU etiology, other inflammatory and non-inflammatory conditions are associated with cutaneous and digital ischemia that affects the individual's quality of life and is a handicap. In this chapter, we review DUs and distal gangrene etiologies other than SSc, focusing more specifically on DUs associated with vasculitides and some inflammatory conditions, in which they are mostly the consequence of an ischemic process and often associated with gangrene.

Skin and Ischemic Manifestations of Systemic Necrotizing Vasculitis (SNV)

Cutaneous ischemia is a rare manifestation of SNV. In the retrospective study organized by the French Vasculitis Study Group, only 65 (5%) of the 1304 SNV patients had them [2]. DUs and digital necrosis (DN) are uncommon cutaneous manifestations of SNV [3]. The authors of three published series [3–5] of patients with cutaneous manifestations of granulomatosis with polyangiitis (Wegener's) (GPA) reported skin ulcers in 6–27% of them, rates which seem to be high. Notably, those series came from dermatology departments where DUs are more common, but the DU frequency in the general SNV population is probably lower. Ulcers were not located exclusively on the digits but also occurred in unusual sites, e.g., the perineal area [6], trunk, face, and neck [4, 5, 7]. Ulcers and other cutaneous ischemias can be the first manifestation of SNVs in 1–5% of patients [8].

Granulomatous manifestations associated with necrotic papules, like in GPA or eosinophilic granulomatosis with polyangiitis (Churg-Strauss) (EGPA), must be differentiated from ulcers caused by ischemic necrotizing vasculitis located in small- or medium-sized skin vessels [3]. DN is a less frequent manifestation, mainly described in case reports that also emphasized the poor outcomes of DN in GPA, polyarteritis nodosa (PAN), and EGPA in adults [7, 9] and children [10, 11], with a higher amputation rate (67%) than in our personal series (25%) [2]. The condition affects mainly, but not exclusively, the fingertips. DN frequency is roughly the same in SNV. We observed digital ischemia in 7.1% of our MPA [12], 3.7% of our EGPA [13], and 6% of our PAN patients [14].

Cutaneous ischemia mechanisms in SNV are not fully understood. Causes may include necrotizing inflammatory obliteration of small-sized vessels, primary thrombus formation in a medium- or small-sized artery simultaneously affected with vasculitis, acquired thrombophilia, vasculitis-induced or

B. Chaigne · L. Guillevin (✉)
National Referral Center for Rare Systemic Autoimmune Diseases,
Department of Internal Medicine, Hôpital Cochin, Assistance
Publique-Hôpitaux de Paris (APHP), Université Paris Descartes,
Paris, France

© Springer Nature Switzerland AG 2019
M. Matucci-Cerinic, C. P. Denton (eds.), *Atlas of Ulcers in Systemic Sclerosis*, https://doi.org/10.1007/978-3-319-98477-3_17

preexisting endothelial dysfunction, and/or vasomotor disturbances. The case of a 12-year-old girl also suggested a role of vasospasm in digital ischemia and its reversibility with nifedipine [15]. Bessias et al. described multiple recurrent thromboses in femoral, popliteal, posterior tibial, anterior tibial, and peroneal arteries as signs of GPA onset that required a pregnant patient's below-the-knee amputation [16]. A patient with cryofibrinogenemia [10] and another with EGPA associated with antiphospholipid antibodies were also described [17].

Atherosclerosis plays a role, too. An association of subclinical atherosclerosis or artery dysfunction, e.g., SNV-induced endothelial dysfunction or arterial stiffness, was previously reported [18]. In addition, cutaneous ischemia has been associated with coronary atherosclerosis, smoking, and hypertension. Preexisting endothelial dysfunction secondary to well-known cardiovascular risk factors may worsen limb ischemia in SNVs. For DN, urging patients to stop smoking is still strongly warranted, even essential, in those SNVs. Inflammation, in turn, favors the atherosclerotic process, and its attenuation restores endothelial function [19].

DUs and digital ischemia are independent of the presence or absence of antineutrophil cytoplasmic antibodies (ANCA), as suggested by our results showing similar frequencies in patients with ANCA-associated vasculitides and PAN with or without vascular symptoms (Table 17.1) [2].

Table 17.1 Characteristics of systemic necrotizing vasculitis patients with or without cutaneous ischemia

Characteristic	With cutaneous ischemia ($n = 65$)	Without cutaneous ischemia ($n = 1239$)	P value
Age at diagnosis, mean ± SD years	54.6 ± 14.7	51.5 ± 17.0	0.23
First symptom to diagnosis, mean ± SD months	6.6 ± 8.0	7.1 ± 12.3	0.74
Diagnosis, n (%)			0.72
Microscopic polyangiitis	15 (23.1)	234 (18.9)	
Granulomatosis with polyangiitis (Wegener's)	18 (27.7)	372 (30)	
Polyarteritis nodosa	21 (32.3)	370 (29.9)	
Eosinophilic granulomatosis with polyangiitis (Churg-Strauss)	11 (16.9)	263 (21.2)	
Cutaneous manifestations, n (%)	65 (100)	471 (38.0)	<0.0001
Nodules	8 (12.3)	134 (10.8)	0.71
Purpura	33 (50.8)	245 (19.8)	<0.0001
Livedo	13 (20)	98 (7.9)	0.001
Raynaud's phenomenon	11 (16.9)	40 (3.2)	<0.0001
Associated factors, n (%)			
Gastrointestinal perforation(s)	4 (6.2)	22 (1.8)	0.004
Smoker (current or former)	22 (33.8)	282 (22.8)	0.04
Hypertension or smoking	33 (50.8)	419 (33.8)	0.005
Coronary artery disease	6 (9.2)	59 (4.8)	0.04

Data from Lega et al. [2]

Prognosis and Outcomes

Distal ischemic manifestations were not considered a poor-prognosis factor and were not items included in the 1996 and 2011 revisited five-factor score (FFS) [20, 21]. Although patients' outcomes did not differ according to the presence or absence of cutaneous involvement [3], that does not exclude the potential severity of these rare manifestations; it just means that they do not impact the final FFS. In our recent personal study, a link was found between cutaneous ischemia and poor long-term SNV outcomes [2]. DN was associated with an increased risk of gastrointestinal perforation, relapse with digital ischemia, other systemic manifestations, and vasculitis-related death. However, despite significantly increased frequencies of prior coronary artery disease, smoking, and arterial hypertension in patients with cutaneous ischemia, their survival rate did not indicate increased cardiovascular mortality.

Treatment

Because these clinical manifestations are severe and patients have poor outcomes, it seems reasonable to combine corticosteroids and an immunosuppressant or rituximab to treat patients with ANCA-associated vasculitides. When patients do not improve under this regimen, plasma exchange can be prescribed [22]. For limb ischemia caused by medium-to-large-sized artery disease, thrombectomy or bypass has been proposed [16, 23]. If either intervention is done, it should be combined with a general systemic regimen, as described above. Moreover, anticoagulation is recommended during the acute phase to treat and prevent thrombosis formation favored by endothelial injury and subsequent dysfunction. However, that recommendation has not been proven by prospective study or case series. Prostacyclin, mainly iloprost, can be added for ischemia but not for tissue necrosis, whose reversibility cannot be expected [11].

Rheumatoid Arthritis (RA)

DU is not a common RA feature; its presence characterizes rheumatoid vasculitis (RV). Even though RV is a rare phenomenon, whose frequency ranges from 15% to 31% of RA patients, some authors consider ischemic focal digital lesions a very common RV sign and a classical RA symptom [24]. RV occurs mainly in patient seropositive for rheumatoid factor and/or anti-cyclic citrullinated peptide. RV is considered to be an immune-complex disease. In addition, a relationship between it and three specific genotypes, *0401/*0401, *0401/*0404, and *0101/*0401, of the HLA-DRB1 shared epitope has been described [25] and a link with HLA-C3 [26].

Histological examination usually shows small-sized vessel vasculitis, but in some patients, RV can affect medium-sized arteries and mimic PAN. Fibrinoid necrosis of the media and leukocytoclastic vasculitis are common, with disruption of the internal and external elastic laminae.

Clinical manifestations are ubiquitous and all organs can be affected. However, skin disease is one of the most common, with nail fold capillaritis, purpura, livedo, and, more rarely, nodules. Digital microinfarcts are frequently seen, usually subungual and visible through the nail, but they also can be periungual in the digital pulp. They are frequently associated with subcutaneous skin nodules. These microinfarcts are not considered factors of poor RV prognosis, unless they are associated with systemic manifestations. Some patients also have leg arterial ulcers that respond to vasculitis treatment. Livedo reticularis, purpura, and digital gangrene can occur, with the latter being considered to carry a poor prognosis. Among the other clinical manifestations, mononeuritis multiplex [27], poor general condition, and visceral involvements, e.g., gastrointestinal or cardiac manifestations, can be observed.

RV is diagnoses based on the skin, nerve, or muscle biopsy findings. RV incidence was estimated at 1–5% of RA patients, but its prevalence has dramatically decreased since more effective drugs, like methotrexate, antitumor necrosis factor (TNF), abatacept, and anti-CD20, have been widely used, with subsequent control of inflammation, which seems to be a major factor contributing to vascular injury. According to the recent analysis of the French Autoimmunity and Rituximab registry, 17/1994 RV patients have been described [28]; 82% of them responded to rituximab. However, it is too early to recommend this agent for systematic use in the RV therapeutic strategy. Voskuyl et al. reported the clinical characteristics of 31 patients with histologically proven RV: 4 had superficial skin ulcers, and 1 had gangrene. Among the 50 other patients with RA and extra-articular manifestations, 9 had superficial skin ulcers and 1 gangrene [29]. Still, arteriograms of three patients with leg ulcers and/or gangrene revealed occlusion of arteries, suggesting vessel disorders, even in the absence of RV [30]. One case report also advanced the possible implication of cryofibrinogenemia in DU pathogenesis in RV [31].

The RV prognosis was poor before the advent of "modern" therapeutic strategies. However, when this vasculitis occurs despite these treatments, outcome can be poor. A possible explanation could be RV-cause persistence because RA can remain active or at least persist in such patients. Only the RV form characterized by nail fold petechia has a good prognosis. For the other forms, including patients with digital ischemia, a combination of corticosteroids and cyclophosphamide (six to nine pulses, as described above), followed by azathioprine (2–3 mg/kg/day) or methotrexate (0.3 mg/kg/week) for 12 to 18 months, is recommended. Despite the lack of controlled studies, anti-TNFα and rituximab have successfully treated RV. Mounting evidence suggests that TNF plays a central role in RV pathophysiology, and thus, anti-TNFα can be a therapeutic option [32]. Only case reports indicated efficacy of drugs commonly used to treat RA, e.g., methotrexate and anti-TNF (i.e., infliximab, adalimumab, etanercept) [30, 31]. The latter study provided evidence that anti-TNFα and corticosteroids achieved remission in six/ nine patients with active refractory RV, thereby allowing notable corticosteroid sparing; however, the infection rate was high for those severely ill patients.

Although to date no argument supports the systematic prescription of plasma exchanges, they might be useful as second-line therapy for patients with severe RV and vascular gangrene or leg arterial ulcers who are rheumatoid factor- and cryoglobulinemia-positive.

Rituximab is also able to induce remissions: complete RV remission was obtained in most patients receiving rituximab, thereby enabling significant decreases of their daily predni- sone doses along with an acceptable toxicity profile. In the French Autoimmunity and Rituximab registry [28], 12 (71%) of the 17 RV patients, among the 1994 RA patients entered, achieved complete vasculitis remissions after 6 months of rituximab administration, 4 had partial responses, and 1 died of uncontrolled vasculitis. The relapse rate was higher under methotrexate than rituximab, when one or the other was required as maintenance therapy for every patient. Notably, rituximab made it possible to lower corticosteroid doses. Some authors have also prescribed empirical rituximab suc- cessfully [33].

Behçet's Disease (BD)

BD is associated with bipolar aphthosis and thromboem- bolism. The International Study Group for Behçet's Disease described cutaneous lesions as a major criterion for the diagnosis [34]. Furthermore, BD comprises a wide variety of cutaneous lesions [35]. Hence, BD could be expected to be associated with DUs. To the best of our knowledge, only case reports on digital lesions of BD patients have been published. They mostly showed digital vasculitis with toe involvement [36], gangrene of the hand [37], or necrosis of the fifth foot digit [38]. Exceptional nodular lesions may also occur. Indeed, Cantini et al. described a unique case of a patient with recurrent, multi- ple, papulonodular, roundish, erythematous, painful, blu- ish-red nodules, 0.5–1 cm in diameter, on the palms and fingers of both hands [39].

Mucocutaneous Lesions of Behçet's Disease [35]

Oral ulcers
Genital ulcers
Erythema nodosum-like
Papulopustular
Superficial thrombophlebitis
Extragenital ulceration
Pathergy reaction
Cutaneous vasculitic
    Sweet's syndrome
    Pyoderma gangrenosum-like
    Erythema multiforme-like
    Palpable purpura
    Subungual infarctions
    Hemorrhagic bullae
    Furuncles
    Abscesses
    Pernio-like
    Polyarteritis-like
    Acral purpuric papulonodular

However, hand involvement in BD is not that uncommon. A 2006 study reported BD patients' hand manifestations: among the 57 BD patients with specific hand examination, 32 had clinical findings, but no patient had DUs. Clinical hand involvement was associated with disease duration (OR = 3.4; $P < 0.05$). Pulp atrophy, observed in 17 patients, was the most frequent clinical finding [40].

Movasat et al. analyzed the nail fold capillaroscopies of 127 BD patients. Although findings were abnormal for 40% of them, no DUs were reported [41].

DU is a rare BD symptom and, unsurprisingly, caused by a vasculitic process. That process might be underestimated in the pathogenesis of skin lesions, as revealed by a histopatho- logical study of 48 skin biopsy specimens from 42 BD patients [42]. In that study, 20 (48%) patients had cutaneous vasculitis, predominantly venulitis or phlebitis, with 17% leukocytoclastic vasculitis and 31% lymphocytic vasculitis. Clinical manifestations were mainly erythema nodosum-like eruptions, infiltrated erythema, and papulopustular lesions; only six patients had ulcerations.

No gold standard currently exists for BD treatment, and no randomized-controlled trial has examined reduction of vessel wall inflammation in BD [43]. Evidence-based rec- ommendations concerning BD skin-mucosa involvement depend on the dominant or codominant lesions present [43]. Colchicine is widely used, because it was associated with fewer mucocutaneous lesions, e.g., genital ulcers ($P = 0.004$) and erythema nodosum ($P = 0.004$) in women [44]. To treat leg ulcers, the European League Against Rheumatism task force advocated treatment selected according to the ulcer cause, which includes post-thrombotic, venous stasis, or vasculitic phenomena in BD, and highlighted the lack of controlled evidence for vascular involvement. Treatment of resistant cutaneous lesions relies on azathioprine, thalidomide, interferon-α, and/or TNFα antagonists [43].

Alibaz-Oner et al. recently investigated the therapeutic approach to vascular BD in Turkey based on their retrospective study on 936 patients: 363 (38.7%) had mucocutaneous disease, and 260 (27.7%) had vascular involvement [45], with the latter being the first sign of the disease for 149 (57.3%). Notably, vascular involvement was not held responsible for any mucocutaneous lesions. Vascular BD was treated with immunosuppressants (e.g., corticosteroids, methotrexate, azathioprine, cyclophosphamide, infliximab, or interferon-α) and an anticoagulant, like warfarin and conventional or low-molecular-weight heparin. Immunosuppressants, given to 88.8% after the first vascular event, were negatively correlated with vascular manifestation relapse. Adjunction of an anticoagulant to an immunosuppressant was not associated with a positive effect on vascular relapse.

Overall, DUs in BD are rare and mainly associated with vascular involvement of the disease, which is mostly treated with immunosuppressants, despite the lack of consensus.

DU-Associated Thrombosis

Antiphospholipid Syndrome

Although SSc is a main cause of DUs, the latter could be masking something else, and antiphospholipid syndrome (APS) can also be associated with DUs in this setting. Indeed, Küçükşahin et al. described a patient with limited cutaneous SSc complicated by treatment-resistant digital ischemia [46]. The lack of response to conventional therapy led to biological analyses and proof of APS; warfarin was added and the digital lesion regressed.

Digital manifestations of APS include acute ischemia and gangrene [47–49]. In a European cohort of 1000 APS patients, the estimated frequency of leg ulcers, pseudovasculitic lesions, and digital gangrene, respectively, was 5.5%, 3.9%, and 3.3% [50]. At disease onset, 1.9% of the patients had digital gangrene [50]. A few years later, Francès et al. reported the dermatological characteristics and symptoms of 200 APS patients. Among the 15 (7.5%) APS patients with DN, it was the presenting sign for 5 [51]. Digital lesions can occur at any age [52–54], at any time during APS evolution, and are rarely an isolated symptom [55]. They occur in primary and secondary APS, such as systemic lupus erythematous (SLE)-associated APS [56]. Nail fold capillaroscopy can be a useful tool in APS to detect microscopic abnormalities, mainly hemorrhages, edema, or bushy capillaries [57], or suggest differences between primary APS- and SLE-associated APS by showing more microhemorrhages in the latter than the former [58].

Possible pathogenic mechanisms include an ischemic process, due to fibrin microthrombi forming in the vessels [59], and a vasculitic process [60]. In the series reported by Francès et al., digital gangrene was related to medium- or large-sized vessel occlusion [51].

Notably, digital ischemia and APS can reveal anecdotal situations, for example, familial APS [61] or malignancy-associated APS and metastatic colon cancer or poorly differentiated metastatic epithelial carcinoma [53]. Intriguingly, in their retrospective study on 21 APS patients of different national origins who endured limb or digit amputation, Asherson et al. emphasized that livedo reticularis appeared before arterial thrombosis in 9 of them [60].

Digital manifestations of APS must be treated with anticoagulation, the essential cornerstone of its therapy. Moreover, digital gangrene is a severe manifestation of the disease that requires acute anticoagulation with heparin and then long-term warfarin [51]. Iloprost and plasma exchange have also been reported to be effective, when heparin failed to impact skin lesions [51, 62, 63]. Oral non-vitamin K antagonist anticoagulants are currently being evaluated for APS [64].

Thromboangiitis Obliterans (TAO)

TAO, also known as Buerger's disease, is a non-atherosclerotic segmental inflammatory disease of small- and medium-sized arteries of the distal extremities of predominantly young male smokers. The diagnosis, mainly clinical, is suspected when ischemic lesions of the distal limbs are present [65]. Common onset symptoms include gangrene, acral ulcer, ischemic rest pain, subungual and/or skin infection(s), phlegmon(s), claudication, acral skin discoloration and coldness, Raynaud's phenomenon (RP), and thrombophlebitic nodules [66]. TAO ulcers are distal and associated with clubbing, pain, and bluish discoloration of the fingers when exposed to cold [67, 68].

Quitting smoking is a mandatory treatment measure, as it favors ulcer healing and can prevent new ulcer formation and/or amputation [69]. Intravenous iloprost for 28 days effectively heals ulcers and relieves TAO-related pain. In the first randomized, double-blind trial comparing iloprost to aspirin that enrolled 152 TAO patients, Fiessinger et al. showed that 85% of the iloprost-treated patients reached the primary endpoint (ulcer healing or relief of ischemic pain) compared to 17% of those given aspirin [70]. In 2013, Bozkurt et al. confirmed those results in 60% of 158 patients treated with intravenous iloprost for 28 days [71]. Other TAO treatments include antiplatelet agents, anticoagulants, and vasodilating drugs, but there is no evidence of their efficacy [66]. At present, no proven indication supports sympathectomy or immunosuppressive agents for TAO [66]. As for SSc, bosentan has been evaluated for TAO. A pilot study assessed the reoccurrence of ischemic lesions in 12 TAO patients (13 extremities) treated with bosentan in a compassionate use program [72]. In that evaluation, which unfortunately lacked a control group, 11 patients had toe or finger ulcer(s) at study onset. At the end of the study, only 1 patient had developed new ischemic lesions, and 2 of the 13 extremities were amputated. Bosentan for TAO is not currently under evaluation in ant phase III clinical trial (www.clinicaltrial.gov).

Vascular Embolism

Because embolic disease is a well-recognized cause of acute digital ischemia, every potential embolism etiology should be considered when managing a patient with digital ischemia, especially when the patient has a pulseless, unilateral acute lesion. Arterial stenosis or aneurysm can cause acral emboli, which clinically give rise to a blue finger syndrome, which requires endovascular intervention [73]. Aneurysms of ulnar [74], axillary or subclavian arteries, and other thrombotic conditions, e.g., a descending thoracic aorta mass [75] or arteriovenous fistula [76], have been reported. Other etiologies of digital embolic lesions include cholesterol embolism [77], bacterial septic embolism [78], atrial fibrillation, myxoma, and intracardiac thrombosis [79].

Conditions favoring a procoagulant state, such as thrombocythemias, thrombophilia, paraproteinemia, and cancer, should also be sought for the differential diagnosis of digital embolic lesions [80].

Vascular Spasms

Raynaud's Phenomenon

Maurice Raynaud first characterized RP in 1862. Its hallmark is ischemia of the digits in response to cold. RP is diagnosed clinically. It is then subclassified into primary or secondary RP. Primary RP diagnostic criteria include those for RP and exclusion of secondary causes, as assessed by a capillaroscopy, physical examination, history of connective tissue disease, and antinuclear antibody serology [81]. Secondary RP causes include vasoconstrictive medication, autoimmune disorders (SSc, mixed connective tissue disease, RA, SLE, dermatomyositis, Sjögren's syndrome), vasculitis, arteriopathies, dysthyroidea, acromegalia, malignancies, and professional wrist trauma [82]. Primary RP is usually not associated with DUs, but exceptional fingertip necrosis has been reported [83, 84]. In Landry et al.'s longitudinal study, 7.7% of 585 patients with vasospastic RP had DUs at their initial evaluations, and 14% of 50 patients had them after 10 years of follow-up. Nine (1.5%) patients initially and only two (4%) after 10-year follow-up underwent digital or phalangeal amputation [85].

RP treatment includes patient education, warmth maintenance, cold avoidance, and various pharmacological therapies, among which, calcium channel blockers are widely prescribed [86].

Ergotism

Ergot alkaloids are metabolites of fungus species of the genus *Claviceps*, most commonly *Claviceps purpurea*. The *Claviceps* fungus and, thus, ergotism might have been responsible for one of the plagues of Egypt, as it could have contaminated grain and storage facilities opened by the oldest sons just before dying of arterial ischemia [87]. Ergotism is also called Saint Anthony's fire, which refers to the intense inflammation caused by eating food prepared with ergot-contaminated rye during the Middle Ages [88].

Nowadays, ergotism is a rare etiology of arterial ischemia that is mainly seen in human immunodeficiency virus-infected patients [89] and/or those treated with ergot alkaloids for migraine [90]. It is mainly due to drug interactions or overexposure to ergot derivatives, e.g., ritonavir or ergotamine [91]. It affects the extremities, causing leg ischemia, ulcers, and gangrene as common manifestations [92]. Treatment requires the discontinuation of all ergot-containing medications, cessation of caffeine intake, and stopping smoking. The prognosis can be poor as for a reported limb amputation [93], but iloprost has also been used effectively [92, 94].

Iatrogenic Spasm

Medications other than ergot-containing drugs can be responsible for vascular spasms, for example, high-dose epinephrine, *coxibs* (e.g., COX-2-selective nonsteroidal anti-inflammatory drugs) [95], and nonsteroidal anti-inflammatory drugs like diclofenac [96], nabumetone [97], and naproxen [98].

Other Causes

Other possible DU causes (e.g., congenital, tunnel syndrome, frostbite, local trauma, drugs or mercury injections, psychological parasitophobia, infections) that should also be considered in the differential diagnosis of DUs are summarized below, which concludes this overview of the differential diagnoses of DU.

Other Uncommon Causes of Digital Ulcers

Congenital
   Porphyria [99]
   Aicardi-Goutières syndrome [100]
   Familial chilblain lupus [101]
Mechanical
   Carpal tunnel syndrome [102]
   Local microtrauma
   Self-injections (drugs, mercury) [103, 104]
Frostbite [105]
Infectious
   Bacteria: purpura fulminans [106], *Bacillus anthracis*, *Neisseria gonorrhoeae*, *Treponema pallidum*, pyogenic granuloma, bacillary angiomatosis [107]
   Mycobacteria: tuberculosis, atypical mycobacteria, leprosy
   Viruses: human immunodeficiency virus, herpes simplex virus, human herpesvirus-8, *Parapoxvirus*, orf virus
   Fungi: sporotrichosis [108]
   Parasites: leishmaniasis [109], trypanosomiasis
Malignancies and Kaposi's syndrome [110–115]

References

1. Nitsche A. Raynaud, digital ulcers and calcinosis in scleroderma. Reumatol Clin. 2012;8(5):270–7.
2. Lega JC, Seror R, Fassier T, Aumaître O, Quere I, Pourrat J, et al. Characteristics, prognosis, and outcomes of cutaneous ischemia and gangrene in systemic necrotizing vasculitides: a retrospective multicenter study. Semin Arthritis Rheum. 2014;43(5):681–8.
3. Francès C, Dû LT, Piette JC, Saada V, Boisnic S, Wechsler B, et al. Wegener's granulomatosis. Dermatological manifestations in 75 cases with clinicopathologic correlation. Arch Dermatol. 1994;130(7):861–7.
4. Daoud MS, Gibson LE, DeRemee RA, Specks U, el-Azhary RA, Su WP. Cutaneous Wegener's granulomatosis: clinical, histopathologic, and immunopathologic features of thirty patients. J Am Acad Dermatol. 1994;31(4):605–12.
5. Hu CH, O'Loughlin S, Winkelmann RK. Cutaneous manifestations of Wegener granulomatosis. Arch Dermatol. 1977;113(2):175–82.
6. Aymard B, Bigard MA, Thompson H, Schmutz JL, Finet JF, Borrelly J. Perianal ulcer: an unusual presentation of Wegener's granulomatosis. Report of a case. Dis Colon Rectum. 1990;33(5):427–30.
7. Choi SW, Lew S, Cho SD, Cha HJ, Eum EA, Jung HC, et al. Cutaneous polyarteritis nodosa presented with digital gangrene: a case report. J Korean Med Sci. 2006;21(2):371–3.
8. Reed WB, Jensen AK, Konwaler BE, Hunter D. The cutaneous manifestations in Wegener's granulomatosis. Acta Derm Venereol. 1963;43:250–64.
9. Otani Y, Anzai S, Shibuya H, Fujiwara S, Takayasu S, Asada Y, et al. Churg–Strauss syndrome (CSS) manifested as necrosis of fingers and toes and liver infarction. J Dermatol. 2003;30(11):810–5.
10. Shimbo J, Miwa A, Aoki K. Cryofibrinogenemia associated with polyarteritis nodosa. Clin Rheumatol. 2006;25(4):562–3.
11. Zulian F, Corona F, Gerloni V, Falcini F, Buoncompagni A, Scarazatti M, et al. Safety and efficacy of iloprost for the treatment of ischaemic digits in paediatric connective tissue diseases. Rheumatology (Oxford). 2004;43(2):229–33.
12. Guillevin L, Durand-Gasselin B, Cevallos R, Gayraud M, Lhote F, Callard P, et al. Microscopic polyangiitis: clinical and laboratory findings in eighty-five patients. Arthritis Rheum. 1999;42(3):421–30.
13. Comarmond C, Pagnoux C, Khellaf M, Cordier J-F, Hamidou M, Viallard J-F, et al. Eosinophilic granulomatosis with polyangiitis (Churg–Strauss): clinical characteristics and long-term follow-up of the 383 patients enrolled in the French Vasculitis Study Group cohort. Arthritis Rheum. 2013;65(1):270–81.
14. Pagnoux C, Seror R, Henegar C, Mahr A, Cohen P, Le Guern V, et al. Clinical features and outcomes in 348 patients with polyarteritis nodosa: a systematic retrospective study of patients diagnosed between 1963 and 2005 and entered into the French Vasculitis Study Group Database. Arthritis Rheum. 2010;62(2):616–26.
15. Kejriwal R, Lim TM, Kumar S. Wegener's granulomatosis and acute upper limb digital ischemia. Int J Rheum Dis. 2008;11(2):185–7.
16. Bessias N, Moulakakis KG, Lioupis C, Bakogiannis K, Sfyroeras G, Kakaletri K, et al. Wegener's granulomatosis presenting during pregnancy with acute limb ischemia. J Vasc Surg. 2005 Oct;42(4):800–4.
17. Ferenczi K, Chang T, Camouse M, Han R, Stern R, Willis J, et al. A case of Churg–Strauss syndrome associated with antiphospholipid antibodies. J Am Acad Dermatol. 2007;56(4):701–4.
18. Pagnoux C, Chironi G, Simon A, Guillevin L. Atherosclerosis in ANCA-associated vasculitides. Ann N Y Acad Sci. 2007;1107:11–21.
19. Raza K, Thambyrajah J, Townend JN, Exley AR, Hortas C, Filer A, et al. Suppression of inflammation in primary systemic vasculitis restores vascular endothelial function: lessons for atherosclerotic disease? Circulation. 2000;102(13):1470–2.
20. Guillevin L, Lhote F, Gayraud M, Cohen P, Jarrousse B, Lortholary O, et al. Prognostic factors in polyarteritis nodosa and Churg–Strauss syndrome. A prospective study in 342 patients. Medicine (Baltimore). 1996;75(1):17–28.
21. Guillevin L, Pagnoux C, Seror R, Mahr A, Mouthon L, Le Toumelin P. The Five-Factor Score revisited: assessment of prognoses of systemic necrotizing vasculitides based on the French Vasculitis Study Group (FVSG) cohort. Medicine (Baltimore). 2011;90(1):19–27.
22. Leung A, Sung CB, Kothari G, Mack C, Fong C. Utilisation of plasma exchange in the treatment of digital infarcts in Wegener's granulomatosis. Int J Rheum Dis. 2010;13(4):e59–61.
23. Maia M, Brandão P, Monteiro P, Barreto P, Brandão D, Ferreira J, et al. Upper limb ischemia in a patient with Wegener's granulomatosis. Interact Cardiovasc Thorac Surg. 2008;7(6):1137–40.
24. Genta MS, Genta RM, Gabay C. Systemic rheumatoid vasculitis: a review. Semin Arthritis Rheum. 2006;36(2):88–98.

25. Gorman JD, David-Vaudey E, Pai M, Lum RF, Criswell LA. Particular HLA-DRB1 shared epitope genotypes are strongly associated with rheumatoid vasculitis. Arthritis Rheum. 2004;50(11):3476–84.

26. Turesson C, Schaid DJ, Weyand CM, Jacobsson LT, Goronzy JJ, Petersson IF, et al. Association of HLA-C3 and smoking with vasculitis in patients with rheumatoid arthritis. Arthritis Rheum. 2006;54(9):2776–83.

27. Puéchal X, Said G. Necrotizing vasculitis of the peripheral nervous system: nonsystemic or clinically undetectable? Arthritis Rheum. 1999;42(4):824–5.

28. Puéchal X, Gottenberg JE, Berthelot JM, Gossec L, Meyer O, Morel J, et al. Rituximab therapy for systemic vasculitis associated with rheumatoid arthritis: results from the AutoImmunity and Rituximab Registry. Arthritis Care Res (Hoboken). 2012;64(3):331–9.

29. Voskuyl A, Hazes J, Zwinderman A, Paleolog E, van der Meer FJM, Daha M, et al. Diagnostic strategy for the assessment of rheumatoid vasculitis. Ann Rheum Dis. 2003;62(5):407–13.

30. Hasegawa M, Nagai Y, Sogabe Y, Hattori T, Inoue C, Okada E, et al. Clinical analysis of leg ulcers and gangrene in rheumatoid arthritis. J Dermatol. 2013;40(12):949–54.

31. Soyfoo MS, Couturier B, Cogan E. Cryofibrinogenaemia with vasculitis: a new overlap syndrome causing severe leg ulcers and digital necrosis in rheumatoid arthritis? Rheumatology. 2010;49(12):2455–7.

32. Puéchal X, Miceli-Richard C, Mejjad O, Lafforgue P, Marcelli C, Solau-Gervais E, et al. Anti-tumour necrosis factor treatment in patients with refractory systemic vasculitis associated with rheumatoid arthritis. Ann Rheum Dis. 2008;67(6):880–4.

33. Bartels CM, Bridges AJ. Rheumatoid vasculitis: vanishing menace or target for new treatments? Curr Rheumatol Rep. 2010;12(6):414–9.

34. Criteria for diagnosis of Behçet's disease. International Study Group for Behçet's Disease. Lancet. 1990;335(8697):1078–80.

35. Alpsoy E, Zouboulis CC, Ehrlich GE. Mucocutaneous lesions of Behçet's disease. Yonsei Med J. 2007;48(4):573–85.

36. Travis SP, Czajkowski M, McGovern DP, Watson RG, Bell AL. Treatment of intestinal Behçet's syndrome with chimeric tumour necrosis factor alpha antibody. Gut. 2001;49(5):725–8.

37. Gera C, Jose W, Malhotra N, Malhotra V, Dhanoa J. Radial artery occlusion, a rare presentation of Behçet's disease. J Assoc Physicians India. 2008;56:643–4.

38. Ateş A, Karaaslan Y, Aşlar ZÖ. A case of Behçet's disease associated with necrotizing small vessel vasculitis. Rheumatol Int. 2006;27(1):91–3.

39. Cantini F, Salvarani C, Niccoli L, Senesi C, Truglia MC, Padula A, et al. Behçet's disease with unusual cutaneous lesions. J Rheumatol. 1998;25(12):2469–72.

40. Yurtkuran M, Yurtkuran M, Alp A, Sivrioglu K, Dilek K, Tamgaç F, et al. Hand involvement in Behçet's disease. Joint Bone Spine. 2006;73(6):679–83.

41. Movasat A, Shahram F, Carreira PE, Nadji A, Akhlaghi M, Naderi N, et al. Nail fold capillaroscopy in Behçet's disease, analysis of 128 patients. Clin Rheumatol. 2009;28(5):603–5.

42. Chen KR, Kawahara Y, Miyakawa S, Nishikawa T. Cutaneous vasculitis in Behçet's disease: a clinical and histopathologic study of 20 patients. J Am Acad Dermatol. 1997;36(5 Pt 1):689–96.

43. Hatemi G, Silman A, Bang D, Bodaghi B, Chamberlain AM, Gul A, et al. EULAR recommendations for the management of Behçet disease. Ann Rheum Dis. 2008;67(12):1656–62.

44. Yurdakul S, Mat C, Tüzün Y, Ozyazgan Y, Hamuryudan V, Uysal O, et al. A double-blind trial of colchicine in Behçet's syndrome. Arthritis Rheum. 2001;44(11):2686–92.

45. Alibaz-Oner F, Karadeniz A, Ylmaz S, Balkarl A, Kimyon G, Yazc A, et al. Behçet disease with vascular involvement: effects of

different therapeutic regimens on the incidence of new relapses. Medicine (Baltimore). 2015;94(6):e494.

46. Küçükşahin O, Ateş A, Okoh AK, Kulahcioglu E, Turgay M, Kınıklı G. Treatment resistant severe digital ischemia associated with antiphospholipid syndrome in a male patient with systemic sclerosis. Case Rep Rheumatol. 2014;2014:291382.

47. Crome CR, Rajagopalan S, Kuhan G, Fluck N. Antiphospholipid syndrome presenting with acute digital ischaemia, avascular necrosis of the femoral head and superior mesenteric artery thrombus. BMJ Case Rep. 2012;2012:bcr2012006731.

48. Jou IM, Liu MF, Chao SC. Widespread cutaneous necrosis associated with antiphospholipid syndrome. Clin Rheumatol. 1996;15(4):394–8.

49. Hai A, Aslam M, Ashraf TH. Symmetrical peripheral gangrene: a rare presentation of antiphospholipid syndrome. Intern Emerg Med. 2012;7(Suppl 1):S71–3.

50. Cervera R, Piette J-C, Font J, Khamashta MA, Shoenfeld Y, Camps MT, et al. Antiphospholipid syndrome: clinical and immunologic manifestations and patterns of disease expression in a cohort of 1,000 patients. Arthritis Rheum. 2002;46(4):1019–27.

51. Francès C, Niang S, Laffitte E, Le Pelletier F, Costedoat N, Piette JC. Dermatologic manifestations of the antiphospholipid syndrome: two hundred consecutive cases. Arthritis Rheum. 2005;52(6):1785–93.

52. Wollina U, Verma SB. Acute digital gangrene in a newborn. Arch Dermatol. 2007;143(1):121–2.

53. Grossman A, Gafter-Gvili A, Green H, Ben Aharon I, Stemmer SM, Molad Y, et al. Severe digital ischemia – a presenting symptom of malignancy-associated antiphospholipid syndrome. Lupus. 2008;17(3):206–9.

54. Méchinaud-Lacroix F, Jehan P, Debré MA, Prieur AM, Sizun J, Harousseau JL. Thrombotic manifestations and acute distal ischemia in primary antiphospholipid syndrome in children. Arch Fr Pediatr. 1992;49(Suppl 1):257–9.

55. Rezende SM, Franco R. Multiple peripheral artery occlusions in antiphospholipid syndrome. Am J Hematol. 2007;82(6):498.

56. Bouaziz JD, Barete S, Le Pelletier F, Amoura Z, Piette JC, Francès C. Cutaneous lesions of the digits in systemic lupus erythematosus: 50 cases. Lupus. 2007;16(3):163–7.

57. Vayssairat M, Abuaf N, Deschamps A, Baudot N, Gaitz JP, Chakkour K, et al. Nail fold capillary microscopy in patients with anticardiolipin antibodies: a case–control study. Dermatology (Basel). 1997;194(1):36–40.

58. Candela M, Pansoni A, De Carolis ST, Pomponio G, Corvetta A, Gabrielli A, et al. Nail fold capillary microscopy in patients with antiphospholipid syndrome. Recenti Prog Med. 1998;89(9):444–9.

59. Szodoray P, Hajas A, Toth L, Szakall S, Nakken B, Soltesz P, et al. The beneficial effect of plasmapheresis in mixed connective tissue disease with coexisting antiphospholipid syndrome. Lupus. 2014;23(10):1079–84.

60. Asherson RA, Cervera R, Klumb E, Stojanovic L, Sarzi-Puttini P, Yinh J, et al. Amputation of digits or limbs in patients with antiphospholipid syndrome. Semin Arthritis Rheum. 2008;38(2):124–31.

61. Jelušić M, Starčević K, Vidović M, Dobrota S, Potočki K, Banfić L, et al. Familial antiphospholipid syndrome presenting as bivessel arterial occlusion in a 17-year-old girl. Rheumatol Int. 2013;33(5):1359–62.

62. Francès C, Tribout B, Boisnic S, Drouet L, Piette AM, Piette JC, et al. Cutaneous necrosis associated with the lupus anticoagulant. Dermatologica. 1989;178(4):194–201.

63. Zahavi J, Charach G, Schafer R, Toeg A, Zahavi M. Ischaemic necrotic toes associated with antiphospholipid syndrome and treated with iloprost. Lancet. 1993;342(8875):862.

64. Cohen H, Doré CJ, Clawson S, Hunt BJ, Isenberg D, Khamashta M, et al. Rivaroxaban in antiphospholipid syndrome (RAPS) protocol: a prospective, randomized controlled phase II/III clini-

cal trial of rivaroxaban versus warfarin in patients with thrombotic antiphospholipid syndrome, with or without SLE. Lupus. 2015;24(10):1087–94.

65. Dargon PT, Landry GJ. Buerger's disease. Ann Vasc Surg. 2012;26(6):871–80.

66. Klein-Weigel PF, Richter JG. Thromboangiitis obliterans (Buerger's disease). Vasa. 2014 Sep;43(5):337–46.

67. Rosencrance G, Thistlewaite T. Images in clinical medicine. Thromboangiitis obliterans. N Engl J Med. 1996;334(14):891.

68. Sims JR, Hanson EL. Images in clinical medicine. Thromboangiitis obliterans (Buerger's disease). N Engl J Med. 1998;339(10):672.

69. Ohta T, Ishibashi H, Sugimoto I, Iwata H, Kawanishi J, Yamada T, et al. The clinical course of Buerger's disease. Ann Vasc Dis. 2008;1(2):85–90.

70. Fiessinger JN, Schäfer M. Trial of iloprost versus aspirin treatment for critical limb ischaemia of thromboangiitis obliterans. TAO Study Lancet. 1990;335(8689):555–7.

71. Bozkurt AK, Cengiz K, Arslan C, Mine DY, Oner S, Deniz DB, et al. A stable prostacyclin analogue (iloprost) in the treatment of Buerger's disease: a prospective analysis of 150 patients. Ann Thorac Cardiovasc Surg. 2013;19(2):120–5.

72. De Haro J, Acin F, Bleda S, Varela C, Esparza L. Treatment of thromboangiitis obliterans (Buerger's disease) with bosentan. BMC Cardiovasc Disord. 2012;12:5.

73. Gaines PA, Swarbrick MJ, Lopez AJ, Cleveland T, Beard J, Buckenham TM, et al. The endovascular management of blue finger syndrome. Eur J Vasc Endovasc Surg. 1999;17(2):106–10.

74. Haesler P, Hoffmann U, Meyer VE, Bollinger A. Cutaneous micro167embolisms in aneurysm of the distal ulnar artery. Vasa. 1994;23(2):–70.

75. Bansal RC, Pauls GL, Shankel SW. Blue digit syndrome: transesophageal echocardiographic identification of thoracic aortic plaque-related thrombi and successful outcome with warfarin. J Am Soc Echocardiogr. 1993;6(3 Pt 1):319–23.

76. Lacombe M. Digital microembolism after thrombosis of an arteriovenous fistula. Presse Méd. 1989;18(31):1525.

77. Cardani R, Pileggi A, Ricordi C, Gomez C, Baidal DA, Ponte GG, et al. Allosensitization of islet allograft recipients. Transplantation. 2007;84(11):1413–27.

78. Acar P, Emmerich J, Acar C, Capron L, Fiessinger JN. Staphylococcus aureus endocarditis: an unusual clinical picture. Rev Méd Interne. 1993;14(7):733–6.

79. Chanudet X, Clément R, Brunetti G, Ollivier JP, Bauduceau B, Celton H, et al. Digital microembolism disclosing intracardiac thrombosis. Ann Cardiol Angeiol (Paris). 1986;35(2):107–10.

80. Poppe H, Poppe LM, Bühler C, Machann W, Solymosi L, Dlaske H, et al. Painful cyanotic discoloration of the distal phalanges IV and V of the left hand in a 53-year-old female smoker. J Dtsch Dermatol Ges. 2013;11(9):887–91.

81. Maverakis E, Patel F, Kronenberg DG, Chung L, Fiorentino D, Allanore Y, et al. International consensus criteria for the diagnosis of Raynaud's phenomenon. J Autoimmun. 2014;48–49:60–5.

82. CEDEF. Item 327—Raynaud phenomenon. Ann Dermatol Venereol. 2012;139(11 Suppl):A223–6.

83. Senel S, Zorlu P, Dogan B, Acar M. Successfully treated fingertip necrosis in an infant with primary Raynaud phenomenon. Indian J Pediatr. 2014;81(12):1399–400.

84. Uygur S, Tuncer S. Partial fingertip necrosis following a digital surgical procedure in a patient with primary Raynaud's phenomenon. Int Wound J. 2014;11(6):581–2.

85. Landry GJ, Edwards JM, McLafferty RB, Taylor LM, Porter JM. Long-term outcome of Raynaud's syndrome in a prospectively analyzed patient cohort. J Vasc Surg. 1996;23(1):76–85; discussion 85–86

86. Valdovinos ST, Landry GJ. Raynaud syndrome. Tech Vasc Interv Radiol. 2014;17(4):241–6.

87. Marr JS, Malloy CD. An epidemiologic analysis of the ten plagues of Egypt. Caduceus. 1996;12(1):7–24.

88. Craig AM, Klotz JL, Duringer JM. Cases of ergotism in livestock and associated ergot alkaloid concentrations in feed. Front Chem. 2015;3:8. Available from: http://www.ncbi.nlm.nih.gov/pmc/articles/PMC4332362/

89. Liaudet L. Severe ergotism associated with interaction between ritonavir and ergotamine. BMJ. 1999;318(7186):771.

90. Ayarragaray JEF. Ergotism: a change of perspective. Ann Vasc Surg. 2014;28(1):265–8.

91. Acle S, Roca F, Vacarezza M, Álvarez RA. Ergotism secondary to ergotamine-ritonavir association. Report of three cases. Rev Med Chil. 2011;139(12):1597–600.

92. Brancaccio G, Celoria GM, Falco E. Ergotism. J Vasc Surg. 2008;48(3):754.

93. Musikatavorn K, Suteparuk S. Ergotism unresponsive to multiple therapeutic modalities, including sodium nitroprusside, resulting in limb loss. Clin Toxicol (Phila). 2008;46(2):157–8.

94. Piquemal R, Emmerich J, Guilmot JL, Fiessinger JN. Successful treatment of ergotism with Iloprost – a case report. Angiology. 1998;49(6):493–7.

95. Schmutz J-L, Barbaud A, Trechot P. Pseudoporphyria and coxib. Ann Dermatol Venereol. 2006;133(2):213.

96. Turnbull N, Callan M, Staughton RCD. Diclofenac-induced pseudoporphyria; an under-recognized condition? Clin Exp Dermatol. 2014;39(3):348–50.

97. Cron RQ, Finkel TH. Nabumetone induced pseudoporphyria in childhood. J Rheumatol. 2000;27(7):1817–8.

98. Maerker JM, Harm A, Foeldvari I, Höger PH. Naproxen-induced pseudoporphyria. Hautarzt. 2001;52(11):1026–9.

99. Roche M, Daly P, Crowley V, Darby C, Barnes L. A case of porphyria cutanea tarda resulting in digital amputation and improved by anastrozole. Clin Exp Dermatol. 2007;32(3):327–8.

100. Prendiville JS, Crow YJ. Blue (or purple) toes: chilblains or chilblain lupus-like lesions are a manifestation of Aicardi–Goutières syndrome and familial chilblain lupus. J Am Acad Dermatol. 2009;61(4):727–8.

101. Lee-Kirsch MA, Gong M, Schulz H, Rüschendorf F, Stein A, Pfeiffer C, et al. Familial chilblain lupus, a monogenic form of cutaneous lupus erythematosus, maps to chromosome 3p. Am J Hum Genet. 2006;79(4):731–7.

102. Perdan-Pirkmajer K, Praprotnik S, Tomšič M. Digital ulcers as the first manifestation of carpal tunnel syndrome. Rheumatol Int. 2011;31(5):685–6.

103. Simonnet N, Marcantoni N, Simonnet L, Griffon C, Chakfe N, Wertheimer J, et al. Puffy hand in long-term intravenous drug users. J Mal Vasc. 2004;29(4):201–4.

104. Cowan NC, Kane P, Karani J. Case report: metallic mercury embolism – deliberate self-injection. Clin Radiol. 1992;46(5):357–8.

105. Johnson-Arbor K. Images in clinical medicine. Digital frostbite. N Engl J Med. 2014;370(2):e3.

106. Ashokkumar GK, Madhu R, Shaji M, Singh BR. Bilateral symmetrical digital gangrene of upper and lower limbs due to purpura fulminans caused by Streptococcus pyogenes: a rare entity. Indian J Crit Care Med. 2015;19(5):290–1.

107. Alves JV, Matos DM, Furtado CM, Fernandes Bártolo EA. Bacillary angiomatosis presenting as a digital ulcer. Indian J Dermatol Venereol Leprol. 2015;81(4):398–400.

108. Akhtar N, Begum M, Saleh AA, Paul HK, Uddin MJ, Chowdhury AQ. Cutaneous sporotrichosis. Mymensingh Med J. 2010;19(3):458–61.

109. Chaabane H, Turki H. Images in clinical medicine. Cutaneous leishmaniasis with a paronychia-like lesion. N Engl J Med. 2014;371(18):1736.

110. Bouchentouf R, Benjelloun A, Aitbenasser MA. Digital ulcers revealing lung carcinoma. Rev Pneumol Clin. 2012;68(6):367–9.

111. Allen D, Robinson D, Mittoo S. Paraneoplastic Raynaud's phenomenon in a breast cancer survivor. Rheumatol Int. 2010; 30(6):789–92.
112. Pronk WG, Baars JP, De Jong PC, Westermann AM. Some unusual paraneoplastic syndromes. Case 2. Digital ulceration as a paraneoplastic syndrome in ovarian cancer. J Clin Oncol. 2003;21(13):2620–2.
113. Ohtsuka T, Yamakage A, Yamazaki S. Digital ulcers and necroses: novel manifestations of angiocentric lymphoma. Br J Dermatol. 2000;142(5):1013–6.
114. Field J, Lane IF. Carcinoma of the lung presenting with digital ischaemia. Thorax. 1986;41(7):573–4.
115. Hladunewich M, Sawka C, Fam A, Franssen E. Raynaud's phenomenon and digital gangrene as a consequence of treatment for Kaposi's sarcoma. J Rheumatol. 1997;24(12):2371–5.

Part VII

The Local Treatment of Skin Ulcers in Systemic Sclerosis

The Local Treatment: Methodology, Debridement and Wound Bed Preparation

Guya Piemonte, Laura Benelli, Francesca Braschi, and Laura Rasero

The Assessment

The local treatment of ulcers is based on a methodological approach that considers the type of lesion and any variables (infection, associated pain, localization, dimensions) that can be present at baseline, or it can occur subsequently. Therefore, a preliminary assessment is always necessary to develop an effective treatment.

The classification of upper and lower limb systemic sclerosis (SSc) ulcers [1, 2] defines the ulcer type and provides the fundamental elements to decide the type of local treatment (e.g. removal of calcinotic deposits in DU or the curettage of DPS) and also the information necessary to make a prognosis defining the risk of recurrences.

Ulcers and Pain

Ulcers are often a source of moderate/severe pain, which may cause functional impairment and deeply affect patient's health-related quality of life (HRQoL) [3]. Ulcer-related pain must be always analysed and classified (WUWHS classification, 2004) [4] (see Table 18.1).

Assessing skin ulcers' related pain is crucial to verify the effectiveness of the therapeutic approach and to plan a correct local treatment.

At baseline, the clinician must evaluate pain to decide an antalgic therapy which should be changed if the previous therapy was ineffective. An increased amount of necrotic tissue, infection and a not suitable dressing may be potential sources of pain. Therefore, the local approach should start by the removal of the dead or infected tissue. Moreover, an adequate dressing is mandatory to maintain the wound bed moist and protect the tissue. It is also important to assess the onset of critical ischaemia which can cause pain and need a systemic therapeutic approach to prevent its evolution to necrosis and/or gangrene.

During the change of the dressing, the detersion and the debridement of the wound bed, some procedural problems may be encountered. First, if the dressing is adherent to the wound bed, it is useful to use warm sterile saline solution to moist the attached medication and remove it gently. The use of medications that provide a warm moist environment without sticking to the wound bed is always recommended.

The detersion must be performed using warm (37 °C) sterile saline solution to avoid tissue thermal shock using a 10 ml syringe to reduce rinsing pressure on DU.

At least 15 min before debridement, the application of lidocaine/prilocaine ointments (cream 2.5%/2.5%) or gauze with lidocaine solution (2–4%) to control pain and to perform a safe and effective debridement is fundamental.

G. Piemonte
Department of Health Science, University of Florence, Florence, Italy

L. Benelli
Nurse Independent Contractor, Florence, Italy

F. Braschi (✉)
Health Professions Department, Azienda Ospedaliera Universitaria Careggi, Florence, Italy
e-mail: braschif@aou-careggi.toscana.it

L. Rasero
Department of Health Sciences, University of Florence – Careggi of Hospital, Florence, Italy

M. Matucci-Cerinic, C. P. Denton (eds.), *Atlas of Ulcers in Systemic Sclerosis*, https://doi.org/10.1007/978-3-319-98477-3_18

Table 18.1 DU-related pain, classification, definitions and evaluation tools

Type of pain	Definition	Assessment tools
Background pain	Background pain can be described as a continuous sharp and/or throbbing sensation which is present at rest and is relatively constant. It is generally associated with DU aetiology and other local factors (ischaemia, infection, eventual reaction to a medication) A severe and intense pain spreading from the ulcer to the whole arm may indicate a critical infection	1. Tools for subjective evaluation VAS (visual analogue scale) NRS scale (numeric rating scale) 2. Tools for subjective evaluation suitable for children, cognitively impaired patients, subjects with speech and language disorders VRS
Episodic (breakthrough) pain	Transitory flare of pain generally occurring during the daily activities	Wong-Baker scale McGill questionnaire
Procedural pain	Transitory pain occurring during a specific therapeutic procedure (dressing change, DU detersion, debridement)	3. Tools for objective evaluation FLACC scale (face, legs, activity, cry, consolability scale)

> **Instructions to Control DU-Related Pain**
>
> **Background Pain**
> - Initiate/change antalgic therapy.
> - Assess new onset of infection.
> - Assess new onset of critical ischaemia.
> - Evaluate RP severity and intensity (Raynaud's Condition Score – RCS) [5].
> - Assess efficacy of local therapy (change type of medication/gauze).
>
> **Procedural Pain**
> *During Dressing Change*
> - Remove gently the previous dressing using warm sterile saline solution.
> - Use nonadhesive medications.
> - Use hydrogel which hydrates viable tissue and protects cutaneous nerve endings.
> - Assess efficacy of local therapy (change type of medication/gauze).
>
> *During DU Detersion*
> - Rinse and irrigate the ulcer with warm (37°C) sterile saline solution.
> - Reduce rinsing pressure using 10 ml syringe.
>
> *Before Sharp Debridement*
> - Application of lidocaine/prilocaine ointments (cream 2.5%/2.5%)
> - Application of gauze with lidocaine solution (2–4%)

Ulcer Dimension and Depth

The ulcer dimension should be monitored over time to assess the healing process. Experts agree on the fact that a reduction of wound area from 20% to 40% in 2–4 weeks of treatment is a sign of a good healing process [6].

However, due to the small DU dimensions, it is difficult to ensure a reliable measurement. Therefore, to assess the DU dimension, it is necessary to use photographic records with standard anatomical reference points and unit of measurement adequately defined. Photographic records can be stored and used for research purposes only with patient's written consent. Figure 18.1 reports DU measurement.

The following staging of ulcers has been proposed:

- Superficial: partial thickness skin loss involving epidermis (Fig. 18.2).
- Intermediate: full thickness skin loss involving damage to, or necrosis of, subcutaneous tissue that may extend down to, but not through, the underlying fascia (Fig. 18.3).
- Deep: full thickness skin loss with extensive destruction or damage to muscle down over the fascia to the bone. All the structures, tendon, joint capsule and bone are usually involved (Fig. 18.4).

All these types of ulcers must be considered as potentially critical due to the high risk of infection and the evolution to severe complications as necrosis and gangrene [1].

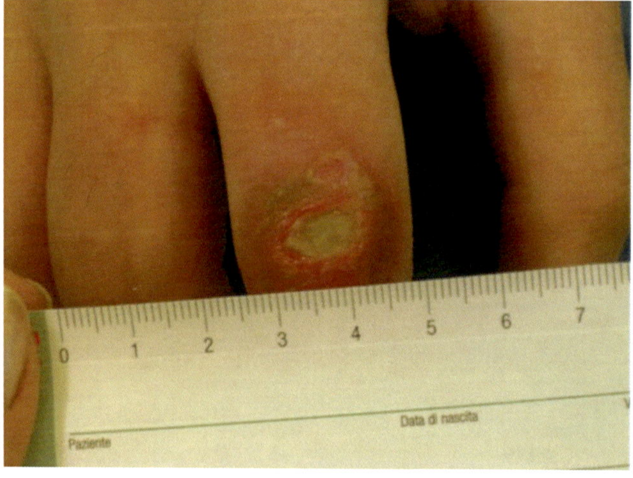

Fig. 18.1 DU measurement

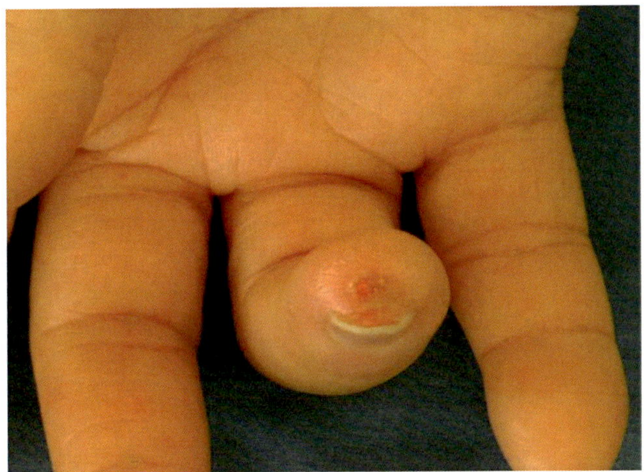

Fig. 18.2 Superficial – partial thickness skin loss involving the epidermis only

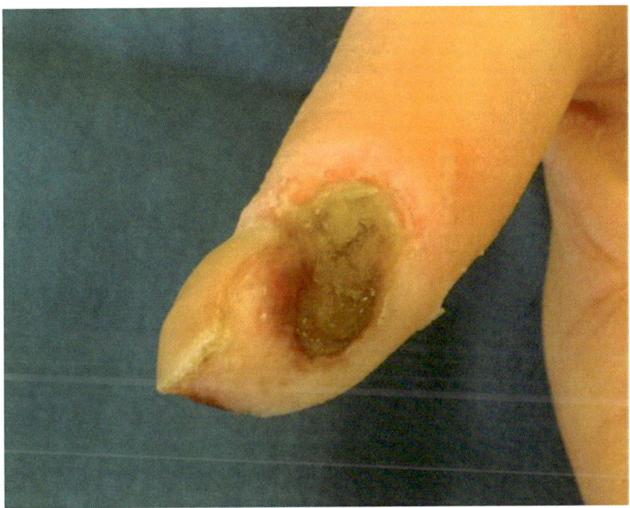

Fig. 18.3 Intermediate – full thickness skin loss involving necrosis of subcutaneous tissue

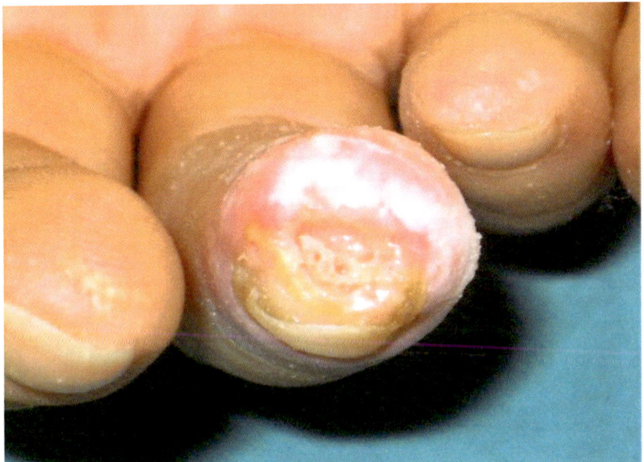

Fig. 18.4 Deep – full thickness skin loss down to the bone

The Wound Bed Preparation (WBP)

In SSc, the local therapy of ulcers is based on the principles of WBP, which has gained international recognition as a structured approach to the management of chronic wounds (a chronic wound is defined as a wound which lasts more than 6 weeks) [7]. The definition of WBP is "the management of an ulcer in order to accelerate endogenous healing or to facilitate the effectiveness of other therapeutic measures".

To explain the correct strategy to approach an ulcer, the acronym TIME was developed in 2002 by a group of experts as a practical guide to summarize the four main components of WBP [8]:

- *T*: *T*issue management
- *I*: Control of infection and inflammation
- *M*: *M*oisture imbalance
- *E*: Advancement of the epithelial edges of the wound

The TIME approach is a strategical framework which is a useful and practical tool to identify the main elements that should be considered to achieve a steady healing and to carry out a plan of care apt to promote wound healing.

Tissue Management "T"

The assessment of the tissue consists in a careful observation of the characteristics of the ulcer considering its bed, edges and the perilesional skin. The primary goal of this step is the identification of the main barriers to a steady healing that are the biofilm, the bioburden, the slough and the nonviable or deficient tissue (Table 18.2).

The treatment of tissue is carried out following two different steps:

1. The first step is *detersion* – the mechanical removal of dirt, cellular debris, necrotic tissue, remnants of previous dressings and other wastes present on the wound bed and on the surrounding skin [14, 15]. It can be performed by irrigating with a warm (37 °C) saline solution (NaCl 0.9%) and using a 35 ml syringe and 19 G needle for lower limb ulcers and a 10 ml syringe and a 19G needle cannula for all the other types of ulcers, modulating the strength applied on the plunger (Fig. 18.5).

Table 18.2 Barriers to healing in SSc cutaneous ulcers

Barriers to healing	Definition
Biofilm	A biofilm is defined as a structured conglomerate of microbial cells encompassed by polymer matrix produced by the host [9]. Fibrin, platelets or immunoglobulins may be present into the biofilm [10]
Bioburden	The concept of bioburden includes the following dimensions: the microbial load, the pathogenicity, the virulence and the diversity of the microorganisms across the wound bed [11]
Slough	Nonviable tissue which facilitates the development of biofilm [12]
Nonviable or deficient tissue	Ischaemic tissue, no longer viable [13]

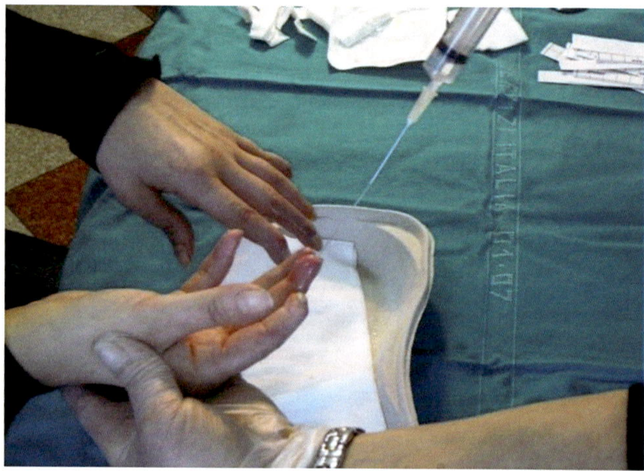

Fig. 18.5 Detersion of a fingertip digital ulcer in a SSc patient

Instructions for Detersion

- Detersion – irrigation of the wound with saline solution (NaCl 0.9%) and applying a pressure ranging from 8 to 15 psi (using a 35 ml syringe and a 19G needle). This procedure allows an efficient detersion without damaging the granulating tissue.
- The detersion may be extremely painful for SSc patients; in these situations it is mandatory to decrease remarkably the irrigating pressure. This is possible using a 10 ml syringe and a 19G needle cannula modulating the strength applied on the plunger.
- In order to avoid vasospastic attacks, the irrigating solution must be warmed (37°C).
  2. The second step is *debridement* which is defined as follows: "The removal of necrotic material, eschar, nonviable tissue, infected tissue, slough, pus, foreign bodies, cellular debris, bone fragments or any other kind of bioburden from a wound in order to promote its healing" [8]. Thus, debridement mainly consists in the removal of nonviable material, foreign bodies and necrotic tissue from a wound. Surgical resection of viable tissue or surgical amputation is not included in the debridement procedure. Debridement procedure must be carried out also on wound edges and perilesional skin. There are five types of debridement:

- *Passive debridement* – It is based on the enhancement of the physiological and endogenous processes of debridement naturally occurring in a healing wound.

- *Active debridement* – It is carried out by a physician using specific surgical tools.
- *Selective debridement* – It consists on the selective removal of nonviable tissue, preserving viable material and granulating tissue.
- *Nonselective debridement* – It consists on the removal of healthy or/and nonviable tissue.
- *Maintenance debridement* [7] – In chronic wounds, in which the normal process of healing has been disrupted, the necrotic burden continually accumulates on the ulcer surface. In these cases, it may be more appropriate to perform regular or even continuous debridement. In SSc, the maintenance debridement is mandatory on fingertip DU, due to the continuous and fast production of bioburden.

The debridement is recommended in all types of SSc wounds. The assessment of the clinical features of a wound (e.g. presence/absence of biofilm, slough, infection, etc.) is essential to choose the adequate type of debridement. In addition many other factors have to be taken into account such as the patient's general health status, the ability of the caregiver and the presence and intensity of wound-related pain, patient's age and HRQoL [8].

Table 18.3 shows the most frequent methods of debridement in SSc. They are frequently performed in association. In Table 18.4, the instructions for an efficacious debridement are displayed.

Principal Goals of Debridement in SSc Ulcers
- Removing all barriers to healing
- Decreasing the amount of exudate
- Decreasing wound smell
- Reducing the risk of infection
- Decreasing the pain intensity (necrotic/nonviable tissue produces algogenic toxins)
- Promoting the proliferation of viable and granulating tissue
- Improving patient's HRQoL

Table 18.3 Methods of debridement in SSc ulcers

Methods of debridement	Tools (dressings/surgical instruments)	Description
Autolytic debridement is a physiological and highly specific process by which endogenous proteolytic enzymes break down necrotic tissue. Every healing wound naturally experiences this kind of process in some level. This debridement method takes advantage of the moist and warm environment present on the interface between the wound bed and the dressing. Autolytic debridement doesn't cause pain or discomfort to the patient, but it is a slow method of nonviable tissue removal. Owing to this characteristic autolytic debridement is often combined with other types of debridement or in case of minimal production of bioburden [8, 16]	*Hydrogel*	Hydrated carboxymetil-cellulose polymer dressings, containing 90% water in a gel base, which helps regulate fluid exchange from the wound surface. Hydrogels are used in association with sharp debridement
	Hydrocolloids	Occlusive or semi-occlusive dressings composed of carboxymethyl cellulose, pectin, and elastomers. They jellify absorbing the wound exudate This type of dressing is rarely used in SSc, owing to its occlusive nature Hydrocolloids may cause discomfort and harm perilesional sclerotic skin
Sharp debridement – It is a minor surgical debridement which is usually carried out using scalpels, courgettes and scissors. It is a bedside procedure, which main goal is the removal of nonviable tissue. It is considered as a selective debridement, and it causes severe procedural pain. This problem could be overcome with the use of topically applied local anaesthetics (lidocaine), applied 30–45 min prior to debridement The real surgical debridement is a procedure performed by surgeons using general anaesthesia. It is the fastest way to remove wide patches of nonviable tissue especially in areas where there is a significant risk of lesion of major anatomical structures or in case of severe infections [17, 18]	*Scalpel and forceps*	It is used if the necrotic tissue is markedly separated from viable one This procedure must follow a thorough evaluation of patient's general health condition to rule out clotting disorders The tissue removed should be evaluated to assess eventual infectious processes The surgical site must be treated with antiseptics

Table 18.4 Instructions for debridement

Instructions	Rationale
A. Preliminary treatments and detersion	
1. Observe thoroughly the previous dressing	To notice and record signs of excessive exudation
2. Remove atraumatically the previous dressing, stretching the edges of the bandage in parallel to the skin. If the bandage was stuck to the perilesional skin and/or to the wound bed, it would be necessary to wet it with warm (37 °C) sterile saline solution or Ringer's lactate solution	Remove the dressing atraumatically
3. Clean the wound bed and the perilesional skin as summarized in *instructions for detersion* (above)	To remove foreign bodies, bioburden and exudate poorly adherent to the wound without damaging the granulating tissue
4. Get a compress with a gauze wet with 0.1% undecylenamidopropyl betaine/0.1% polyamide water solution for about 15 min	To remove the biofilm and prepare the wound for debridement
5. *Local analgesia* – it is recommended in case of sharp debridement. It would be useful in case of painful dressing removal. The antalgic effect must be verified before debridement The analgesic method is chosen based on the pain score previously recorded: 2.5% lidocaine/2.5% prilocaine cream compress (for 15 min) [19] Lidocaine hydrochloride, 2% water solution compress (for 15 min) [20] Lidocaine hydrochloride, 4% water solution compress (for 15 min)	To reduce the procedural pain Contraindications: allergy to the analgesic medication
B. Debridement	

Sharp debridement: the debridement is carried out by a sterile scalpel (blade 15 or 10) or a sterile courgette
The wound bed and the perilesional skin must be both debrided (Fig. 18.6). Calcium deposits –*calcinosis* (stone, mousse, web) must be removed by sharp debridement (Fig. 18.7)
A specific training is recommended to perform sharp debridement and to avoid damaging of granulating tissue
Figure 18.8 shows a fingertip digital ulcer covered by slough.
Figure 18.9 shows the same lesion after several sessions of local treatment
	To remove necrotic tissue, slough, exudate and calcium deposits
	Sharp debridement must be performed on hyperkeratotic areas too (DPS)
	This type of debridement must not be carried out in case of clotting disorders
	Sharp debridement is not recommended in the following situations:
	    When it's not possible the local analgesia
	    If the patient can't tolerate the procedure itself
	Calcification in a wound creates chronic foreign body inflammatory reaction that contributes to a non-healing ulcer if calcific deposits are not removed. The removal of these deposits is essential to promote healing

Table 18.4 (continued)

Instructions	Rationale
Autolytic debridement: the type of primary dressing has to be chosen considering the amount of exudate and the dryness of the wound bed: Heavily exuding wounds: alginate dressing, hydrofibers Dried lesions/poorly exuding wounds/necrotic wounds: hydrogels, hydrocolloids The dressing has to be shaped based on the DU size *Secondary dressings*: secondary dressing provides several important functions such as holding the primary dressing in the correct position, protecting the wound site from traumatic events or environmental factors (temperature/moisture) and camouflaging the dressing and providing treatment to the wound in synergy with primary dressing For DU it is important to apply protective secondary dressings (foams) A protective secondary dressing is shaped and based on the DU size; secondly we put on the top a TNT gauze stripe (15 × 100 mm), paying attention to keep the primary dressing in the correct place Cut three stripes of adhesive tape: n. 2 stripes 10 × 40 mm 8 (to place on the fingertip forming a cross) n. 1 stripe 10 × 100 mm (to cover the TNT gauze wrapping the fingertip). Figure 18.10 shows how to apply an adequate secondary dressing for a DU	Autolytic debridement can be used combined with sharp debridement or as primary treatment Hydrogel is often applied to the wound bed after the sharp debridement to carry on the removal of bioburden (*maintenance debridement*) and to moisture and to keep the granulating tissue healthy A specific training is not necessary to perform autolytic debridement. It is an easy procedure that can be performed by a caregiver too Foams (secondary dressing) are useful to protect the DU from traumatic events and to reduce episodic pain too The TNT gauze protects the primary dressings and holds them in the correct position The secondary dressing must not be tight, in order to allow the digital perfusion The overall thickness of the dressing (primary +secondary dressing) has to be as thin as possible in order not to interfere with finger movements and to allow to wear protective gloves

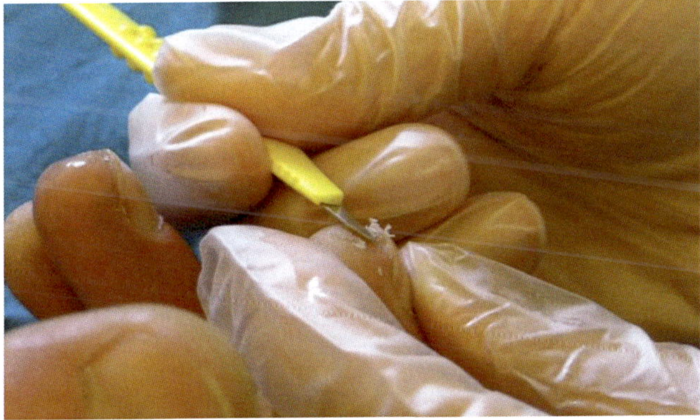

Fig. 18.6 Sharp debridement in a DU

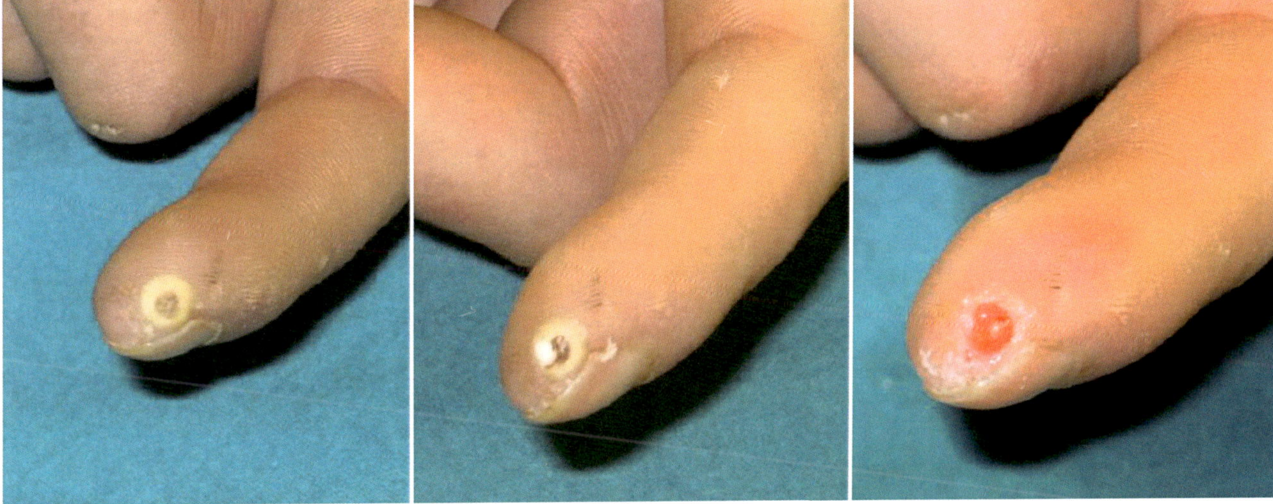

Fig. 18.7 Sharp debridement in a calcinosis

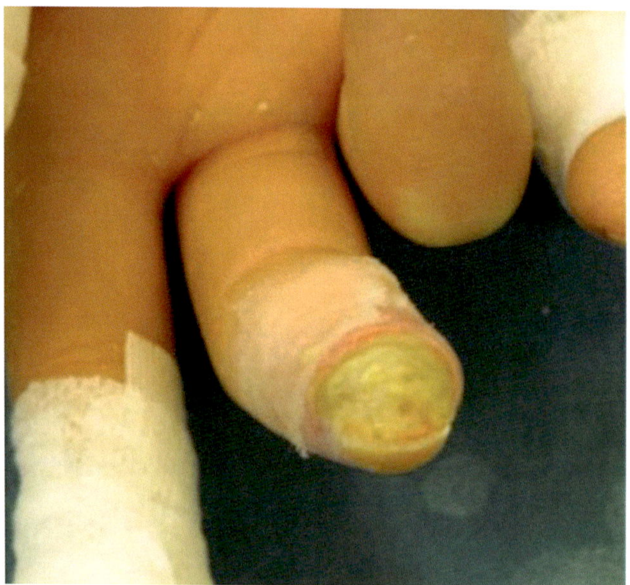

Fig. 18.8 DU covered by slough

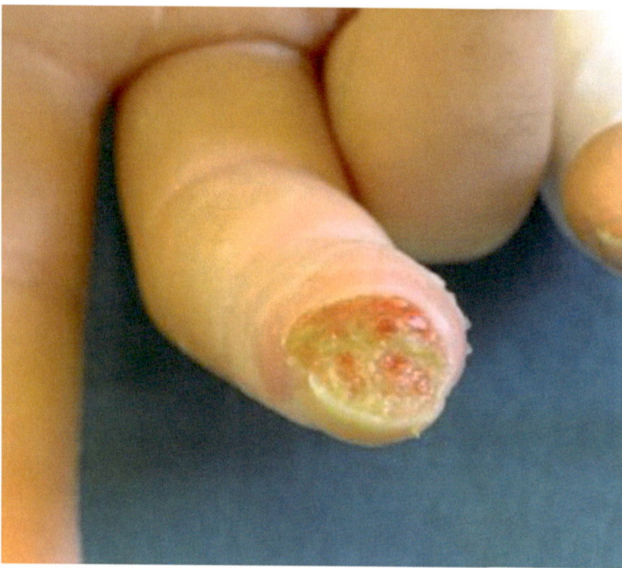

Fig. 18.9 DU after several sessions of local therapy based on sharp debridement and application of adequate dressings

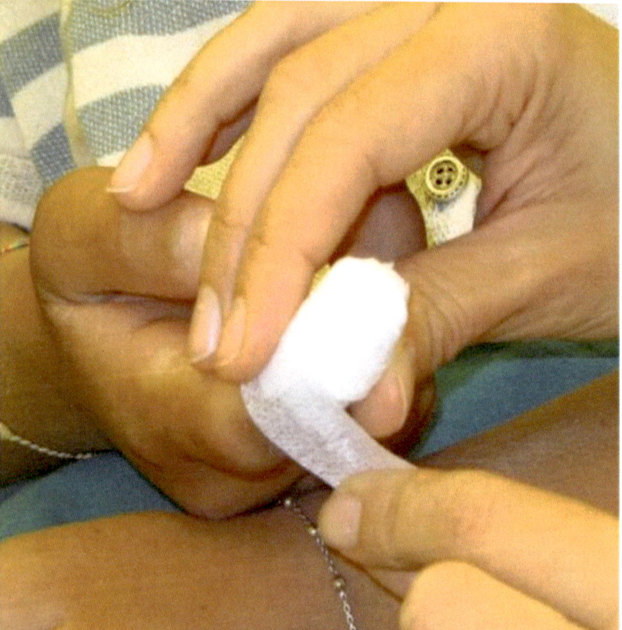

Fig. 18.10 Secondary dressing – application

Identification of Signs and Symptoms of Infection and Treatment "I"

In WBP, the correct approach to an inflamed or/an infected ulcer is pivotal to avoid the delay or even the block of the healing process.

Inflammation

It is a physiological response to tissue damage and it leads the way to wound healing. However, excessive or inappropriate inflammatory response – common in infection – can have serious consequences for the patient. Inflammation is not only related to physiological healing or to infection process. A persistent inflammation can lead to a stall of the healing process, favouring its chronicization and the block of wound healing. In chronic wounds, studies underline the fact that inflammation phase may become a disrupting event: in fact, fibroblasts from chronic wounds are dysfunctional; they show a premature senescence, and they are not responsive to growth factors. Fibrin on the wound bed seems to block the production of growth factors. The exudate of chronic wound exudate shows an increased activity of matrix metalloproteinases (MMPs), elastases and cytokines [19, 21, 22]. All these elements hinder the covering movement of the wound edges thus worsening the wound conditions.

Infection

Definition of "infection" is one of the most debated topics as there are many factors that take part in the development of infection where there is a critical bacterial wound colonization.

The infection process depends on the following:

- Bacterial burden (number of microorganism on the wound bed)
- Pathogen virulence (ability to produce toxins, invasiveness)
- Host resistance (capability to resist to bacterial growth through an effective immune response)

The presence of microorganism on wound's surface does not necessarily mean the presence of injury to the host. Contamination at wound site is common in any ulcer, and a constant number of bacteria are present on the wound bed usually not slowing the healing process. A real infection is a characterized by a critical bacterial colonization of the ulcer that can spread over the surrounding tissue: this is due to some concomitants, and usually this process follows a typical time continuum.

Biofilm

Most recent studies about the management of wound bed underlines the increasing importance of assessing and treating biofilms [23]. A biofilm is a complex microbial community, consisting of bacteria endowed in a protective matrix of sugars and proteins (glycocalyx). Biofilms are known to form on the surface of medical devices and are also found in wounds. Bacteria communities embedded within biofilm are partially protected from antimicrobials, environmental stresses and host's immune responses. The interaction between those microorganisms and host tissue is parasitical: bacteria get stable attachment and nutrition. Biofilms are a major contributing factor to chronic inflammatory changes in the wound bed. The chronic inflammation benefits the organisms in the biofilm which gains a higher resistance against antimicrobial and immune activity (phagocytosis, immune complex). Biofilm removal is fundamental to improve wound condition and to lead towards healing: it can be eradicated through debridement, though it can be treated with less invasive techniques such combinations of surfactant and products with antimicrobial activity.

Diagnosis

Diagnosis of infection in chronic skin ulcer is based upon bacteriological examination after the removal of biological material from the wound. Culture is indicated to identify the microorganisms and to guide antibiotic therapy. Swab culture is the most frequently employed method for confirming wound infection.

In everyday clinical practice, when infection is suspected, a prompt action must be taken, without waiting for the culture response, in order to prevent progression. The clinical evaluation of the lesion and the general conditions of the patient are sufficient to set a therapeutic plan on empirical basis in order to quickly stop the infection process and the deterioration of the wound. Afterwards, the result of the culture will be useful to confirm the infection and to set up an antimicrobial therapy.

Local Treatment of Infected Ulcer

Infections in DU have to be prevented or treated as soon as possible because they can lead to gangrene, osteomyelitis or self-amputation [24]. For this reason, local treatment in chronic wounds can be undertaken also as prevention or when an infection is probable because of the presence of typical signs and symptoms but without the evidence of an infection in the culture. Local therapy is based on broad-spectrum antimicrobial dressings and does not cause micro-bial resistance [25]. Table 18.5 reports the most frequent antimicrobial local treatments.

In SSc, DUs are often infected because of their specific localization (touching people, objects, surfaces). Poor patient's general conditions (malnutrition) and their hand disability increase the risk of infection. Moreover, the impairment of the immune response and sclerodactyly reduces the capacity to keep the hands clean [28]. In Table 18.6 the instructions for an efficacious management of infected ulcers are displayed.

Table 18.5 Main antimicrobial local treatments and their characteristics

Chlorine-based disinfectant (sodium hypochlorite in 0.05% water solution)	Before managing debridement it is useful to make a poultice with chlorine-based disinfectant for at least 10 min.
Antimicrobial dressings [26]	
1. Silver dressings	Silver has a long history of use as a topical antimicrobial in wound care Silver is a broad-spectrum antimicrobial. Although there is no scientific evidence supporting this recommendation, it is broadly used in everyday practice. Anyway some studies underline its efficacy in promoting the healing process [20]. Silver is incorporated into dressings either as nanocrystalline silver or ionized silver; this is the most common type of silver dressing
2. DACC dressings (dial carbamoyl chloride)	DACC encourages a natural hydrophobic interaction whereby hydrophobic organisms are attracted and irreversibly bound in the dressing hydrous environment. It seems that this process is effective on a variety of bacteria and some fungi. DACC dressing have a lighter antimicrobial effect than silver ones, but they have almost any cytotoxicity, and they cause no resistance
3. Iodine dressings	Iodine-based preparations have a long history of use in surgery and wound care. Some studies and a review demonstrate the effectiveness of cadexomer iodine in the healing of venous ulcers burdened by infection [27]
4. PHMB dressings	The polyhexamethylene biguanide (PHMB) is a broad-spectrum antimicrobial agent which is effective in both decreasing bacterial load and preventing bacterial penetration of the dressing. It also has a low cellular toxicity. PHMB dressings can be found as foams or gel

Table 18.6 Instructions for proper management of infected ulcers

Instructions	Rationale
1. Assessment of patient general health conditions noticing systemic signs and symptoms of infection/inflammation: appearance or increase of pain, uneasiness, fever	An infected ulcer can cause systemic effects. Suspect osteomyelitis in presence of fever, severe pain worsening with limb irradiation, oedema spread to the whole hand or leg and disability
2. Remove and check old dressing	Assess signs of moisture imbalance and changes in its components: wound smell/colour
3. Observe the ulcer in all its characteristics (signs and symptoms of topical infection/inflammation – Fig. 18.11)	Appearance of these signs can be related to a phlogistic or infective process that has to be assessed and marked down in nursing clinical records
4. *Wound bed*: granulating tissue fragile and hyperemic, unusual bleeding, change in wound bed colour, areas of necrosis, increasing fibrinous tissue, increased/purulent exudate. Notice possible presence of slime (opaque film spread all over the wound)	
5. *Wound edges:* no progression nor viability of wound edges. Take account of undermined edges	
6. *Perilesional skin*: rush, swelling and heat, tenderness	
7. *In general terms:* healing delay and further deterioration of the wound	
8. Measurement and photography of the ulcer	This allows comparing images and data before and after
9. Cleansing of the wound following the *instructions for detersion* (above)	Removal of dirt, shreds of previous dressings, debris and metabolic wastes
10. When there are clear signs of local or global infection (fever, aching of the whole limb, oedema, rush, purulent exudate, characteristic smell, functional impairment), perform a poultice for at least 10 min with a gauze soaked in a 0.025% hydrous solution of sodium hypochlorite. After the poultice removing the solution from wound bed with saline	Antisepsis method is chosen based on wound conditions: using sodium hypochlorite solution is the most aggressive method; it is chosen in case of clear infection. After application of this solution, it is important to wash it away from the wound bed through detersion, so that you can get rid of antiseptic residues that may have cytotoxic effects on granulation tissue

Table 18.6 (continued)

Instructions	Rationale
11. Analgesia and debridement by following the instructions in Table 18.4.	Eliminate/reduce procedural pain
12. Proper choice of dressing:	
(a) *Infected wound or systemic signs of infection (fever, pain widespread to the limb, oedema, redness, purulent exudate, characteristic odour, reduced functionality)* Semiquantitative swab. Ask the physicians for an eventual antibiotic therapy Apply iodine or silver dressings Warn the patient that mild local pain symptoms are common with silver dressings Choose combined dressings if necessary for the management of exudate and odour	When infection is highly suspected, the antibiotic therapy can be prescribed based upon the semiquantitative swab Silver and iodine have antimicrobic characteristics. Sometimes these dressings can lead to the development of resistance Gain information about eventual patient sensitivity to silver If iodine dressing is chosen, it is important to assess eventual thyroid diseases because of the possibility of systemic absorption of iodine Activated charcoal dressings reduce foul odour from the ulcer Restrict the use of silver dressings only in cases of overt infection to reduce the risk of resistance
(b) *Swollen wound with specific signs (increase in fibrin production and exudate, hypergranulation, bleeding, discoloration)* Recommendation of the following dressings: silver dressings, DACC dressings, PHMB dressings, honey or hypertonic saline dressings	These dressings have a less aggressive antimicrobic property but a higher tolerability
(c) *Not progressing wound without signs of infection/inflammation* Apply DACC or PHMB dressings but also saline or honey dressings	Often the delay in healing is the first sign of infection. Not healing wounds suspect infection; therefore, antimicrobic dressing can be used even if only for preventive purpose
1. Assess the need for a secondary dressing with absorbent or protective function.	Proper exudate management. Reducing risk of injuries and occasional pain
2. Wound closure following the instructions in Table 18.4	

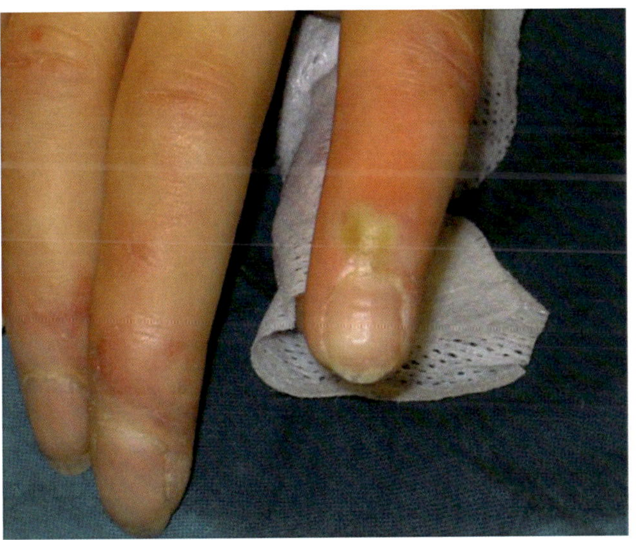

Fig. 18.11 A periungual-infected ulcer

Moisture Balance: Maceration or Dryness "M"

Managing exudate in chronic wounds is fundamental: wound epithelialization is stimulated by a moist environment, but an excess of fluid can macerate the healthy skin and delay the healing for the high content of proinflammatory cytokines and metalloproteinases that decrease the healing progression. The increased proteolytic activity of chronic wound exudate is thought to inhibit healing by damaging the wound bed, degrading the extracellular matrix and aggravating the integrity of the peri-wound skin, while the high levels of cytokines promote and prolong the chronic inflammatory response seen in these wounds.

The quantity and quality of wound exudate are associated with several factors:

- Ulcer surface
- Type of wound
- Stage in healing process
- Infection
- Oedema
- Local treatments

High exudate volume is one of the problems of chronic wounds that, with smell too, highly affect the patient quality of life. Excessive exudate production brings to a loss of protein, worsening malnutrition and increasing oedema. Moreover it increases the risk of infection as it favours the conditions for the replication of microorganisms. Wound leakage causes high distress in patients because it makes the wound smelly and it can soil clothes. Wound bed dryness is a relevant problem which blocks wound healing and is frequent in SSc ulcers where it may be due to low blood provision typical of microcirculation pathologies. Table 18.7 shows the adequate management of dry wounds. Table 18.8 shows how to manage the fluid balance in SSc ulcers both for the location, for the microvascular damage and for the dysfunction of the connective tissue (Table 18.9).

Table 18.7 The most frequent medications to treat dry ulcers

Hydrogel: hydrated carboxymetil –cellulose polymer dressings, containing 90% water in a gel base	Because of their structure, they have moisturizing properties. They also bring on the debridement of necrotic tissue
Hydrocolloid dressings (*occlusive dressings*): occlusive or semi-occlusive dressings, in contact with exudate, gel slowly	To be used in wounds not completely dehydrated. They keep the humidity at an optimum level. Contraindicated in case of infection
Paraffin gauze: gauze dressing impregnated with paraffin. These are water-repellent dressings; therefore, they do not absorb the exudate, and they keep it in contact with the wound bed	This kind of dressing is commonly used for the protection of the wound in the phase of re-epithelialization: at this step it is important to promote the maintenance of a moist environment. It is not recommended in case of ulcers "firm" or suspected of being infected
Polyurethane film: these dressings promote the moisture on the wound bed	They are impermeable to liquids but not to gases

Table 18.8 Instructions to balance fluid

Instructions	Rationale
1. Remove the previous dressing. Assess the quantity and quality of exudate	Observe old dressing: you can notice if it has been a good choice An hyperexudating wound could soak the dressing leading to liquid leakage and edges maceration In case of a dry wound bed, the dressing could adhere to the ulcer, and the removal has to be cautious; it is recommended to irrigate with saline
2. Choosing the dressing that is appropriate to the quantity/quality of exudate	Effective management of exudate

Table 18.9 Instructions to assess and treat the lesion edges and the perilesional skin in scleroderma ulcers

Instructions	Rationale

Assess the functionality of the edges:
  Measure the area of lesion to check if re-epithelialization is progressing (see instructions in *ulcer dimension and depth* section)
  Observe the ratios of new epithelium to granulation tissue, the outline of the edge in relation to the wound bed
  Observe the morphological characteristics of the new epithelium (hyperproliferation of the edges, discoloration and fragility of the new tissue)
  Detect and point out the presence of hyperkeratosis in the edge
	Monitor the healing process advancement
	In the DU the survey of the area may be difficult owing to the small size of the lesion

Assess the perilesional skin: its colour, temperature, dryness/maceration, integrity, pain
1. Interventions on the edges:
  Removal of the nonvital tissue which blocks re-epithelialization and maintains inflammation (debridement of the edges)
  Protection of wound edges from maceration or from agents attacking the new epithelium (collagenase-based preparations, sticking plaster)
  Promotion of the re-epithelialization process with dressings containing metalloprotease-modulating agents, hyaluronic acid, purified collagen
2. Interventions on the skin: protection and hydration
	Detect anomalies in the perilesional skin
	Create the environment which most favours wound closure
	The application of ointment containing vitamin e makes the skin elastic and trophic and appears to reduce recovery time [34]

Epidermis and Epithelial Edges "E"

The evolution of the healing process is shown by the growth of the epithelial edges. Assessing the characteristics of the epithelial growth allows understanding whether the ulcer is moving or is "blocked" into the state of chronic lesion. In a healing ulcer, actively proliferating keratinocytes form a line which progressively degrades in the bed made up of ripe granulation tissue. In chronic ulcers with a reduced tendency to recovery, epithelial cells often present phenotypic alterations and a reduced capacity of proliferation and migration [29]. Frequently, the chronic wound edge appears thickened with a typical "clifflike" outline. In addition, hyperproliferation of the edges interfering with the normal cell migration on the wound bed may be observed [30]. The hyperproliferation might be due to the inhibition of apoptosis (programmed cellular death) of keratinocytes and fibroblast [9].

The assessment of the outline of the edges has an important diagnostic value in particular when the edges do not adhere to the wound bed and the wound closure does not take place. The "undermining" of the edges should be always checked out following the "clock" method: the depth of the edges is probed clockwise with a sterile swab along the whole ulcer perimeter [31].

Digital pitting scars (DPS) are frequent and may manifest in the form of microareas of pinhole-sized depression and corneous deposit. The DU secondary to DPS often presents phenomena of undermining as well as a marked thickening and hardening of edges and perilesional skin.

The functionality of the edges also depends from the trophism and conditions of perilesional skin. For the perilesional skin, the following aspects are considered:

- Colour: red/erythematous skin (infection/inflammation), pale skin (ischemia), yellowish skin (hyperkeratosis), cyanotic skin (hypoperfusion)
- Temperature: warm skin (infection/inflammation), cold skin (hypoperfusion)
- Dryness: callosity, hyperkeratosis, hardening
- Maceration: white-greyish skin, softening, wrinkling
- Integrity: epithelial stripping, microlesions (skin tear)
- Pain and tenderness

Education of SSc Patients Affected by Ulcers

The optimal medical strategy for an SSc patient affected by ulcers includes a local and a systemic approach. This synergism promotes skin perfusion and trophism leading to a marked improvement of the patient's condition and to the ulcers' healing.

Nevertheless, to assure lasting results and to properly manage chronic wounds, it is necessary to achieve full patient participation and adherence to the treatments. This means that the clinicians must provide therapeutic educational interventions about dressing, protection of the extremities, self-management and measures to prevent the onset of new DUs. The therapeutic education process includes a thorough evaluation of the patient and its caregivers to assess their skills in self-management.

Basic instructions for skin care and DU prevention and treatment are listed below. These basic skills must be provided to patients and their caregivers.

Moreover the therapeutic education must be focused on the practical skills for DU self-management. Information materials (brochures, videos and educative sessions) could be extremely useful.

A direct helpline led by rheumatology nurses specialized in wound care allows home dweller patient to manage DU treatment and to recognize severe complications on time. Information and support about DU prevention and systemic therapy are given if necessary.

All those measures allow patients' active involvement in DU care and prevention to reduce hospital admission costs.

Life-Style Modifications for SSc Patients

- Wear gloves to reduce the intensity and the frequency of RP attacks when the temperature is cold (below 20 °C).
- Use cotton gloves in warm season too if the temperature is below 20 °C or in air-conditioned rooms [32].
- Protect dressings and medications on DUs using PVC or latex gloves to keep them clean, dry and in the correct position.
- It is mandatory to keep the hands clean.
- Check your hands' conditions daily in order to point out dyschromic areas or any signs of inflammation. Inform wound care nurses about:
  - RP frequency, duration and related pain
  - Itch, erythema or any other kind of cutaneous manifestation
- Don't smoke and don't assume vasoconstrictive agents (caffeine) [33].
- Keep the skin moisturized (with ointments/creams).
- Don't use aggressive soaps or detergents.

References

1. Amanzi L, Braschi F, Fiori G, et al. Digital ulcers in scleroderma: staging, characteristics and sub-setting through observation of 1614 digital lesions. Rheumatology (Oxford). 2010;49:1374–82.

2. Blagojevic J, Piemonte G, Benelli L, et al. Assessment, definition, and classification of lower limb ulcers in systemic sclerosis: a challenge for the rheumatologist. J Rheumatol. 2016;43(3):592–8. https://doi.org/10.3899/jrheum.150035. Epub 2016 Feb 1

3. Galluccio F, Matucci-Cerinic M. Two faces of the same coin: Raynaud phenomenon and digital ulcers in systemic sclerosis. Autoimmun Rev. 2011;10:241–3.

4. World Union of Wound Healing Societies, Principles of Best Practice. Minimising Pain at Wound Dressing-Related Procedures: A Consensus Document. London: Medical Education Partnership; 2004.

5. Pope J. Measures of systemic sclerosis (scleroderma): Health Assessment Questionnaire (HAQ) and Scleroderma HAQ (SHAQ), physician- and patient-rated global assessments, Symptom Burden Index (SBI), University of California, Los Angeles, Scleroderma Clinical Trials Consortium Gastrointestinal Scale (UCLA SCTC GIT) 2.0, Baseline Dyspnea Index (BDI) and Transition Dyspnea Index (TDI) (Mahler's Index), Cambridge Pulmonary Hypertension Outcome Review (CAMPHOR), and Raynaud's Condition Score (RCS). Arthritis Care Res (Hoboken). 2011;63 Suppl 11:S98–111. https://doi.org/10.1002/acr.20598. Review

6. Kantor J, Margolis DJ. A multicenter study of percentage change in venous leg ulcer area, as a prognostic index of healing at 24 weeks. Br J Dermatol. 2000;142(5):960–4.

7. Cutting KF, Tong A. Wound Physiology and Moist Wound Healing. Clinical Education in Wound Management Series. Holsworthy Medical Communication UK Ltd. 2003.

8. Schultz GS, Sibbald RJ. Wound bed preparation: a systematic approach to wound management. Wound Rep Reg. 2003;11:1–28.

9. Hall-Stoodley L, Stoodley P, Kathju S, Hoiby N, Moser C, Costerton JW, Moter A, Bjarnsholt T. Towards diagnostic guidelines for biofilm-associated infections. FEMS Immunol Med Microbiol. 2012;65:127–45.

10. Hoiby N, Bjarnsholt T, Moser C, Bassi GL, et al. ESCMID guideline for the diagnosis and treatment of biofilm infections 2014. Clin Microbiol Infect. 2015;21:S1–25.

11. Grice EA, Segre JA. Interaction of the microbiome with the innate immune response in chronic wounds. Adv Exp Med Biol. 2012;946:55–68.

12. Percival SL, Suleman L. Slough and biofilm: removal of barriers to wound healing by desloughing. J Wound Care. 2015;24(11):498, 500–3, 506–10. https://doi.org/10.12968/jowc.2015.24.11.498.

13. Kirshen C, Woo K, Ayello EA, Sibbald RG. Debridement: a vital component of wound bed preparation. Adv Skin Wound Care. 2006;19:506–17.

14. Strohal R, Apelqvist J, Dissemond J, et al. EWMA Document: Debridement. J Wound Care. 2013;22(Suppl. 1):S1–S52.

15. Rodeheaver GT. Wound cleansing, wound irrigation, wound disinfection. In: Krasner D, Kane D, editors. Chronic wound care: a clinical source book for healthcare professionals. Wayne, PA: Health Management Publications, Inc.; 1997. p. 97–108.

16. Caula C, Apostoli A. Cura e Assistenza al Paziente con Ferite Acute e Ulcere Croniche: Maggioli Editore; 2011.

17. Ramundo J, Gray M. Enzymatic wound debridement. J Wound Ostomy Continence Nurs. 2008;35(3):273–80.

18. Preece J. Sharp debridement: the need for training and education. Nurs Times. 2003;99(5):54–5.

19. Lukashev ME, Werb Z. ECM signalling: orchestrating cell behaviour and misbehaviour. Trends Cell Biol. 1998;8:437–41.

20. Cutting KF, Harding KG. Criteria for identifying wound infection. J Wound Care. 1994;3(4):198–201.

21. Harding KG, Moore K, Phillips TJ. Wound chronicity and fibroblast senescence--implications for treatment. Int Wound J. 2005;2:364–8.

22. Gibson D, Cullen B, Legerstee R, Harding KG, Schultz G. MMPs made easy. Wounds Int. 2010;1:1–6.

23. Bianchi T, Wolcott RD, Peghetti A, Leaper D, et al. Recommendations for the management of biofilm: a consensus document. J Wound Care. 2016;25(6):305–17.

24. Giuggioli D, Manfredi A. Scleroderma digital ulcers complicated by infection with fecal pathogens. Arthritis Care Res. 2012;64(2):295–7.

25. International consensus. Appropriate use of silver dressings in wounds. London: Wounds International; 2012.

26. Lipsky BA, Dryden M, Gottrup F, Nathwani D, Seaton RA, Stryja J. Antimicrobial stewardship in wound care: a Position Paper from the British Society for Antimicrobial Chemotherapy and European Wound Management Association. J Antimicrob Chemother. 2016;71:3026–35. https://doi.org/10.1093/jac/dkw287. Advance Access publication 25 July 2016

27. Leaper DJ. Silver dressings: their role in wound management. Int Wound J. 2006 Dec;3(4):282–94.

28. O'Meara S, Al-Kurdi D, Ovington LG. Antibiotics and antiseptics for venous leg ulcers. Cochrane Database Syst Rev. 2008;1:CD003557.

29. Lawton S, Langøen A. Assessing and managing vulnerable periwound skin. World Wide Wounds http://www.worldwidewounds.com/2009/October/Lawton-Langoen/vulnerable-skin-2.html. Accessed 4 Nov 2015.

30. Falanga V. The chronic wound: impaired healing and solutions in the context of wound bed preparation. Blood Cells Mol Dis. 2004 Jan-Feb;32(1):88–94.

31. Al-Najjar M, Jackson MJ. Non-healing leg ulcers in a patient with dystrophic calcification and crest syndrome: a challenging clinical case. Int Wound J. 2011;8:537–41.

32. Woo K, Ayello EA, Sibbald RG. The edge effect: current therapeutic options to advance the wound edge. Adv Skin Wound Care. 2007;20(2):99–117.

33. Fiori G, Galluccio F, Braschi F, et al. Vitamin E gel reduces time of healing of digital ulcers in systemic sclerosis. Clin Exp Rheumatol. 2009;54:51–4.

34. Fiori G, Amanzi L, Moggi Pignone A, Braschi F, Matucci-Cerinic M. The treatment of skin ulcers in patients with systemic sclerosis. Reumatismo. 2004;56:225–34.

Silvia Bellando-Randone, Tiziana Pucci, Laura Rasero, Christopher P. Denton, and Marco Matucci-Cerinic

Introduction

Wound healing is a complex process regulated by a pattern of events including coagulation, inflammation, formation of granulation tissue, epithelialization, and tissue remodeling. The first injury damages blood vessels, triggers coagulation, and provokes an acute local inflammatory response. It is followed by mesenchymal cell recruitment, proliferation, and extracellular matrix generation which allow scar formation [1]. In systemic sclerosis (SSc), the reduction of the flow through the microcirculation involves a state of chronic tissue hypoxia, which slows down the wound healing process, affecting quality of life (QoL) and potentially leading to therapeutic failure. The most common skin lesions are represented by digital ulcers (DUs) that develop in poorly oxygenated tissues, compounded by the presence of infection, epidermal thinning, and tightly stretched skin and contractures [2]. In SSc, the treatment of DUs should improve tissue integrity and viability, promote ulcer healing, and reduce the

formation of new DU. The healing of the digital ulcerations may lead to scarring and/or digital resorption; most seriously, chronic ulcers can become infected and can be complicated by osteomyelitis and/or gangrene needing amputation [2–4] requiring hospitalizations for aggressive treatment with high socioeconomic cost [5, 6].

A multidisciplinary approach to management of DUs is required, including both systemic and local treatment, using a combination of non-pharmacological care, antibiotics if an infection is suspected [7–9], and surgical intervention in most severe cases. Furthermore, educational aspects are of paramount importance to make patient active in the healing process of DU [10–12].

Systemic therapy is crucial both for disease treatment, with immunosuppressive therapy that should help to control immune system dysregulation, and for improving vascular dilatation with the use of vasoactive drugs as calcium channel blockers, phosphodiesterase type 5 (PDE-5) inhibitors, prostanoids (iloprost), and endothelin receptor antagonist (ERA) (bosentan) [13].

The local treatment of ulcers is based on a methodological approach that considers the type of lesion and any variables (dimension, depth, presence of exudates, smell and/or other signs of infection) that can be present at baseline or it can occur subsequently, as reported in Chap. 18. Besides an accurate evaluation of DU characteristics, it is fundamental to assess local pain in the area of wound and surrounding tissue. Patients with skin wounds almost invariably need analgesic treatment for long lasting because of chronic pain as well as procedural pain management caused by local wound treatment [14] such as removal and replacing dressing and bandages. In particular, extensive and in-depth debridement of slough and necrotic tissue is an extremely painful procedure [15, 16].

A topical anesthetic drug suitable for use in skin ulcer debridement should have a documented evidence of clinical efficacy, low systemic toxicity and potential for sensitization, and no adverse effects on healing process [17].

S. Bellando-Randone (✉) · M. Matucci-Cerinic
Department of Experimental and Clinical Medicine,
University of Florence, Florence, Italy

Department of Geriatric Medicine, Division of Rheumatology
AOUC, Florence, Italy

T. Pucci
Department of Geriatric Medicine, Division of Rheumatology
AOUC, Florence, Italy

L. Rasero
Department of Health Sciences, University of Florence – Careggi
of Hospital, Florence, Tuscany, Italy

C. P. Denton
Division of Medicine, University College London, Centre for
Rheumatology, Royal Free Hospital, London, UK

© Springer Nature Switzerland AG 2019
M. Matucci-Cerinic, C. P. Denton (eds.), *Atlas of Ulcers in Systemic Sclerosis*, https://doi.org/10.1007/978-3-319-98477-3_19

Wound Bed Preparation

The structured approach to management of chronic wounds (a chronic wound is defined as a wound which lasts more than 6 weeks) in SSc is represented by *wound bed preparation* (WBP), as indicated in Chap. 18, and its definition "the management of an ulcer in order to accelerate endogenous healing or to facilitate the effectiveness of other therapeutic measures" well summarized the characteristic and the aim of local therapy of DUs in SSc.

The first step is *detersion* – defined as the mechanical removal of dirt, cellular debris, necrotic tissue, and other wastes present on the wound bed [18]. It can be performed irrigating with a warm (37 °C) saline solution (NaCl 0.9%) and using a 35 ml syringe and 19 G needle for lower limbs ulcers and a 10 ml syringe and a 19G needle cannula for all the other types of ulcers. The second step is debridement, recommended in all types of SSc wounds, mainly consists in the removal of nonviable material, foreign bodies, and necrotic tissue from a wound, that is a fundamental step to foster healing, prevent chronicity, and reduce the risk of bacterial infection [19]. The removal of foreign material and devitalized or contaminated tissue from or adjacent to the lesion is important because it is well known that tissue necrosis and slough may release cytokines that can frequently determine pain and worsen the status of DU. Debridement can be achieved through surgical, enzymatic, autolytic, mechanic, or biological methods. When the removal of devitalized tissue in DU is performed using scalpels and surgical instruments, the procedure is usually painful. Therefore, it is essential to carefully remove necrotic tissue while maintaining the highest patient comfort possible [17].

There are five types of debridement (passive debridement, active debridement, selective debridement, *nonselective debridement, and maintenance debridement*) as reported in Chap. 18.

Debridement can be mechanical, via curette or scalpel, or chemical, via enzyme-debriding agents [20]. Autolitic debridement, using endogenous proteolytic enzymes, takes advantage of the moist and warm environment present on the interface between the wound bed and the dressing. This kind of debridement does not cause pain to the patient, but it is a slow method of nonviable tissue removal. The most common dressings used are hydrogel and hydrocolloids as reported in Chap. 18.

Hydrogel includes hydrated carboxymetil-cellulose polymer dressings, containing 90% water in a gel base, which helps regulate fluid exchange from the wound surface. Hydrogel is used in association of sharp debridement.

Hydrocolloids are occlusive or semiocclusive dressings composed by carboxymetil-cellulose, pectin, and elastomers. They jellify absorbing the wound exudate. This type of dressing is rarely used in SSc, owing to its occlusive nature. Hydrocolloids may cause discomfort and harm perilesional sclerotic skin.

Wound Dressing in the Different Healing Phase

New research on wound care has focused on the "advanced" dressings that can help the operator with difficult/chronic lesions. These products are able to trigger the healing process of a lesion during the different phases, keeping a moist environment in the lesion.

In presence of:

- *Necrosis or fibrin:* proteolytic enzymes, maggots, silvers dressings, and alginate may be used.
- *Granulation:* foams and hydrogels should be used.
- *Epithelization:* hydrocolloid, foams, and impregnated gauzes are helpful.

There are more than 1000 different dressings to choose in the different stages of the ulcers:

- *Transparent film dressings* provide a moist, healing environment, promote autolytic debridement, protect the wound from mechanical trauma and bacterial invasion, and act as a blister roof or "second skin." Because they're flexible, these dressings can conform to wounds located in awkward locations such as the elbow. The transparency makes it easy to visualize the wound bed. Transparent film dressings are waterproof and impermeable to bacteria and contaminants. Although these dressings can't absorb fluid, they're permeable to moisture – allowing one-way passage of carbon dioxide and excess moisture vapor away from the wound. Indicated for partial-thickness wounds with little or no exudate, wounds with necrosis, and as both primary and secondary dressing. Also used to cover IV sites, donor sites, lacerations, abrasions, and second-degree burns. Available in a wide variety of sizes, both sterile and bulk.
- *Barrier cream:* Protect perilesional skin from maceration due to excess exudate.
- *Oil solution fatty acids:* Includes hyperoxygenated essential fatty acids (EFA) that help to maintain skin elasticity and donate moisture to promote skin repair. Pleasant odor. Quick absorption. Easy spray application.
- *Hydrogel:* The amorphous gel may contain CMC, calcium alginate versus sodium, starch polyglycosides, and sodium chloride. It is used for surface wounds or cavities or in combination with other dressings.
- *Non-adherent dressing (medicazioni non aderenti)*: Impregnated gauze with gel, vaseline, paraffin, and

silicone. Gauzes are useful in avoiding pain from trauma during dressing removal.

- *Hydrocolloids dressing:* The active surface of the dressing is coated with a cross-linked adhesive mass containing a dispersion of gelatin, pectin, and carboxy-methylcellulose together with other polymers and adhesives forming a flexible wafer. In contact with wound exudate, the polysaccharides and other polymers absorb water and swell, forming a gel. The gel may be designed to drain or to remain within the structure of the adhesive matrix. The moist conditions produced under the dressing are intended to promote fibrinolysis, angiogenesis, and wound healing, without causing softening and breaking down of tissue. The gel, which is formed as a result of the absorption of wound exudate, is held in place within the structure of the adhesive matrix. Most hydrocolloid dressings are waterproof, allowing normal washing and bathing. They can be used in poorly exuding lesions to favor an autolytic debridement.
- *Polyurethane foams:* Multilayer absorbing dressing with or without adhesive edges, with or without adherent contact, may have a gelificant component. This type of dressing could be useful in certain anatomic sites (heels) and for mild/moderate exudate.
- *Alginate:* Medications based on calcium or sodium salts of alginic acid, a polysaccharide extract from seaweed. They are used as dressing of cavity lesions with moderate to abundant exudate that need debridement.
- *Hydrophilic dressing:* Dressings made of carbohydrate methyl cellulose pure sodium with a high degree of absorption, gelling in contact with the exudate by holding it without releasing it. They are used for superficial or deep lesions, with high exudate, under bandage.
- *Collagen and cellulose dressing:* Matrix based on collagen packed in tampons, particles, and gel; they are useful in presence of granulation tissue or mild exudate, and they should be associated to a subocclusive medication.
- *Hyaluronic acid dressing:* Dressings are as cream, spray, transparent film, and microgranules. Medications are useful in lesions with difficulty in healing, requiring debridement, or lesions with granulation tissue with moderate exudate.
- *Modulators of protease metal:* Medications made up of an oxidized cellulose matrix and collagen favoring the formation and organization of new collagen fibers modulating growth factors. They are used on superficial and deep, well-detached, deep-fractured lesions with delay in healing.
- *Hydrophobic dressings for controlling bacterial charge:* Medications made up of acetate gauze and a hydrophobic compound. They are used as primary dressings for critically colonized lesions, even cavities or infestations, in intolerant antiseptic patients.

- *Dressings with silver:* Of various technologies, polyurethane foam, hydrocolloid, alginate, and hydrophobic with silver addition in ionic form or nanocrystals or antiseptic. They are used in lesions with mild and moderate exudate, smelly; they can also be used under bandage.

Semiocclusive wound dressings prevent evaporation and water loss thus retaining warmth, which improves wound healing [19]. Antiseptics should be avoided because of the known cytotoxic effects on cells, and local antibiotics may induce the emergence of resistance to the entire class of antibiotics used topically. Ulcers must be cleaned with physiologic water. The use of systemic antibiotics should be reserved only for clinically infected ulcers and not for bacterial colonization [19].

Conclusions

The management of ulcers is a real challenge for physicians and nurses. The observation of the ulcer characteristics is fundamental to choose the strategy which will drive the WBP in the effort to heal the wound as soon as possible. Obviously, infections necrosis and gangrene can complicate the scenario. For this reason, the physician must foster vascularization as much as possible, while the nurse will choose the most appropriate dressings for the wound characteristics. This combined approach may significantly accelerate wound healing and improve the quality of life of SSc patients.

References

1. Goss JR. Regeneration versus repair. In: Cohen IK, Diegelmann RF, Lindblad WJ, editors. Wound healing biochemical and clinical aspects. Philadelphia: WB Saunders; 1992. p. 40–62.
2. Korn JH, Mayes M, Matucci Cerinic M, et al. Digital ulcers in systemic sclerosis: prevention by treatment with bosentan, an oral endothelin receptor antagonist. Arthritis Rheum. 2004;50:3985–9.
3. Ferri C, Valentini G, Cozzi F, et al. Systemic sclerosis: demographic, clinical, and serologic features and survival in 1,012 Italian patients. Medicine. 2002;81:139–53.
4. Denton CP, Korn JH. Digital ulceration and critical digital ischaemia in scleroderma. Scleroderma Care Res. 2003;1:12–6.
5. Botzoris V, Drosos AA. Management of Raynaud's phenomenon and digital ulcers in systemic sclerosis. Joint Bone Spine. 2011;78:341–6.
6. Barr WG, Robinson JA. Systemic sclerosis and digital gangrene without scleroderma. J Rheumatol. 1988;15:875–7.
7. Chung L, Fiorentino D. Digital ulcers in patients with systemic sclerosis. Autoimmun Rev. 2006;5:125–8.
8. Korn JH. Scleroderma: a treatable disease. Cleve Clin J Med. 2003;70:954–8.
9. Denton CP, Black CM. Scleroderma and related disorders: therapeutic aspects. Baillieres Best Pract Res Clin Rheumatol. 2000;14:17–35.

10. Steen V, Denton CP, Pope JE, Matucci-Cerinic M. Digital ulcers: overt vascular disease in systemic sclerosis. Rheumatology (Oxford). 2009;48(Suppl 3):iii19–24.2.
11. Abraham S, Steen V. Optimal management of digital ulcers in systemic sclerosis. Ther Clin Risk Manag. 2015;11:939–47.
12. Schiopu E, Impens AJ, Phillips K. Digital ischemia in scleroderma spectrum of diseases. Int J Rheumatol. 2010;2010:1.
13. Kowal-Bieleck O, Fransen J, Avouac J, et al. Update of EULAR recommendations for the treatment of systemic sclerosis. Ann Rheum Dis. 2017;76:1327–39.
14. Giuggioli D, Manfredi A, Vacchi C, Sebastiani M, Spinella A, Ferri C. Procedural pain management in the treatment of scleroderma digital ulcers. Clin Exp Rheumatol. 2015;33:5–10.
15. Moffatt CJ, Franks PJ, Hollinworth H. Understanding wound pain and trauma: an international perspective. EWMA Position Document: Pain at wound dressing changes; 2002.
16. Hollinworth H. Pain and wound care. Wound care society educational leaflet. Wound Care Society: Huntingdon; 2000.
17. Braschi F, Bartoli F, Bruni C, Fiori G, Fantauzzo C, Paganelli L, De Paulis A, Rasero L, Matucci-Cerinic M. Lidocaine controls pain and allows safe wound bed preparation and debridement of digital ulcers in systemic sclerosis: a retrospective study. Clin Rheumatol. 2017 Jan;36(1):209–12.
18. International consensus. Per un uso corretto delle medicazioni all'argento nelle ferite. Consenso di un panel di esperti. London: Wounds International; 2012. http://www.woundsinternational.com/media/issues/588/files/content_10495.pdf
19. Fonder MA, Lazarus GS, Cowan DA, Aronson-Cook B, Kohli AR, Mamelak AJ. Treating the chronic wound: a practical approach to the care of nonhealing wounds and wound care dressings. J Am Acad Dermatol. 2008;58:185–206.
20. Fiori G, Galluccio F, Braschi F, Amanzi L, Miniati I, Conforti ML, et al. Vitamin E gel reduces time of healing of digital ulcers in systemic sclerosis. Clin Exp Rheumatol. 2009;27:51–4.

Part VIII

The Systemic Treatment of Skin Ulcers in Systemic Sclerosis

Ulcer Healing and Prevention in Systemic Sclerosis

20

Cosimo Bruni, Silvia Bellando-Randone, Christopher P. Denton, and Marco Matucci-Cerinic

Digital ulcers (DU) are common in systemic sclerosis (SSc) and have a major clinical impact. Whilst treating established ulcers is important, the most logical and effective approach to DU is to prevent their formation, as this will immediately remove the risk of severe complications and avoid the morbidity that is otherwise inevitable and substantial. Thus, the best therapeutic strategy for DU is *prevention of their occurrence or recurrence*, which is strategically linked to the frequency and severity of Raynaud's phenomenon (RP) episodes. For this reason, it is necessary to achieve RP control and to educate patients regarding its non-pharmacological management [1]. Patients should be taught to avoid cold temperatures by means of proper garments and gloves, hats and heavy socks, whenever there is exposure to different external temperature (e.g., cold temperature in hot seasons due to sudden weather changes, conditionated air, refrigerators in a supermarket, etc.). Stress is also an impacting trigger for vasospasm in RP [2], requiring careful examination of the psychologic conditions of SSc patients and, if necessary, counseling or prescription for antidepressants or anxiolytics. Patients should also be taught to treat dry skin with simple topical lubricating products and emulsifying ointments, in order to prevent dry skin from cracking or fissuring. Patients should be suggested to avoid nicotine [3] and any substances that cause vasoconstriction (caffeine, cephalosporins, b-blockers), and whenever possible, also to avoid trauma to the digits, such as those related to repetitive hand actions (e.g. typing or manual work) [1].

Given the impossibility to primarily prevent SSc and DU onset, DU secondary prevention begins with the identification and detection of risk factors. A recent systematic literature review identified male gender, early diffuse cutaneous SSc, in particular associated with anti-topoisomerase I antibody positivity and previous history of DU, as the predominant SSc-related features increasing the risk for DU appearance [4]. Moreover, circulating biomarkers studies identified high placental growth factor levels and low endothelial progenitor cells levels were associated with increased risk for future DU appearance, in particular for patients with history of previous digital ulcers [5]. Another study also identified Interleukin-6 levels as a predictor for future DU development, representing systemic inflammation [6]. Nail fold video capillaroscopy has an additional value in identifying patients at risk for vascular worsening: this was demonstrated for both qualitative evaluation with the late scleroderma pattern or evolution in the microvascular signs of vasculopathy [7] and for a composite videocapillaroscopic parameters score, named CSURI, derived from the combination of capillary number, maximum loop diameter and the number of giant capillaries, with a 2.9 score cut-off predicting high risk for DU development at 3 months [8].

Given these early high-impact disease-related features, the prompt initiation of background treatment could prevent new DU onset, which is strongly based on immunosuppression [9] and vasoactive-vasodilating treatments [10].

It is pivotal to understand how the concepts of healing and prevention are strongly linked and imbricated when taking care of SSc-DU patients. In fact, tertiary prevention starts once DU are manifested, in order to promote and determine their

C. Bruni (✉)
Department of Experimental and Clinical Medicine,
Division of Rheumatology, University of Florence, Florence, Italy

S. Bellando-Randone · M. Matucci-Cerinic
Department of Experimental and Clinical Medicine,
University of Florence, Florence, Italy

Department of Geriatric Medicine, Division of Rheumatology,
AOUC, Florence, Italy

C. P. Denton
Division of Medicine, University College London, Centre for Rheumatology, Royal Free Hospital, London, UK

M. Matucci-Cerinic, C. P. Denton (eds.), *Atlas of Ulcers in Systemic Sclerosis*, https://doi.org/10.1007/978-3-319-98477-3_20

healing, avoid recurrency and positively influence patient reintroduction in daily social, working and family life. Therefore, a drug that helps DU healing can still also be practically considered as a preventive drug (see overview in Table 20.1).

Among vasoactive drugs, Bosentan, a dual endothelin-1 receptor antagonist, was approved for DU *prevention* after two randomized clinical trials (RCT). Its use determined a 30–48% reduction in new DU appearance at 16–24 weeks, more effectively in patients entering the trial with ≥3 DU, although no effect was shown in healing rates of already present DU [29, 30]. The positive short-term RCT results were also confirmed in various real-life studies: in particular, drug effects were evident also when the drug was primarily prescribed for pulmonary arterial hypertension treatment [18], and these effects maintained for at least 12 months [17] up to 3 years for both safety [15] and efficacy [14]. Moreover, Fanauchi et al. hypothesized possible extravascular effects on the drug, in particular antifibrotic properties [16].

The DU-preventing properties of anti-ET1 bosentan could be at least partially explained by its effect on microvasculature: in particular, it was shown to determine deremodeling effects of nailfold videocapillaroscopy changes, both alone [31] and when used in combination with prostanoids [32].

These results have not been reproduced for other members of this pharmacological class, such as macitentan [33] and ambrisentan. Conversely, ambrisentan has shown efficacy in DU healing, both in combination with iloprost [11] and alone: although a definite placebo-controlled study has not been fully performed, Chung et al. showed a complete healing of all baseline DUs in 14/20 patients [12].

Healing of DUs is possible and easier if early detected. Treatment should be started promptly, and, although pharmacologic systemic treatment is pivotal, it is not the only possible approach. DU treatment is mostly based on vasodilating agents, which take into account various pharmacological entities, characterized by different mechanisms of action, routes of administration and direct/indirect costs. Calcium-channel blockers are commonly used for the treatment of both primary and secondary RP and have been anecdotally used for treating DUs [34]. Intravenous prostaglandin analogue alprostadil has shown effect in treating SSc-DU [35] and is still commonly used, in particular, when other treatments are not easily available [36]. Prostacyclin analogues are frequently prescribed for treating pulmonary arterial hypertension, and, given the pathogenetic link with DU, their use has been exported to DU treatment. Intravenous iloprost, infused continuously for 6 h 0.5–2.0 ng/kg/min on 5 consecutive days, has been extensively used for RP and DU treatment: it was shown to determine DU healing in both open-label [21] and double-blinded [19] studies. Iloprost has shown to be comparably effective for both low and high dosages (0.5 and 2.0 ng/kg/min) [20] also characterized by long-term efficacy in preventing new DU appearance [37]. Recent data have also shown the possibility of avoiding hospitalization using a portable siring pump [38]. Among other prostacyclin analogues, treprostenil showed initial significant impact on DU healing in a small open-label pilot study [39] and the worsening of the DU status after its withdrawal [40]. A recent double-blind RCT did not show any significant effect in reducing DU net burden and impacting healing and prevention [41]. Similarly, oral beraprost and intravenous epoprostenol showed only a trend to improvement of DU prevention and healing, although data seem to be less supportive compared to iloprost [42, 43].

Table 20.1 Summary of available positive evidences for DU healing and preventing drugs

Drug	Study	Year	n	Description
Ambrisentan	Parisi et al. [11]	2013	6	Preliminary, open-label
	Chung et al. [12]	2014	20	Prospective, open-label
Atorvastatin	Abou-Raya et al. [13]	2008	84	Single centre, placebo-controlled
Bosentan	RAPIDS-1 [11]	2004	122	*Double-blind*, placebo-controlled, multicentre
	RAPIDS-2 [12]	2010	188	*Double-blind*, placebo-controlled, multicentre
	Tsifetaki et al. [14]	2009	26	Prospective, 3-year follow-up
	Garcia de la Pena Lefebvre et al. [15]	2008	15	Prospective, observational
	Funauchi et al. [16]	2009	8	Single centre, observational
	Roman Ivorra et al. [17]	2011	67	Multicentre, retrospective cohort
	Cozzi et al. [18]	2013	30	Retrospective, case control
Iloprost	Wigley et al. [19]	1992	35	*Double-blind*, placebo-controlled
	Kawald et al. [20]	2008	50	Randomized, open label
	Zachariae et al. [21]	2009	14	Open label, observational
N-acetylcysteine	Sambo et al. [22]	2001	22	Multicentre, open-label
	Rosato et al. [23]	2009	50	Prospective, observational
Sildenafil	Brueckner et al. [24]	2010	19	Single centre, pilot study
	Kumar et al. [25]	2012	16	Prospective, open label, uncontrolled
	SEDUCE [26]	2015	83	*Double-blind*, placebo-controlled, multicentre
Tadalafil	Agarwal et al. [27]	2010	53	Placebo-controlled, multicentre
	Shenoy et al. [28]	2010	25	Placebo-controlled, single centre

Phosphodiesterase 5 inhibitors are also commonly prescribed vasodilators in SSc-related RP and DU, in particular sildenafil, supporting initial promising results in case series [24, 25]. The SEDUCE study showed a trend for higher DU healing rate and a significantly lower DU number after 8 and 12 weeks of treatment with sildenafil vs placebo [26]. In this RCT, 28 patients received bosentan concomitantly with sildenafil: in this subgroup *time to healing was shorter in the sildenafil group* than in the placebo group [26]. From the same class, Tadalafil also proved some beneficial effect on RP and DU in two small double-blinded placebo-controlled studies [27, 28].

Among other IV treatments, intravenous administration of N-acetyl cysteine has shown beneficial effects on both SSc-related RP and DU, both in short-term [22] and long-term [23] treatment duration.

Combined with above-mentioned systemic treatments, *local topical treatment* is also crucial: in fact, a careful management is important to prevent further complications, i.e. infection, osteomyelitis and/or gangrene needing amputation. Among wound healing procedures, the use of different advanced dressings is supported and needs to be adapted to the changing DU status [44]. Vitamin E gel application, in combination with local wound healing procedures and dressings, was shown to significantly reduce time to DU healing [45].

The association of local and systemic treatment is of pivotal importance, and the combination of vasoactive and vasodilating drugs is frequently used to have higher impact on DU healing [46].

Case reports and case series also show promising positive effect of other medical or surgical treatments. Botulin A toxin injection, for example, is a minimally invasive and relatively safe local vasodilating treatment: it has shown beneficial effects in improving blood flow and RP and promoting DU healing in both a case series [47] and a single-blinded placebo-controlled study [48]. Beneficial effects were also demonstrated in a placebo-controlled double-blind trial of atorvastatin for 4 months, determining significant reduction in overall DU number and new DU development [13].

Regenerative medicine is also a possible approach for treating patients who are resistant to medical treatment. Autologous platelet-rich gel is a hemo-component containing numerous growth factors, which has been shown to determine improvement to healing in few case reports and an Italian case series [49]. Bone-marrow mononuclear cells have also been administered into the DU affected limb, improving pain and reducing risk of amputation/ischaemia recurrence [50, 51]. Autologous adipose-derived stromal vascular fraction and autologous adipose tissue-derived cells fractions are other source of regenerative factors: fat can be derived from patient body and then reinjected after an extraction procedure. Their use has been tested in some case series with interesting reports regarding DU number decrease [52] and reduced time to healing, also associated with pain reduction and increase in capillary number on nailfold videocapillaroscopy [53]. RCTs are currently ongoing to definitively support fat grafting use in clinical practice.

Among other medical options, tocilizumab [54], rituximab [55], recombinant human erythropoietin [56], hyperbaric oxygen therapy [57], vacuum-assisted closure therapy [58] and extracorporeal shock wave therapy [59] can be listed. Regarding surgical approaches, digital sympathectomy [60] and skin grafting [61] could be also considered but further studies are needed before being routinely performed. They can however be used for refractory DU cases or when conventional treatments are contraindicated.

Whatever the treatment choice, chronic wounds management requires full patient participation. It is therefore crucial to provide therapeutic educational interventions to increase and ensure treatment adherence and compliance. This starts from either DU-related [62] and procedures-related [63] pain control, as among the most patient perceived DU features. Patient collaboration is indeed a key aspect for achieving maximum results.

References

1. Herrick AL. Recent advances in the pathogenesis and management of Raynaud's phenomenon and digital ulcers. Curr Opin Rheumatol. 2016;28(6):577–85.
2. Raynaud's Treatment Study Investigators. Comparison of sustained-release nifedipine and temperature biofeedback for treatment of primary Raynaud phenomenon. Results from a randomized clinical trial with 1-year follow-up. Arch Intern Med. 2000;160(8):1101–8.
3. Caramaschi P, Martinelli N, Volpe A, et al. A score of risk factors associated with ischemic digital ulcers in patients affected by systemic sclerosis treated with iloprost. Clin Rheumatol. 2009;28(7):807–13.
4. Silva I, Almeida J, Vasconcelos C. A PRISMA-driven systematic review for predictive risk factors of digital ulcers in systemic sclerosis patients. Autoimmun Rev. 2015;14(2):140–52.
5. Avouac J, Meune C, Ruiz B, et al. Angiogenic biomarkers predict the occurrence of digital ulcers in systemic sclerosis. Ann Rheum Dis. 2012;71(3):394–9.
6. Alivernini S, De Santis M, Tolusso B, et al. Skin ulcers in systemic sclerosis: determinants of presence and predictive factors of healing. J Am Acad Dermatol. 2009;60(3):426–35.
7. Smith V, Riccieri V, Pizzorni C, et al. Nail fold capillaroscopy for prediction of novel future severe organ involvement in systemic sclerosis. J Rheumatol. 2013;40(12):2023–8.
8. Sebastiani M, Manfredi A, Vukatana G, et al. Predictive role of capillaroscopic skin ulcer risk index in systemic sclerosis: a multicentre validation study. Ann Rheum Dis. 2012;71(1):67–70.
9. Cappelli S, Bellando-Randone S, Guiducci S, et al. Is immunosuppressive therapy the anchor treatment to achieve remission in systemic sclerosis? Rheumatology (Oxford). 2014;53(6):975–87. Review
10. Guiducci S, Bellando Randone S, Bruni C, et al. Bosentan fosters microvascular de-remodelling in systemic sclerosis. Clin Rheumatol. 2012;31(12):1723–5.

11. Parisi S, Peroni CL, Laganà A, et al. Efficacy of ambrisentan in the treatment of digital ulcers in patients with systemic sclerosis: a preliminary study. Rheumatology (Oxford). 2013;52(6):1142–4.

12. Chung L, Ball K, Yaqub A, et al. Effect of the endothelin type A-selective endothelin receptor antagonist ambrisentan on digital ulcers in patients with systemic sclerosis: results of a prospective pilot study. J Am Acad Dermatol. 2014;71(2):400–1.

13. Abou-Raya A, Abou-Raya S, Helmii M. Statins: potentially useful in therapy of systemic sclerosis-related Raynaud's phenomenon and digital ulcers. J Rheumatol. 2008;35(9):1801–8.

14. Tsifetaki N, Botzoris V, Alamanos Y, et al. Bosentan for digital ulcers in patients with systemic sclerosis: a prospective 3-year followup study. J Rheumatol. 2009;36(7):1550–2.

15. García de la Peña-Lefebvre P, Rodríguez Rubio S, Valero Expósito M, et al. Long-term experience of bosentan for treating ulcers and healed ulcers in systemic sclerosis patients. Rheumatology (Oxford). 2008;47(4):464–6.

16. Funauchi M, Kishimoto K, Shimazu H, et al. Effects of bosentan on the skin lesions: an observational study from a single center in Japan. Rheumatol Int. 2009;29(7):769–75.

17. Roman Ivorra JA, Simeon CP, Alegre Sancho JJ, et al. Bosentan in clinical practice for treating digital and other ischemic ulcers in Spanish patients with systemic sclerosis: IBER-DU cohort study. J Rheumatol. 2011;38(8):1631–5.

18. Cozzi F, Pigatto E, Rizzo M, et al. Low occurrence of digital ulcers in scleroderma patients treated with bosentan for pulmonary arterial hypertension: a retrospective case-control study. Clin Rheumatol. 2013;32(5):679–83.

19. Wigley FM, Seibold JR, Wise RA, et al. Intravenous iloprost treatment of Raynaud's phenomenon and ischemic ulcers secondary to systemic sclerosis. J Rheumatol. 1992;19(9):1407–14.

20. Kawald A, Burmester GR, Huscher D, et al. Low versus high-dose iloprost therapy over 21 days in patients with secondary Raynaud's phenomenon and systemic sclerosis: a randomized, open, single-center study. J Rheumatol. 2008;35(9):1830–7.

21. Zachariae H, Halkier-Sørensen L, Bjerring P, et al. Treatment of ischaemic digital ulcers and prevention of gangrene with intravenous iloprost in systemic sclerosis. Acta Derm Venereol. 1996;76(3):236–8.

22. Sambo P, Amico D, Giacomelli R, et al. Intravenous N-acetylcysteine for treatment of Raynaud's phenomenon secondary to systemic sclerosis: a pilot study. J Rheumatol. 2001;28(10):2257–62.

23. Rosato E, Borghese F, Pisarri S, et al. The treatment with N-acetylcysteine of Raynaud's phenomenon and ischemic ulcers therapy in sclerodermic patients: a prospective observational study of 50 patients. Clin Rheumatol. 2009;28(12):1379–84.

24. Brueckner CS, Becker MO, Kroencke T, et al. Effect of sildenafil on digital ulcers in systemic sclerosis: analysis from a single centre pilot study. Ann Rheum Dis. 2010;69(8):1475–8.

25. Kumar U, Sankalp G, Sreenivas V, et al. Prospective, open-label, uncontrolled pilot study to study safety and efficacy of sildenafil in systemic sclerosis-related pulmonary artery hypertension and cutaneous vascular complications. Rheumatol Int. 2013;33(4):1047–52.

26. Hachulla E, Hatron PY, Carpentier P, et al. Efficacy of sildenafil on ischaemic digital ulcer healing in systemic sclerosis: the placebo-controlled SEDUCE study. Ann Rheum Dis. 2016;75(6):1009–15.

27. Agarwal V, Parasar G, Aman S, et al. Efficacy of Tadalafil in Raynaud's Phenomenon Secondary to Systemic Sclerosis: A Double Blind Randomized Placebo Controlled Parallel Group Multicentric Study. Arthritis&Rheumatism. 2010;62(10):Supplement.

28. Shenoy PD, Kumar S, Jha LK, et al. Efficacy of tadalafil in secondary Raynaud's phenomenon resistant to vasodilator therapy: a double-blind randomized cross-over trial. Rheumatology (Oxford). 2010;49(12):2420–8.

29. Korn JH, Mayes M, Matucci Cerinic M, et al. Digital ulcers in systemic sclerosis: prevention by treatment with bosentan, an oral endothelin receptor antagonist. Arthritis Rheum. 2004;50(12):3985–93.

30. Matucci-Cerinic M, Denton CP, Furst DE, et al. Bosentan treatment of digital ulcers related to systemic sclerosis: results from the RAPIDS-2 randomised, double-blind, placebo-controlled trial. Ann Rheum Dis. 2011;70(1):32–8.

31. Guiducci S, Bellando Randone S, Bruni C, et al. Bosentan fosters microvascular de-remodelling in systemic sclerosis. Clin Rheumatol. 2012;31(12):1723–5.

32. Cutolo M, Zampogna G, Vremis L, et al. Long term effects of endothelin receptor antagonism on microvascular damage evaluated by nail fold capillaroscopic analysis in systemic sclerosis. J Rheumatol. 2013;40(1):40–5.

33. Khanna D, Denton CP, Merkel PA, et al. Effect of macitentan on the development of new ischemic digital ulcers in patients with systemic sclerosis: DUAL-1 and DUAL-2 randomized clinical trials. JAMA. 2016;315(18):1975–88.

34. Woo TY, Wong RC, Campbell JP, et al. Nifedipine in scleroderma ulcerations. Int J Dermatol. 1984 Dec;23(10):678–80.

35. Baron M, Skrinskas G, Urowitz MB, et al. Prostaglandin E1 therapy for digital ulcers in scleroderma. Can Med Assoc J. 1982;126(1):42–5.

36. Abuowda Y, Almeida RS, Oliveira AA, et al. Treatment of digital ulcers in systemic sclerosis: Case series study of thirteen patients and discussion on outcome. Rev Assoc Med Bras (1992). 2017;63(5):422–6.

37. Colaci M, Lumetti F, Giuggioli D, et al. Long-term treatment of scleroderma-related digital ulcers with iloprost: a cohort study. Clin Exp Rheumatol. 2017;35 Suppl 106(4):179–83.

38. Fraticelli P, Martino GP, Murri M, et al. A novel iloprost administration method with portable syringe pump for the treatment of acral ulcers and Raynaud's phenomenon in systemic sclerosis patients. A pilot study (ILOPORTA). Clin Exp Rheumatol. 2017;35 Suppl 106(4):173–8.

39. Chung L, Fiorentino D. A pilot trial of treprostinil for the treatment and prevention of digital ulcers in patients with systemic sclerosis. J Am Acad Dermatol. 2006;54(5):880–2.

40. Shah AA, Schiopu E, Chatterjee S, et al. The recurrence of digital ulcers in patients with systemic sclerosis after discontinuation of oral Treprostinil. J Rheumatol. 2016;43(9):1665–71.

41. Seibold R, Wigley FM, Schiopu E, et al. Digital ulcers in SSc treated with oral treprostinil: a randomized, double-blind, placebo-controlled study with open-label follow-up. J Scleroderma Relat Disord. 2017;2(1):42–9.

42. Cruz JE, Ward A, Anthony S, et al. Evidence for the use of epoprostenol to treat Raynaud's phenomenon with or without digital ulcers. Ann Pharmacother. 2016;50(12):1060–7.

43. Vayssairat M. Preventive effect of an oral prostacyclin analog, beraprost sodium, on digital necrosis in systemic sclerosis. French Microcirculation Society Multicenter Group for the Study of Vascular Acrosyndromes. J Rheumatol. 1999;26(10):2173–8.

44. Fujimoto M, Asano Y, Ishii T, et al. The wound/burn guidelines - 4: guidelines for the management of skin ulcers associated with connective tissue disease/vasculitis. J Dermatol. 2016;43(7):729–57.

45. Fiori G, Galluccio F, Braschi F, et al. Vitamin E gel reduces time of healing of digital ulcers in systemic sclerosis. Clin Exp Rheumatol. 2009;27(3 Suppl 54):51–4.

46. Kowal-Bielecka O, Fransen J, Avouac J, et al. Update of EULAR recommendations for the treatment of systemic sclerosis. Ann Rheum Dis. 2017;76(8):1327–39.

47. Motegi S, Yamada K, Toki S, et al. Beneficial effect of botulinum toxin A on Raynaud's phenomenon in Japanese patients with systemic sclerosis: a prospective, case series study. J Dermatol. 2016;43(1):56–62.

48. Motegi SI, Uehara A, Yamada K, et al. Efficacy of Botulinum Toxin B injection for Raynaud's Phenomenon and Digital Ulcers in Patients with Systemic Sclerosis. Acta Derm Venereol. 2017;97(7):843–50.

49. Giuggioli D, Colaci M, Manfredi A, et al. Platelet gel in the treatment of severe scleroderma skin ulcers. Rheumatol Int. 2012;32(9):2929–32.

50. Ishigatsubo Y, Ihata A, Kobayashi H, et al. Therapeutic angiogenesis in patients with systemic sclerosis by autologous transplantation of bone-marrow-derived cells. Mod Rheumatol. 2010;20(3):263–72.

51. Takagi G, Miyamoto M, Tara S, et al. Therapeutic vascular angiogenesis for intractable macroangiopathy-related digital ulcer in patients with systemic sclerosis: a pilot study. Rheumatology (Oxford). 2014;53(5):854–9.

52. Daumas A, Magalon J, Jouve E, et al. Long-term follow-up after autologous adipose-derived stromal vascular fraction injection into fingers in systemic sclerosis patients. Curr Res Transl Med. 2017;65(1):40–3.

53. Del Papa N, Di Luca G, Sambataro D, et al. Regional implantation of autologous adipose tissue-derived cells induces a prompt healing of long-lasting indolent digital ulcers in patients with systemic sclerosis. Cell Transplant. 2015;24(11):2297–305.

54. Fernandes das Neves M, Oliveira S, Amaral MC, et al. Treatment of systemic sclerosis with tocilizumab. Rheumatology (Oxford). 2015;54(2):371–2.

55. Khor CG, Chen XL, Lin TS, et al. Rituximab for refractory digital infarcts and ulcers in systemic sclerosis. Clin Rheumatol. 2014;33(7):1019–20.

56. Ferri C, Giuggioli D, Sebastiani M, Colaci M. Treatment of severe scleroderma skin ulcers with recombinant human erythropoietin. Clin Exp Dermatol. 2007;32(3):287–90.

57. Mirasoglu B, Bagli BS, Aktas S. Hyperbaric oxygen therapy for chronic ulcers in systemic sclerosis - case series. Int J Dermatol. 2017;56(6):636–40.

58. Pauling JD, Brown SJ, James J, et al. Vacuum-assisted closure therapy: a novel treatment for wound healing in systemic sclerosis. Rheumatology (Oxford). 2011;50(2):420–2.

59. Saito S, Tomonori I, Kenta I, et al. Extracorporeal shock wave therapy for digital ulcers associated with systemic sclerosis. J Scleroderma Relat Disord. 2016;1(2):181–5.

60. Chiou G, Crowe C, Suarez P, et al. Digital Sympathectomy in patients with scleroderma: an overview of the practice and referral patterns and perceptions of rheumatologists. Ann Plast Surg. 2015;75(6):637–43.

61. Barsotti S, Mattaliano V, d'Ascanio A, et al. Systemic sclerosis chronic ulcers: preliminary results of treatment with allogenic skin grafting in a cohort of Italian patients. Int Wound J. 2016;13(5):1050–1.

62. Giuggioli D, Manfredi A, Colaci M, et al. Oxycodone in the long-term treatment of chronic pain related to scleroderma skin ulcers. Pain Med. 2010;11(10):1500–3.

63. Braschi F, Bartoli F, Bruni C, et al. Lidocaine controls pain and allows safe wound bed preparation and debridement of digital ulcers in systemic sclerosis: a retrospective study. Clin Rheumatol. 2017;36(1):209–12.

Surgical Approaches Including Sympathectomy

21

Lindsay Muir and Ariane L. Herrick

General Approach

We believe that the primary care for patients with systemic sclerosis (SSc)-related digital ulcers should be medical. In refractory cases, however, there is a role for surgery. Although at present there is no good evidence base for the different surgical procedures described in this chapter [1], clinical experience suggests that many patients benefit.

A close working relationship between the hand surgery department and the rheumatologists is essential. Open access to the hand trauma clinic ensures that there is never any delay in obtaining a surgical opinion. Patients with SSc and ischemic fingertips are often in a great deal of pain. We try therefore to provide rapid assessment and rapid access to surgery. We perform this on our hand surgery trauma list to ensure prompt treatment and prompt relief of pain.

> **Patients with SSc Present to Hand Surgeons with**
> - Pain.
> - Ulceration.
> - Necrosis.
> - Soft tissue calcification.
> - Joint stiffness and dysfunction; this is outside the scope of this text and will not be considered further.

In our experience the predominant presentation is pain. Ischemic necrosis and ulceration are often present. Dry gangrene may not be so painful.

The primary cause of pain in SSc is tissue ischemia. The primary aim of surgery is therefore to restore pulsatile blood flow to the skin, thereby improving the nutrition of the skin. This will in turn reduce pain and help ulcers to heal.

The situations in which surgery should be considered are as follows:

1. Failure of the ulcer(s) to respond to "nonsurgical" interventions including:
   (a) Intensifying vasodilator therapy, including administration of intravenous (IV) prostanoid infusions
   (b) Antibiotics if there is any suspicion that the ulcer is infected
   (c) Adequate analgesia
   (d) Expert wound care, often including input from a tissue viability team
2. Severe pain and tenderness, suggestive of a collection of pus and/or necrotic tissue requiring incision and drainage (this should be suspected if pressing over the ulcer causes severe pain). Patients are often kept awake at night with pain.
3. Underlying bone infection. Although this can often be treated medically with a prolonged course of antibiotic therapy (especially when the osteomyelitis is diagnosed early, e.g., with magnetic resonance [MR] scanning [2]), this is not always the case, and surgical debridement or amputation may prove necessary.
4. Calcinosis. Ulcers overlying calcinosis can be difficult to heal, with healing times longer than for ulcers unassociated with calcinosis [3]. Debulking the associated calcinosis may facilitate wound healing.

The following case history gives an example of a situation in which surgery was required for refractory SSc-related digital ulceration and puts into context several of the issues and challenges confronting the surgeon (as discussed later).

L. Muir (✉)
Manchester Hand Centre, Salford Royal NHS Foundation Trust, Salford, Lancashire, UK
e-mail: lmuir@tmhc.co.uk

A. L. Herrick
NIHR Manchester Musculoskeletal Biomedical Research Unit, Central Manchester NHS Foundation Trust, Manchester Academic Health Science Centre, Manchester, UK

© Springer Nature Switzerland AG 2019
M. Matucci-Cerinic, C. P. Denton (eds.), *Atlas of Ulcers in Systemic Sclerosis*, https://doi.org/10.1007/978-3-319-98477-3_21

Case History

A 61-year-old woman with a new diagnosis of limited cutaneous SSc (on the basis of a 12-month history of Raynaud's phenomenon and digital ulceration, sclerodactyly, telangiectasias, a positive anticentromere antibody, and abnormal nailfold capillaroscopy with giant capillaries) was referred with digital ulceration and critical ischemia. Specifically, she had painful ulcers of the left index and middle fingertips for approximately 6 months and for several months a "black" area at the tip of the right index finger. Intravenous iloprost infusions did not result in ulcer healing. On examination at the time of first referral, the tip of the right index finger was gangrenous with extreme tenderness extending to just proximal to the distal interphalangeal joint with erythema, suggestive of infection (Fig. 21.1). She had tender ulcers at the tip of the left index and middle fingers (Fig. 21.2).

She was admitted for further intravenous iloprost infusions, intravenous antibiotics, analgesia, and surgical review. Initial surgery comprised amputation of the tip of the right

index finger, debridements of the left index and middle fingers, and botulinum toxin injections to both hands. The right index finger did not heal well, and 2 weeks later, she underwent further amputation of the right index finger, on this occasion through the middle phalanx. She continued to have problems also with the left index and middle fingers and underwent further debridements of the left middle and index fingers 6 weeks after the initial procedure, together with left palmar sympathectomy (Fig. 21.3). Following these further procedures, she made good progress, and when seen 3 months after first referral, all ulcers were healing well.

The case demonstrates how surgical debridements and/or (limited) amputation can, in conjunction with medical therapy, lead to ulcer healing with minimal tissue loss. This was a particularly severe case with long-standing ulceration. The patient was advised to seek urgent medical advice in the event of any new ulcers developing, so that treatment of these could be initiated without delay. We believe that this approach of an "open door" policy for digital ulcers helps obviate the requirement for (in this case further) surgery.

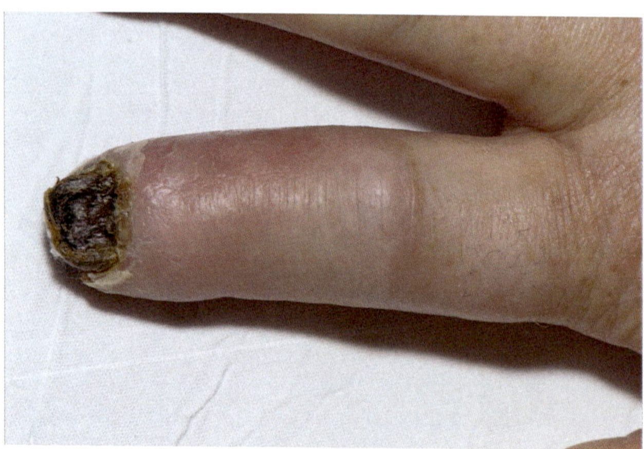

Fig. 21.1 Critical ischemia, with gangrene, of the right index finger, with proximal erythema suggestive of infection. (©Salford Royal NHS Foundation Trust)

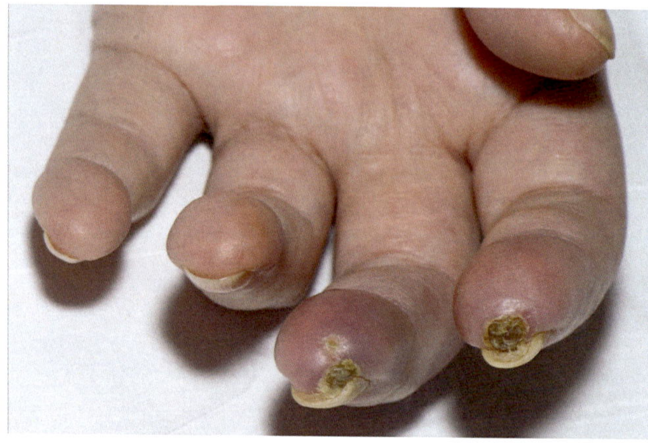

Fig. 21.2 Digital ulcers at tips of left index and middle fingers. (©Salford Royal NHS Foundation Trust)

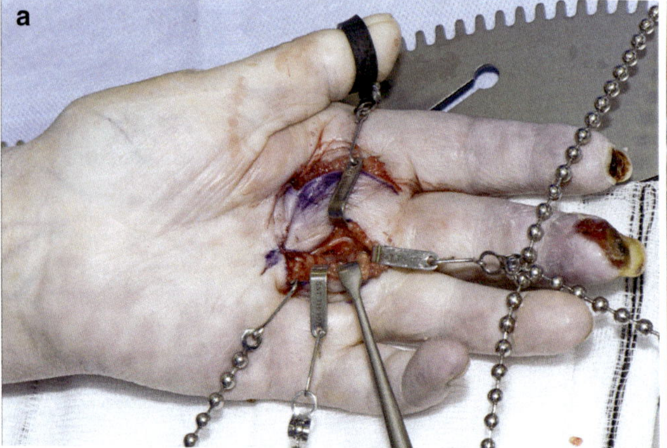
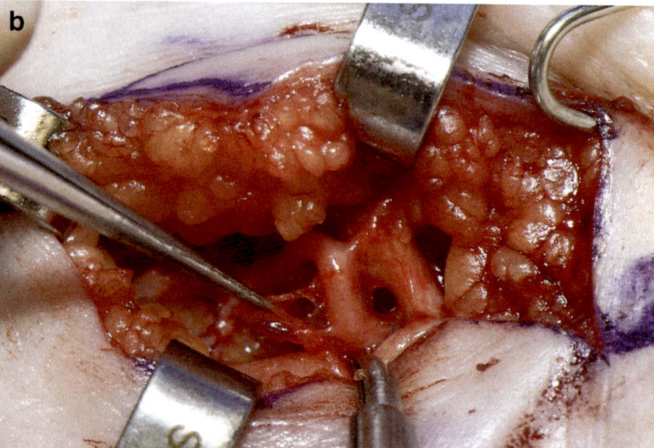

Fig. 21.3 Photographs of the operative field at the time of sympathectomy. (**a**) Widefield view and (**b**) close-up view. The nerve and artery are seen running in parallel in the middle of the field just under the broad retractor at the top of the picture with a bridge of tissue still connecting them. The adventitia is being teased off with the micro forceps on the left of the picture. The adventitia is stripped, and all connections between the nerve and the artery are being divided. (©Salford Royal NHS Foundation Trust)

Prevalence of Surgical Intervention in Reported Series

This varies widely, in part reflecting the very different patient populations reported. In an early study of 118 patients from our own center [4], 101 patients responded to a questionnaire about smoking habits. Of these 17% had surgical debridement of one or more digits, and 15% had surgical amputation of one or more digits. Current smokers were significantly more likely than never smokers to have had debridements (odds ratio 4.5, 95% confidence interval [CI] 1.1–18.3) and more likely to have had amputations (odds ratio 3.4, 95% CI 1.8–15.1) [4]. Of 1168 patients attending the Royal Free Hospital, London [5], 0.9% of patients had auto- or surgical amputation over an 18-month period, and 1.1% was referred for digital sympathectomy during the same period. In an analysis of the Digital Ulcers Outcome (DUO) Registry [6], of patients with SSc and digital ulcer disease, 189/1644 (11.5%) had previous debridement, 158/1661 (9.5%) had previous surgical amputations, 40/1921 (2.1%) had previous digital sympathectomy, and 20/1918 (1.0%) had previous arterial reconstruction. We have become rather less aggressive with our amputations and now make every effort to salvage the digit or at least to minimize the extent of amputation (as exemplified by the case history).

Anatomy

The blood supply of the skin derives from myocutaneous and fasciocutaneous perforators, which in turn give subcutaneous arterioles. These branches form a deep dermal arterial plexus. It is from this level that the hair follicles and sweat glands are supplied.

Also branching from the deep dermal plexus is a subpapillary arterial plexus from which arise ascending arterial and descending venous vessels extending into each papilla [7, 8].

The skin has a major role in thermoregulation [9]. In normal circumstances, only 5–20% of blood flow is through the nutritional beds. Skin blood flow can reach up to 6–8 L/min [10]. The mechanisms of control for this are complex and involve both active vasodilation and active vasoconstriction. Unfortunately, resting blood flow is difficult to measure [11]. The hand is supplied by the radial and ulnar arteries, both branches of the brachial artery. The radial artery forms the deep palmar arch, the ulnar artery forms the superficial palmar arch. The "classical" pattern whereby these two arches link occurs in only 35% of individuals. In 39% the superficial arch derives solely from the ulnar artery. In 4% there is a contribution from the median and ulnar arteries and in 1% from all three arteries. In 16% the radial and ulnar arteries form an incomplete arch and supply the proper digital arteries directly. In the remaining 5%, the three arteries (median, radial, and ulnar) do likewise [7, 9].

Higgins and McClinton [12] point out that these arches are not isolated structures and that there are extensive communications between the various blood supplies. They also point out the importance of the radial artery in the supply of the hand. Dumanian et al. [13] concluded that the radial artery was more important than the ulnar artery for pulsatile flow in the digits and viewed the hand as a single vascular bed rather than two separate systems with a connecting arch.

In SSc the blood vessels are structurally abnormal and may be occluded. This occlusion may occur at any level [14]. In a series of 24 arteriograms in patients with biopsy proven SSc, Janevski [15] demonstrated that the radial artery and deep palmar arch were never affected. The most frequently affected vessels were the proper digital arteries of the index to little fingers, with the thumb vessels often spared. The ulnar artery and superficial palmar arch were totally occluded in 10 (42%).

Kim et al. [14] examined the angiographic findings in 351 hands in 178 patients with Raynaud's phenomenon. 47% of these had an associated systemic disease. They proposed a six-part anatomical classification. This divides the arteries of the hand into level 1 arteries (radial and ulnar), level 2 arteries (palmar arch and common digital), and level 3 (digital) arteries; the classification is as follows:

Type I	Complete occlusion of radial or ulnar artery; decreased flow and narrowing in level 2 and 3 arteries
Type II	As I, but with stenosis of radial or ulnar artery
Type IIIa	The main disorder is in the common digital or digital arteries
Type IIIb	A rare subset characterized by selective occlusion of the digital arteries to the index finger, secondary to vibrating machinery use
Type IV	All levels of vessel are stenotic
Type V	Global ischemia, paucity of vessels, scant flow on angiography

Kim et al. [14] demonstrated stenosis at the ulnar or radial artery in 53.5% of patients. Of these 88.5% of occlusions and 95.7% of stenoses affected primarily the ulnar artery. 27.1% of patients had disease primarily in the palmar arch and common digital vessels. In this they concur with Janevski [15] and with Park et al. [16] who found occlusion of the ulnar artery in 63%. Higgins and McClinton [12] note that by the time patients with collagen vascular disease have ulcers or digit-threatening ischemia, two thirds have ulnar artery thrombosis at the wrist. They believe that recognition and treatment of this can make a worthwhile difference to the vascular status of the hand. Unfortunately reconstruction is not always feasible.

The available procedures include:

Ulcer debridement.

Sympathectomy.

Balloon angioplasty.

Arterial reconstruction.

Excision of calcinotic deposits (for patients in whom subcutaneous calcium deposits are a contributor to digital ulceration or a source of pain or inconvenience).

Amputation.

Botulinum toxin injection (these are not discussed in this chapter as they are included in Chap. 23).

Fat injection.

Joint procedures, specifically proximal interphalangeal (PIP) fusion and metacarpophalangeal (MCP) arthroplasty, may also be helpful.

The indications for surgery are thus:

Refractory ulcers

Rest pain

Calcinosis that is causing functional problems or ulceration

Stiff joints secondary to SSc

Evaluation and Anesthesia

In most instances the patient will be referred to the surgeon by a rheumatologist, and an extensive workup may therefore already have been undertaken. The possibility of concomitant proximal large vessel disease should always be considered (it has been suggested that the prevalence of large vessel disease is increased in patients with SSc [17], although this remains controversial): therefore the peripheral pulses should be carefully assessed. If there is any concern, arterial Doppler studies should be performed and if necessary more invasive vascular assessment.

The vascular supply of the hand may most accurately be assessed by arteriography [9]. Although MR angiography is being increasingly used, if there is any question of arterial reconstruction being required, then most surgeons would request conventional (X-ray) digital subtraction angiography because of the increased detail visualized in the small vessels of the hand [12]. Merritt [18] however cautions that in his experience, arteriography has the potential to cause vasospasm of the ulnar artery and that MR angiography may be more reliable. Other, less invasive, methods of assessing the circulation in the fingers include laser Doppler flowmetry,

laser Doppler perfusion imaging, digital:brachial index measurement, digital plethysmography, and measurement of cutaneous surface temperature, often in association with cold stress testing. However, these are seldom currently used in clinical practice and are mainly used as research tools.

Plain radiology may demonstrate acro-osteolysis. It may be very difficult to differentiate between this and osteomyelitis. MR scanning may be more sensitive in assessing whether there is infection in the terminal phalanx.

Various hand function assessment tools assist in evaluating the results of treatment. These include the Hand Mobility in Scleroderma (HAMIS) test [19], the Scleroderma Health Assessment Questionnaire (SHAQ) [20], the Scleroderma Functional Index [21], and the Cochin Hand Function Scale [22]. None of the standard hand assessment tools such as DASH (Disability of the Arm, Shoulder, and Hand) [23] have been validated in SSc.

Anesthetic Assessment

Patients with SSc may have significant cardiorespiratory dysfunction and thus an increased anesthetic risk. If major surgery is to be undertaken, preoperative anesthetic consultation is advisable. Surgery may however readily be performed under regional anesthesia. We have not experienced any problems with performing surgery under metacarpal block anesthesia, and in a willing patient, this form of anesthesia is ideal for surgery on a single digit. We do not however use epinephrine for metacarpal block anesthesia in patients with SSc.

Surgical Procedures

Ulcer Debridement

Digital ulcers in patients with SSc are often very painful. As highlighted earlier, we recommend that a patient consider surgery if the pain is severe (e.g., disturbing sleep) and if the finger is exquisitely tender. The simple expedient of debriding the ulcer may be surprisingly effective at relieving pain, especially if, as often happens, there is a bead of pus under the scab.

Technique

Surgery may be performed under local, regional, or general anesthesia. A tourniquet is not required. The ulcer is debrided, and the base gently curetted with a No. 15 blade. The surgeon should not anticipate normal bleeding because the fingertip will almost inevitably be relatively avascular. The normal surgical dictum of resecting until healthy tissue is encountered should be resisted in the context of a patient with SSc, because this bleeding will often only occur when a large part of the finger has been amputated. While this may offer a satisfactory result for one finger, the patient may subsequently present with further ulcers requiring surgery, and aggressive amputations may result in the loss of all fingers. The patient should be advised that the ulcer will take some time to heal.

Sympathectomy

Cervical Sympathectomy

Although cervical sympathectomy results in improvement in perfusion in the short term, we do not recommend this in patients with Raynaud's phenomenon and/or digital ulceration. This is in part because sympathetic tone may return within 6–12 weeks and indeed may be increased. Claes et al. [24] noted return of symptoms after 6 months in nine patients with Raynaud's phenomenon.

Periarterial (Digital, Radial, and Ulnar) Sympathectomy

Periarterial sympathectomy may offer some improvement for the patient with refractory SSc-related digital ulcers, especially when these are multiple and recurrent. However, it is a procedure which should be performed only in specialist centers by a surgeon with experience in the technique.

The sympathetic supply to the hand arises not only from the sympathetic chain but also from alternative pathways. Digital sympathectomy was first described by Flatt, who postulated that interrupting the sympathetic nervous supply more distally would be more likely to be effective than central sympathectomy [25]. Morgan and Wilgis [26], using a rabbit ear model, demonstrated that sympathetic fibers in the adventitia have limited capacity for regeneration even after 1 year.

Balogh et al. [27] emphasized that if possible the nerve of Henlé should be identified: the nerve of Henlé sends a consistent branch carrying sympathetic fibers to the ulnar artery [28].

Flatt's original series was of eight patients. The underlying pathology was varied, and Flatt himself describes the difficulty in assessing objectively the results of treatment. Hartzell et al. [29] studied 28 patients with an average follow-up of 96 months (minimum 23 months). The patients in their series had a mixture of autoimmune and arteriosclerotic disease. Their technique was tailored to each patient's pattern of disease and involved surgery at any of the levels described previously. Eleven of the 20 patients with autoimmune disease saw complete healing of ulcers, with 15 experiencing some improvement. However, seven eventually underwent amputation (these are included in the unhealed ulcer group).

Kim et al. [14] undertook a combination of digital sympathectomy of the common digital vessels alone and radical sympathectomy including the proper digital vessels for their patients with type IV and V disease. Of the patients with type IV and type V disease, 66.7% and 53.3%, respectively, experienced an improvement in symptoms. However, 22.9% and 33.3%, respectively, had no change, and 10.4% and 13.3%, respectively, experienced a deterioration.

Koman et al. [30] studied the microvascular physiology in seven hands with refractory pain and ulceration undergoing digital sympathectomy. Following surgery all seven hands achieved a reduction in pain. The ulcers healed in six hands and improved in the remaining one. The results were assessed further by different noninvasive techniques: isolated cold stress testing, digital pulp temperature evaluation, and laser Doppler flowmetry. After sympathectomy, fingertip temperature did not increase (contrary to some other writers' experiences), suggesting that total blood flow was unaffected, although microvascular perfusion and vasomotion increased. On this basis, the authors suggested that the mechanism for the clinical effectiveness of sympathectomy is a preferential increase in flow in nutritional rather than thermoregulatory vessels.

Kotsis and Chung [31] undertook a systematic review of the literature on peripheral sympathectomy; 16 papers met their inclusion criteria. Most, but not all, of the patients studied had SSc. Ulcer healing time took from 2 weeks to 7 months. 15% eventually required amputation despite the sympathectomy, 16% had recurrence/ incomplete healing, and 37% had a postoperative complication. The authors therefore advised that long-term prospective studies are still required and that patients should be warned of the uncertain success rate.

In an early paper, Yee et al. [32] suggested that some of the benefit from digital sympathectomy derived from the adventitial strip/mechanical decompression rather than from the sympathectomy itself.

Technique

Peripheral sympathectomy (Fig. 21.3) may be performed at several different levels: at the level of the ulnar and radial arteries, the common digital arteries, and the proper digital arteries. The surgery is performed with the use of general or regional anesthesia and an exsanguinating tourniquet. The use of loupe magnification or of an operating microscope is advisable. For digital sympathectomy, the common digital artery is approached through a Bruner incision. A 2-cm stretch of the artery is stripped of adventitia. We do not drain the wound; the transverse limb may safely be left open. For radial and ulnar artery sympathectomy, the arteries are approached via a straight 3-cm incision. The adventitia is stripped over a 2-cm stretch of artery.

An extensive sympathectomy of the ulnar artery, superficial palmar arch, and proper digital arteries is described by O'Brien et al. [33]. A radical exposure is also described by Koman et al. [30], in which the superficial palmar arch and the three volar common digital vessels are exposed. Koman et al. also strip a section of the deep branch of the radial artery and the origin of the deep palmar arch through a fourth incision in the anatomic snuffbox. Merritt [18] describes an extensive adventectomy involving the dorsal branch of the radial artery, the ulnar artery from 8 to 10 cm proximal to the wrist, and including the entire superficial palmar arch and the common volar vessels.

Balloon Angioplasty

Kim et al. [14] performed balloon angioplasty in patients with type II disease in whom either the ulnar or radial artery was stenotic. A balloon catheter (2 mm diameter and 14 mm length) was used to dilate the vessels. This was advanced up the ulnar artery as far as the common digital arteries. If balloon angioplasty was not successful, they proceeded to excision of the stenosed segment and interposition vein or arterial graft. They reported overall improvement in 79% of this group with 16% no better and 4% worse. One notable complication was an ulnar artery rupture.

Arterial Reconstruction

Tomaino [34] described arterial reconstruction of the long finger radial digital artery. Kim et al. [14] described tailored surgical intervention. In the case of a thrombosed radial or ulnar artery, the involved segment was excised and replaced with an interposition vein or arterial graft. The preferred donor artery was the deep inferior epigastric artery. If the arteries were only stenotic, a balloon angioplasty was preferred. In the case of an involved superficial palmar arch and spared common digital vessels, Kim et al. [14] advocate reconstruction of the arch with a deep inferior epigastric artery graft anastomosed to the common digital arteries, an approach supported by the work of Higgins and McClinton [12]. These investigators believe that such patients can experience substantial and long-term improvement in the vascular status of their hands with arterial bypass procedures. Trocchia and Hammert [35] also argue that arterial grafts should be studied in more detail in the hand, given the experience of higher patency rates in coronary artery surgery. Kryger et al. [36] describe a reversed lesser saphenous vein graft anastomosed end to side to the radial artery and tunneled to the common digital artery. In a series of six patients, they found that no patient had any further ischemia leading to tissue loss after a follow-up of 4–40 months.

Technique

Angiography is recommended as part of careful preoperative planning. Standard techniques of venous or arterial

grafting are recommended, with careful attention to resection of all diseased artery until normal vessel is found and meticulous microsurgical technique. The exact pattern of the reconstruction depends on the extent of the disease. The graft may be a local interposition graft of a short segment of ulnar artery or may be more complex involving reconstruction of the whole of the palmar arch from the radial artery as described by Kim et al. [14].

Revascularization of the Hand by Retrograde Venous Flow

Kind [37] reported a series of three cases of revascularization of chronically ischemic hands by means of anastomosis of a vein to an artery, thereby arterializing the venous system. The surgical technique is described in detail by Matarrese and Hammert [38]. The cephalic vein is identified and the side branches ligated. Matarrese and Hammert describe anastomosing the vein to the brachial artery, but it may more simply be anastomosed to the radial artery if this latter is patent. The valves of the cephalic vein need to be divided with a valvulotome. The vein is then transected and joined end to side to the parent artery. The authors emphasize that this is a last chance solution and that the long-term results are not clear.

Fat Grafting

Recent interest has been shown in the concept of injecting fat into the palm. Bank et al. [39] studied 21 hands in 13 patients. They injected decanted fat harvested from the abdominal wall and noted a reduction in pain and ulceration. Further recent open-label studies have also suggested that injection of autologous adipose-derived cells confers benefit in patients with SSc-related digital vasculopathy [40, 41], and recent reviews describe the rationale for this therapeutic approach [42, 43]. This treatment must be seen as in the early phases of adoption.

Arthrodesis

The commonest deformity at the proximal interphalangeal (PIP) joint level is one of fixed flexion. This often leads to a compensatory extension at the metacarpophalangeal (MCP) joints. Because the PIP joints remain in this fixed position for a prolonged period, the overlying extensor surface skin and eventually the extensor tendons may necrose, leaving an exposed joint.

In the light of the poor circulation, the standard techniques of skin cover, such as a local flap that one might employ in an otherwise normal joint, are not indicated. Sometimes the joint will heal over if the blood supply can be improved. In recalcitrant cases, the joint may be fused. This allows for shortening and may allow primary healing. Jones et al. [44] described healing of ulcers overlying 53 PIP joints in 12 patients by bone shortening and fixation with K-wires and interosseous wires. Nalebuff [45] also recommends K-wire fixation. Anandacoomarasamy et al. described lengthening the volar surface and using a full-thickness skin graft, albeit in a series of only two patients [46]. Plate fixation seems inadvisable given the bulk of the implant. We currently favor the Apex fusion fixation system (Extremity Medical, Parsippany, NJ). We have rarely found this surgery to be necessary.

Excision of Calcific Deposits

Calcific deposits are often painful and distressing for the patient (Fig. 21.4a, b). They are well visualized on plain radiography and range from being very small (subclinical) to very extensive, whereby the whole finger may become stiff. The skin may ulcerate over a large deposit. Sometimes the deposits extrude in paste form or in small fragments, with some relief of symptoms.

These deposits are similar to gouty tophi; they replace and infiltrate the normal tissues and, despite the tempting radiologic appearance, may not be expressed after blunt dissection as lipomas are. The clinical relevance of this warning is that the digital neurovascular bundle may run through such a calcific mass and is vulnerable to injury. Further, the risk of recurrence of such deposits is significant. Caution should thus be exercised in offering to remove them, and the patient should be warned that surgical intervention can only debulk (and not remove) the calcinosis which may "regrow." In particular, excision of large deposits in the pulp will remove the normal padding and may leave a rather atrophic and unprotected fingertip (Fig. 21.4c). In this circumstance, we recommend careful discussion with the patient to understand his or her hopes for surgery. Gentle debulking of the pulp is preferable to aggressive excision of all palpable calcium.

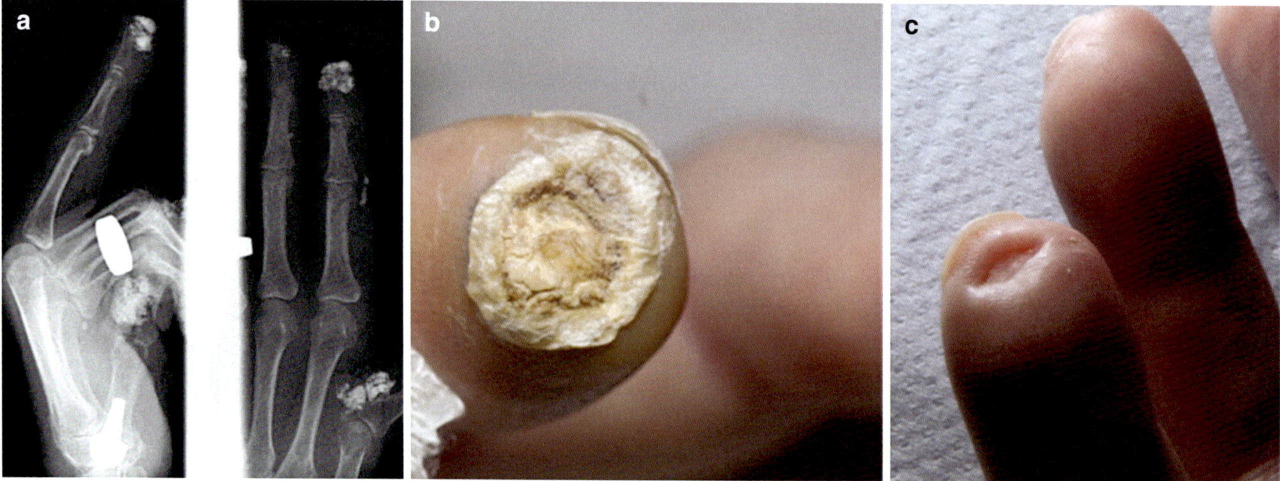

Fig. 21.4 (**a**) Calcific deposits in the index fingertip and (**b**) calcific deposits in the ring fingertip; and (**c**) after excision, the patient is left with a pulp defect. (From: Muir [49]. Reprinted with permission)

Technique

Surgery may be performed with use of local, regional, or general anesthesia. Incisions are planned on the basis of standard hand surgical techniques. After the calcific mass is exposed, this can be scraped away by blunt dissection with a curette or the end of a MacDonald dissector. Some surgeons advocate the use of a power burr [47]. This latter technique may also be used percutaneously, debriding the calcium deposit via a short incision.

Amputation

Amputation may be inevitable when all other measures have failed and may be helpful in cases of refractory infection. Sometimes in cases when an ulcer is associated with dry gangrene, the fingertip mummifies and auto-amputates with relatively little pain. In the case of an ischemic, necrotic, and painful fingertip that has not improved with the preceding treatments (exemplified in the case history), amputation is likely to help the pain. Amputation may be performed at any level. We aim to be as conservative as possible and resect as little tissue as possible, as many patients lose multiple fingertips. General hand surgical procedures should be used, but as the fingers are often abnormal in their movement, and as cosmesis may not be a major priority, we do not always adhere to generally recommended levels of amputation.

Conclusion

A small but significant proportion of patients with SSc-related digital ulcers benefits from surgical treatment. In our opinion the key aspect to successful surgical management is close communication between rheumatologist and surgeon with easy and rapid access to surgery. Fast access to surgical debridement will, in our opinion, often prevent the need for a more extensive surgical debridement. A key point is that surgical and medical approaches to digital ulcer management are complementary, and referral for surgery does not negate the need to continue to pursue all possible medical approaches to therapy.

The main indications for surgery are pain, non-healing, and the presence of underlying calcinosis. Surgical debridement and excision of calcinotic deposits are the two most commonly performed procedures. The use of periarterial sympathectomy is increasing in our own center as well as internationally. Amputation is required when all other measures fail, although it should be recognized that for many patients this offers the most rapid prospect of pain relief, improvement in hand function, and also cosmetic relief from black fingers. The roles of botulinum toxin and of fat grafting are still to be evaluated fully.

There is still room for further detailed investigation into the best treatment for the patient with non-traumatic ischemia of the hand [48]. This will ideally come from larger multicenter investigations.

Summary

The mainstay of treatment for SSc-related digital ulceration is medical.

Surgery may help if medical treatment fails.

Close cooperation between rheumatologist and surgeon will ensure that the patient is offered prompt referral and treatment where surgery may help.

References

1. Herrick A, Muir L. Raynaud's phenomenon (secondary). Systematic review 1125. BMJ Clinical Evidence. http://clinical-evidence.bmj.com/x/systematic-review/1125/overview.html. 2014 October.
2. Zhou AY, Muir L, Harris J, Herrick A. The impact of magnetic resonance imaging in early diagnosis of hand osteomyelitis in patients with systemic sclerosis. Clin Exp Rheumatol. 2014;32(Suppl 86):S-232.
3. Amanzi L, Braschi F, Fiori G, Galluccio F, Miniati I, Guiducci S, et al. Digital ulcers in scleroderma: staging, characteristics and subsetting through observation of 1614 digital lesions. Rheumatology. 2010;49:1374–82.
4. Harrison BJ, Silman AJ, Hider SL, Herrick AL. Cigarette smoking as a significant risk factor for digital vascular disease in patients with systemic sclerosis. Arthritis Rheum. 2002;46:3312–6.
5. Nihtyanova SI, Brough GM, Black CM, Denton CP. Clinical burden of digital vasculopathy in limited and diffuse systemic sclerosis. Ann Rheum Dis. 2008;67:120–3.
6. Denton CP, Krieg T, Guillevin L, Schwierin B, Rosenberg D, Silkey M, et al. Demographic, clinical and antibody characteristics of patients with digital ulcers in systemic sclerosis: data from the DUO registry. Ann Rheum Dis. 2012;71:718–21.
7. Yu HL, Chase RA, Strauch B. In atlas of hand anatomy and clinical implications, 68. St Louis: Mosby; 2004.
8. Koman LA, Paterson Smith B, Smith TL, Ruch DS, Li Z. Vascular disorders. In: Green's operative hand surgery, 2208. Philadelphia: Churchill Livingstone; 2011.
9. Chloros GD, Smerlis NN, Li Z, Smith TL, Smith BP, Koman A. Non invasive evaluation of upper extremity perfusion. J Hand Surg. 2008;33A:591–600.
10. Charkoudian N. Skin blood flow in adult human thermoregulation. How it works, when it does not, and why. Mayo Clin Proc. 2003;78:603–12.
11. Petrovsky JS. Resting blood flow in the skin: does it exist and what is the influence of temperature, aging and diabetes? J Diabetes Sci Technol. 2012;6:674–85.
12. Higgins JP, McClinton MA. Vascular insufficiency of the upper extremity. J Hand Surg. 2010;35A:1545 53.
13. Dumanian GA, Segalman K, Buehner JW, Koontz CL, Hendrickson M, Wilgis EF. Analysis of digital pulse-volume recordings with radial and ulnar artery compression. Plast Reconstr Surg. 1998;102:1993–8.

14. Kim YH, Ng SW, Seo HS, Ahn HC. Classification of Raynaud's disease based on angiographic features. J Plast Reconstr Surg. 2011;64:1503–11.
15. Janevski B. Arteries of the hand in patients with scleroderma. Diagn Imag Clin Med. 1986;55:262–5.
16. Park JA, Sung YK, Bae SC, Song SY, Seo HS, Jun JB. Ulnar artery vasculopathy in systemic sclerosis. Rheumatol Int. 2009;29:1081–6.
17. Ho M, Veale D, Eastmond C, Nuki G, Belch J. Macrovascular disease and systemic sclerosis. Ann Rheum Dis. 2000;59:39–43.
18. Merritt WH. Role and rationale for extended periarterial sympathectomy in the management of severe Raynaud syndrome. Hand Clin. 2015;31:101–20.
19. Sandqvist G, Eklund M. Validity of HAMIS: a test of hand mobility in scleroderma. Arthritis Care Res. 2000;13:382–7.
20. Steen VD, Medsger TA. The value of the Health Assessment Questionnaire and special patient-generated scales to demonstrate change in systemic sclerosis patients over time. Arthritis Rheum. 1997;40:1984–91.
21. Silman A, Akesson A, Newman J, Henriksson H, Sandquist G, Nihill M, et al. Assessment of functional ability in patients with scleroderma: a proposed new disability assessment instrument. J Rheumatol. 1998;25:79–83.
22. Brower LM, Poole JL. Reliability and validity of the Duruoz hand index in persons with systemic sclerosis (scleroderma). Arthritis Care Res. 2004;51:805–9.
23. Hudak P, Amadio PC, Bombardier C, the Upper Extremity Collaborative Group. Development of an Upper Extremity Outcome Measure: The DASH (Disabilities of the Arm, Shoulder, and Hand). Am J Ind Med. 1996;29:602–8.
24. Claes G, Droyt C, Göthberg G. Thoracoscopic sympathectomy for arterial insufficiency. Eur J Surg Suppl. 1994;572:63–4.
25. Flatt AE. Digital artery sympathectomy. J Hand Surg. 1980; 5:550–6.
26. Morgan RF, Wilgis EF. Thermal changes in a rabbit ear model after sympathectomy. J Hand Surg. 1986;11:120–4.
27. Balogh B, Mayer W, Vesely M, Mayer S, Partsch H, Piza-Katzer H. Adventitial stripping of the radial and ulnar arteries in Raynaud's disease. J Hand Surg. 2002;27A:1073–80.
28. Balogh B, Valencak J, Vesely M, Flammer M, Gruber H, Piza-Katzer H. The nerve of Henle: an anatomic and immunohistochemical study. J Hand Surg. 1999;24A:1103–8.
29. Hartzell TL, Makhni EC, Sampson C. Long term results of periarterial sympathectomy. J Hand Surg. 2009;34A:1454–60.
30. Koman AL, Smith BP, Pollock FE, Smith TL, Pollock D, Russell GB. The microcirculatory effects of peripheral sympathectomy. J Hand Surg. 1995;20:709–17.
31. Kotsis AV, Chung KC. A systematic review of the outcomes of digital sympathectomy for treatment of chronic ischaemia. J Rheumatol. 2003;30:1788–92.
32. Yee AMF, Hotchkiss RN, Paget SA. Adventitial stripping: a digit saving procedure in refractory Raynaud's phenomenon. J Rheumatol. 1998;25:269–76.
33. O'Brien BMC, Kumar PAV, Mellow CG, Oliver TV. Radical microarteriolysis in the treatment of vasospastic disorders of the hand, especially scleroderma. J Hand Surg Eur. 1992;17:447–52.
34. Tomaino MM. Digital arterial occlusion in scleroderma: is there a role for digital arterial reconstruction? J Hand Surg Eur. 2000;25:611–3.
35. Trocchia AM, Hammert WC. Arterial grafts for vascular reconstruction in the upper extremity. J Hand Surg. 2011;36A:1534–6.
36. Kryger ZB, Rawlani V, Dumanian GA. Treatment of chronic digital ischaemia with direct microsurgical revascularisation. J Hand Surg. 2007;32:1466–70.
37. Kind GM. Arterialization of the venous system of the hand. Plast Reconstr Surg. 2006;118:421–8.
38. Matarrese MR, Hammert WC. Revascularization of the ischemic hand with arterialization of the venous system. J Hand Surg. 2011;36A:2047–51.
39. Bank J, Fuller SM, Henry GI, Zachary LS. Fat grafting to the hand in patients with Raynaud phenomenon. Plast Reconst Surg. 2014;133:1109.
40. Del Papa N, Di Luca G, Sambataro D, Zaccara E, Maglione W, Gabrielli A, et al. Regional implantation of autologous adipose tissue-derived cells induces a prompt healing of long-lasting indolent digital ulcers in patients with systemic sclerosis. Cell Transplant. 2015;24:2297–305.
41. Guillaume-Jugnot P, Daumas A, Magalon J, Jouve E, Nguyen P-S, Truillet R, et al. Autologous adipose-derived stromal vascular fraction in patients with systemic sclerosis: 12-month follow-up. Rheumatology. 2016;55:301–6.
42. Guillaume-Jugnot P, Daumas A, Magalon J, Sautereau N, Veran J, Magalon G, et al. State of the art. Autologous fat graft and adipose tissue-derived stromal vascular fraction injection for hand therapy in systemic sclerosis patients. Curr Res Translation Med. 2016;64:35–42.
43. Del Papa N, Zaccara E, Di Luca G, Andracco R, Maglione W, Vitali C. Adipose-derived cell transplantation in systemic sclerosis: state of the art and future perspectives. J Scler Relat Dis. 2017;2:33–41.
44. Jones NF, Imbriglia JE, Steen VD, Medsger TA. Surgery for scleroderma of the hand. J Hand Surg. 1987;12A:391–400.
45. Nalebuff EA. Surgery in patients with systemic sclerosis of the hand. Clin Orthop Relat Res. 1999;366:91–7.
46. Anandacoomarasamy A, Englert H, Manolios N, Kirkham S. Reconstructive hand surgery for scleroderma joint contractures. J Hand Surg. 2007;32A:1107–12.
47. Gilbart MK, Jolles BM, Lee P, Bogoch ER. Surgery of the hand in severe systemic sclerosis. J Hand Surg (Eur). 2004;29:599–603.
48. Thibaudeau S, Serebrakian AT, Gerety PA, Levin LS. An algorithmic approach to the surgical treatment of chronic ischaemia of the hand: a systematic review of the literature. Plast Reconstr Surg. 2016;137:818e–28e.
49. Muir L. Surgical management. In: Wigley F, Herrick A, Flavahan N, editors. Raynaud's phenomenon. New York, NY: Springer; 2015.

Jasmin Raja and Voon H. Ong

Introduction

Digital ulceration is common and often recurs [1]. Recent data from the Digital Ulcers Outcome Registry reported that bacterial infection remains as one of the major concerns affecting 36% and 61% of patients with recurrent and chronic DU in SSc [2]. Factors that increase the risk of infection may be disease specific, and these may either be systemic or local to the infected tissue. Systemic factors would include severe gastrointestinal disease and malnutrition, immunosuppressive agents including steroids, duration of disease and ulcer, smoking and coexisting macrovascular disease in addition to other comorbidities including diabetes, while local factors that contribute to infection include history of soft tissue infections, presence of calcinosis, contractures and exposed underlying structures [2–6]. The prolonged healing time of DUs associated with the persistence and chronicity of ulcer in SSc itself also increases the risk of infection.

Features suggestive of an underlying infection include erythema and/or heat at the edge of ulcer, increasing pain and tenderness, presence of discharge, foul odour and breakdown of ulcer (Fig. 22.1). Although concurrent local joint deformity, calcinosis and contractures may cloud assessment, patients are advised to be vigilant of these warning signs and to seek medical review. Infectious complications are particularly detrimental and often contribute to the significant comorbidities with tissue gangrene and amputations (Fig. 22.2) [7]. A global approach including local and systemic treatment with pain management and vasoactive drugs is mandatory, and antibiotic treatment is central to the management of patients with infective DU.

J. Raja
Division of Rheumatology, Department of Medicine, University of Malaya, Kuala Lumpur, Malaysia

V. H. Ong (✉)
Centre for Rheumatology and Connective Tissue Diseases, UCL Medical School Royal Free Campus, London, UK
e-mail: v.ong@ucl.ac.uk

© Springer Nature Switzerland AG 2019
M. Matucci-Cerinic, C. P. Denton (eds.), *Atlas of Ulcers in Systemic Sclerosis*, https://doi.org/10.1007/978-3-319-98477-3_22

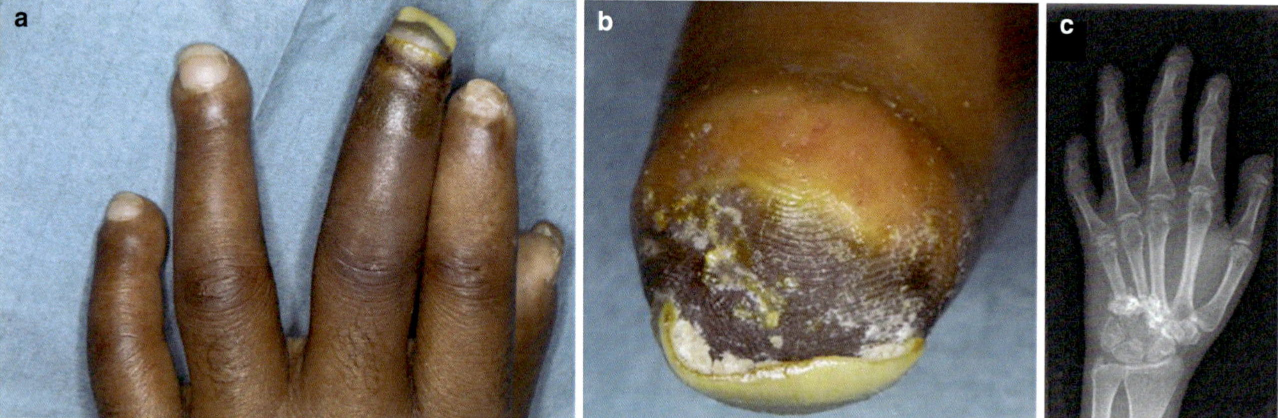

Fig. 22.1 Infected digital tip ulcer. (**a**) Ulcer at the tip of left middle finger with increased swelling and discolouration extending to the proximal interphalangeal joint. Inset (**b**) shows the fingertip ulcer with indistinct ulcer border. (**c**) Radiograph showed acro-osteolysis affecting all distal phalanges of the left five digits with exuberant calcinosis over the carpal bones with no clear loss of soft tissue over the middle finger tip

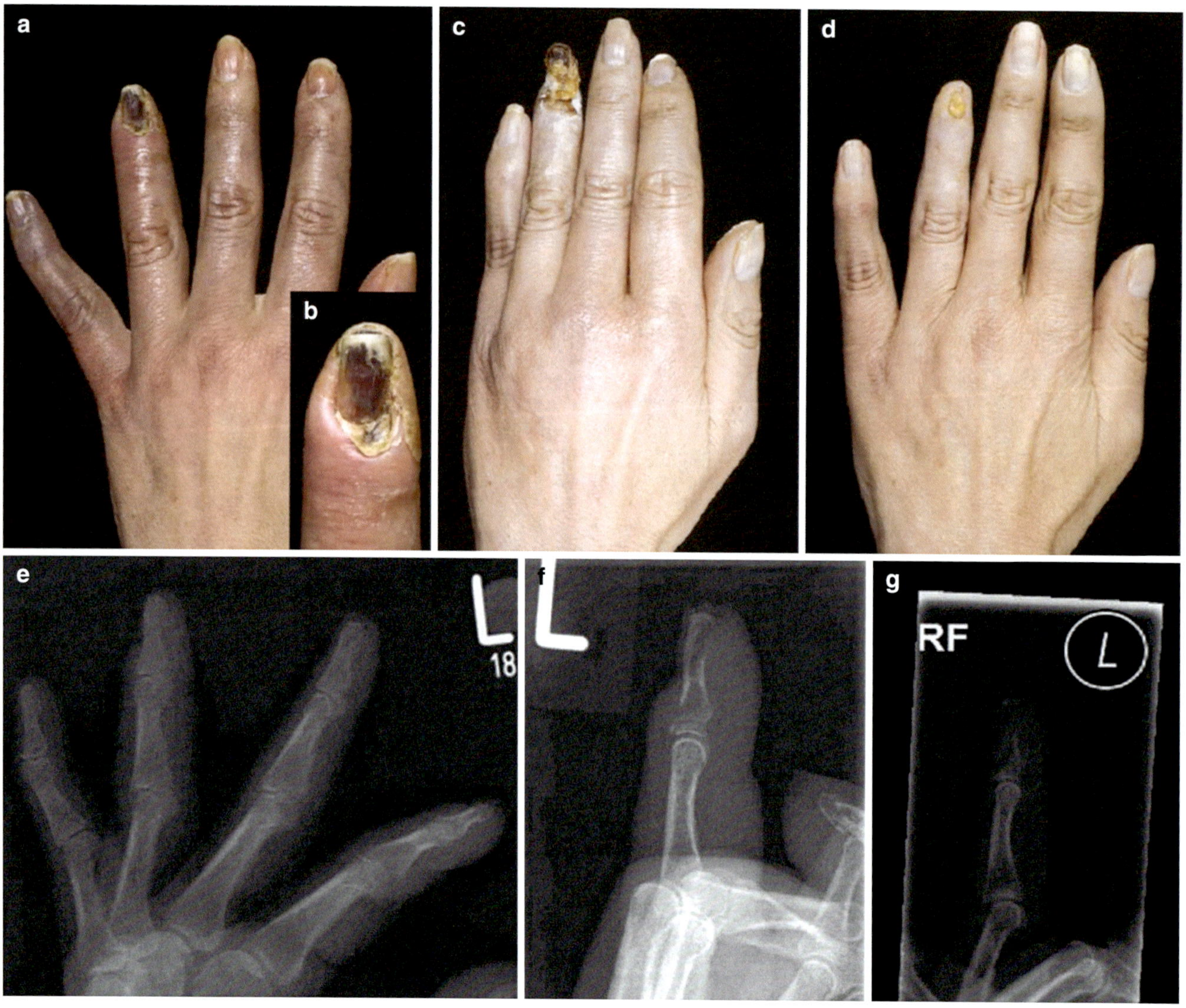

Fig. 22.2 Consequence of severe digital vasculopathy with tissue gangrene and autoamputation. (**a–d**) (with inset **b**): Serial panels showed progressive tissue loss with dry gangrene resulting in autoamputation of the left ring fingertip. (**e–g**) Serial radiographs showed worsening focal area of lucency with cortical erosive irregularity of the distal phalangeal head of the left finger consistent with osteomyelitis

Investigations

All digital ulcers with suspected infection should be evaluated by microbiologic examinations. Wound swabs should be taken routinely. Other potential sources of infections should be excluded in particular indwelling catheters or percutaneous endoscopic gastrostomies/jejunostomies feeding sites. Ideally this should precede the use of systemic antibiotics so that sensitivities can be determined. Empirical treatment can be given once wound swabs have been taken.

Culture of biopsy tissue has been advocated to allow more infections to be identified and to overcome the challenge of overgrowth of commensal or colonising bacteria.

Imaging can be useful to determine the presence of soft tissue infection, extension to involve underlying bone, joint or soft tissue structures. The presence of more invasive infection will necessitate much more intensive antibiotic therapy.

Plain X-ray can be useful, but the impact of acro-osteolysis and calcinosis can make this difficult together with the longer-term effect of bone loss secondary to severe digital ischaemia (Fig. 22.3). In the absence of clear clinical signs of infection, serial plain X-rays may be helpful to monitor evidence of infection. Rapidly progressive osteolysis as evident on serial X-rays may be indicative of osteomyelitis (Fig. 22.4). MR imaging is useful to identify bone marrow oedema that may suggest or confirm the presence of osteomyelitis (Fig. 22.5).

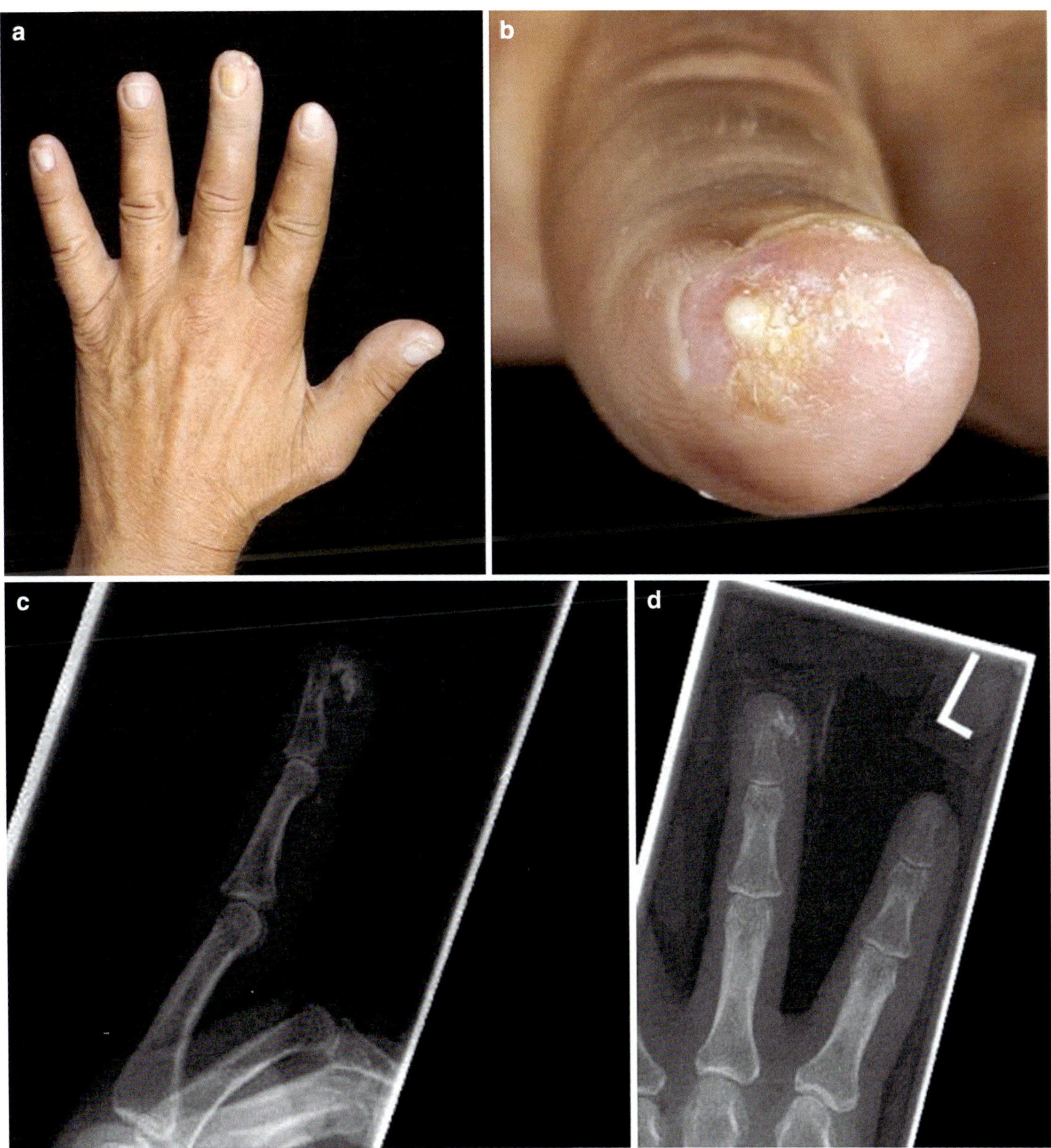

Fig. 22.3 Panel illustrates ulcer at the tip of middle finger associated with calcinosis. (**a**) Left middle finger with digital ulcer at its tip with soft tissue loss. (**b**) The underlying calcinotic nidus at the radial aspect of the digital pulp. (**c**, **d**) Lateral and anterior views of the ulcer with overlying dressing. Multiple calcific foci are shown along the distal tuft of distal phalanx with some associated soft tissue loss with no radiological evidence of osteomyelitis

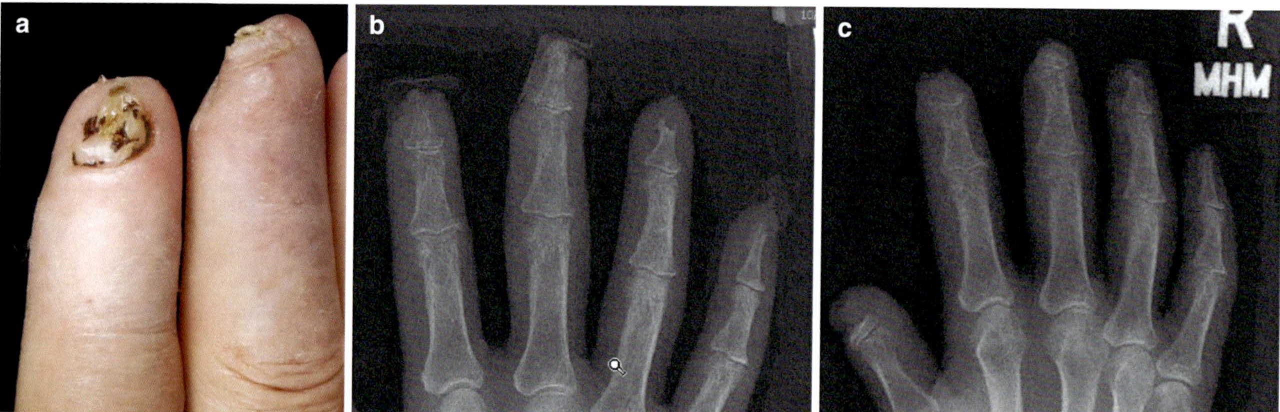

Fig. 22.4 Progressive digital resorption as a consequence of digital vasculopathy. Ulceration of right index and middle digits is shown in panel (**a**). (**b**, **c**) Serial radiographs showed progressive resorption of the affected distal phalanges over a month with irregular and ill-defined cortical erosion suspicious of osteomyelitis over the distal phalanx of the right index finger in panel C. Note the amputation of the distal phalanx of the right thumb as part of the digital vasculopathy in panel C

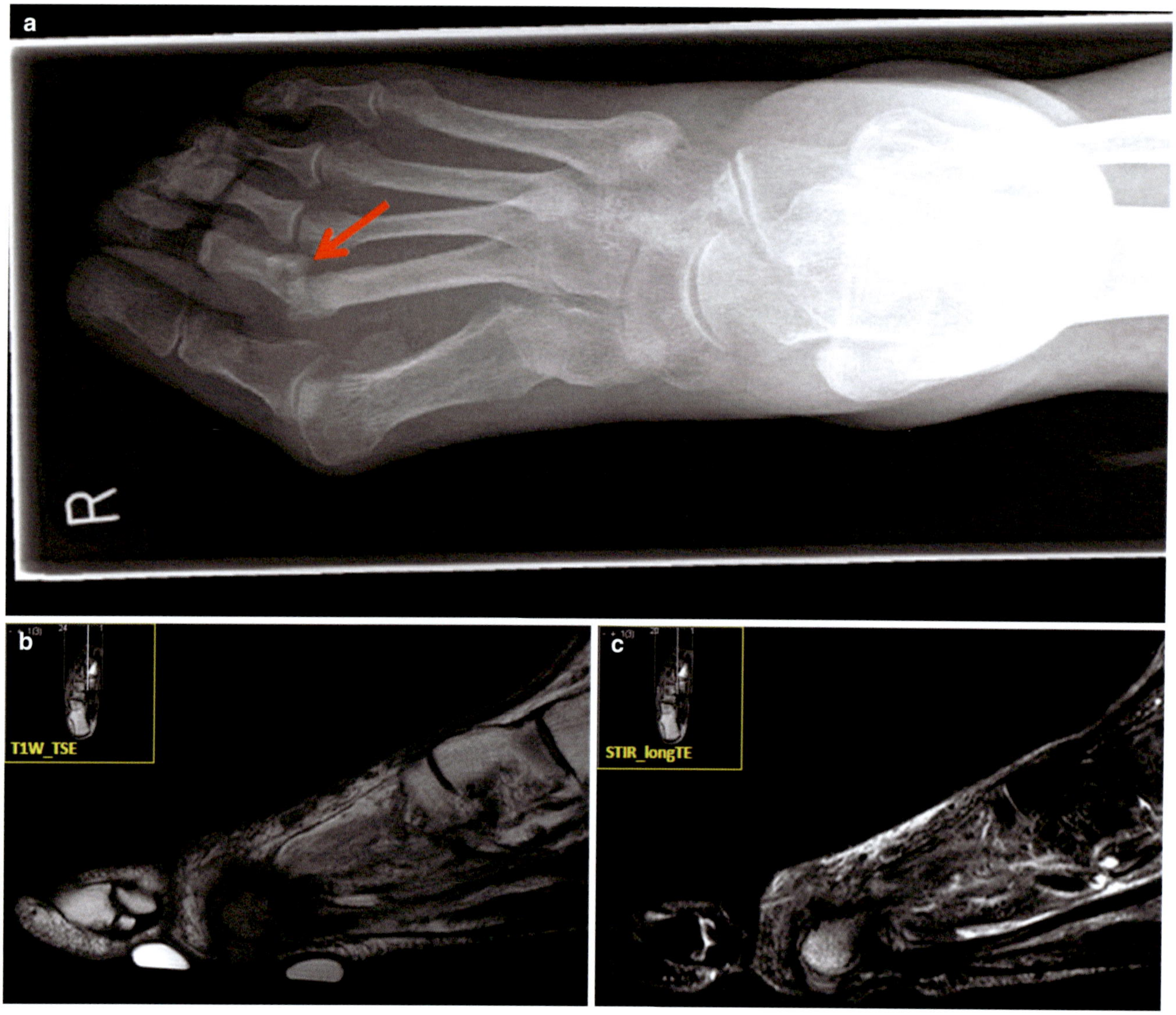

Fig. 22.5 Radiological evidence of osteomyelitis. This patient had an ulcer on the plantar aspect of the right forefoot underlying the head of the second metatarsal. Panel (**a**) showed subluxation of the right second metatarsophalangeal joint in addition to hallux valgus. There is sclero-sis and destruction at this point (red arrow) suspicious of osteomyelitis. Panels (**b**, **c**) showed marked bone marrow oedema within the second metatarsal head extending to involve the distal half of the second metatarsal with cortical destruction of the metatarsal head

Local Treatment

Debridement can be very helpful to remove necrotic tissue to prepare the wound bed to heal. However, this largely depends on local expertise and nature of the DUs. A variety of approaches have been described, and these can be mechanical with either curettage or scalpel under local anaesthetic or chemical or biological techniques with enzymatic agents (including topical D-alpha-tocopheryl acetate) or maggot therapies [8].

Systemic Treatment

Early institution of systemic antibiotics forms the cornerstone of management of infected DU. Up to 50% of patients were reported from various studies to receive systemic antibiotics for soft tissue infections involving digital ulcers [1, 9, 10]. This is most easily administered orally, and the general principle is that higher dose may be required over a prolonged duration due to poor tissue perfusion. This is especially important in ischaemic fingertip invasive ulcers associated with severe secondary Raynaud's. Associated calcinosis can also impact on treatment and makes eradication of associated infection particularly challenging. Intravenous antibiotics are generally used for more severe infections and in association with cellulitis, osteomyelitis or septic arthritis. Choice of antibiotic is governed by results of culture informed by local microbiological expertise.

Supportive Treatment

Other factors to consider include optimal treatment of Raynaud's with vasodilators including advanced therapy with PDE5 inhibitors and endothelin receptor antagonists (ERA). Management is generally in line with the UKSSG management best practice pathway [11, 12].

Concept of Antibiotic Use in Infected Digital Ulcers in SSc

Contamination and colonisation with patients' endogenous flora from the skin, mucous membranes and gastrointestinal tract should be considered carefully as chronic wounds such as SSc are susceptible to colonisation, in the interpretation of swab results in SSc-associated DUs.

The host and local factors related to SSc in particular the immunocompromised state of the individual may predispose these chronic ulcers to be colonised by bacteria. The term critical colonisation describes the clinical state in which bacteria are able to induce the failure of wound healing with formation of biofilm. In fact, there is emerging evidence that biofilm formation is an important virulence factor in contributing to the bacterial persistence and chronicity [13]. As a consequence, these bacteria are difficult to be eradicated. On the other hand, there are also concerns regarding significant excess use of antibiotics in various non-healing ulcers which could contribute to the emergence of antibiotic resistance [14].

The initial choice of antibiotics may be empirical based on local prevalence of the pathogens and should be tailored to the specific needs of each population and institution. The cultures of swab are frequently negative or show mixed growth of microbes; however with cultures demonstrating a predominant bacteria, the choice of antibiotics should be targeted towards that organism depending on the sensitivity of the culture. Further advice from microbiologist on the appropriate antibiotic and the route of administration would be useful.

For mild superficial infection or for prevention of infection, topical antibiotics can be used but with caution as certain topical treatment such as Neosporin and bacitracin can incite irritant contact dermatitis to the already compromised soft tissue. Mupirocin 2% ointment (Bactroban) is a favourable choice instead as it rarely causes dermatitis and protects against MRSA [15]. Antiseptics should also be avoided due to its cytotoxic effects on cells [16].

Intravenous antibiotics should be considered in patients with multiple digital ulcers in particular in those who failed oral therapies. Other circumstances in which intravenous antibiotics may be preferred over oral route include complications of DUs with deep-seated infection and poor tolerability due to comorbidities, for example, gastrointestinal tolerance.

Pathogens Encountered in Infected Digital Ulcers in SSc

Similar to the pathogens identified from common chronic ulcers, digital ulcers in patients with SSc frequently isolate *Staphylococcus aureus* which is found around 50% among the pathogens [6, 10]. In one study involving 42 SSc patients, interestingly intestinal bacteria such as *Escherichia coli* and *Enterococcus faecalis* were detected in 26% from the cultures taken and were the second most common pathogens identified following *Staph aureus* [17]. It is believed that the patient's hand hygiene is often inadequate and the presence of digital ulcers further compromises this after defecation. Hence the importance of effective hand hygiene should be emphasised among patients, relatives and health workers dealing with the ulcers. Other pathogens isolated were *Pseudomonas aeruginosa* (12%) and less frequently *Proteus mirabilis, Streptococcus agalactiae, Citrobacter koseri* and *Stenotrophomonas maltophilia.*

The prevalence of osteomyelitis was invariably found (42%) in the setting of infected SSc digital ulcers in a follow-up study [18]. The most frequently isolated pathogens from the digital ulcers complicated with osteomyelitis were *Staph aureus* and Gram-negative enterofaecal bacteria. Other less commonly identified microorganisms were *Pseudomonas aeruginosa, Streptococcus agalactiae, Staphylococcus epidermidis, Enterobacter aerogenes, Stenotrophomonas maltophilia, Proteus mirabilis* and *Serratia marcescens.* Standard radiographic examinations in chronic infected SSc digital ulcers is important to exclude osteomyelitis as the treatment offered would be variable in terms of the choice, route of administration and duration of antibiotics.

The predominant clinical manifestation of *S. aureus* is colonisation, rather than infection. Both methicillin-sensitive *S. aureus* (MSSA) and methicillin-resistant *S. aureus* (MRSA) infections are directly or indirectly caused by skin colonisation by these microbes. The difficult challenge faced by clinicians treating the infected digital ulcers is infection caused by drug-resistant *Staphylococcus aureus*, particularly MRSA. In the USA, MRSA was seen in 59% out of 320 patients with staphylococcal infection in a study of patients with skin and soft tissue infection attending the emergency departments [19]. Inappropriate use of antibiotics contributes to the emergence of antibiotic resistance in the community resulting in difficulty and complexity in treating this condition. The presence of MRSA infection can occur in soft tissue infection alone or together with osteomyelitis in the setting of digital ulcer.

Choice of Antibiotic

The choice of antibiotic needs consideration of several factors, even though it depends primarily on culture growth and sensitivity. Factors need to be considered include drug tolerability and adverse effects (existing scleroderma-related gastrointestinal symptoms may dictate choice of antibiotics), complications in particular osteomyelitis, drug interaction, predicted duration of therapy, route of administration, cost, toxicity and monitoring and soft tissue and bone penetration profile. SSc patients most often will need prolonged length of antibiotic course due to diminished vascular supply and immunocompromised state. In complex soft tissue infection, 1–4-week length of treatment is recommended, while for cases of osteomyelitis, the predicted treatment course would be from 6 to 12 weeks. The length of treatment is variable between individuals even though similar pathogen is encountered. Therefore, clinical response is the best measure of treatment success. Regular review and monitoring of the ulcer would be necessary to assess the response. Besides antibiotics, debridement of non-viable tissue and drainage of accompanying abscess, if any, for example, would facilitate the resolution of an infection.

It is advisable for the GP and health practitioner to start the patient on a course of oral antibiotics when infection of the digital ulcer is suspected, while swab cultures are taken. The likely pathogen for most digital ulcer-associated infection is *Staph aureus*. It is important to recognise that normal skin flora, e.g. *Pseudomonas* species, is often detected on wound swab and clinical correlation is critical. Subject to local microbiological practice, the recommended antibiotic during initial review of an infected digital ulcer is oral flucloxacillin 500 mg four times daily for a minimum of 2 weeks. Another option would be oral co-amoxiclav 625 mg three times daily. If allergic to penicillin, alternatives such as macrolides, erythromycin or clarythromycin may be considered. Cephalexins and doxycycline are also suitable for this indication [20]. In cases of chronic non-healing, persistently recurring infections, prolonged and/or rotating courses and parenteral administration may be required. Multidisciplinary approach with an expert advice of a microbiologist and infectious disease physician with local wound care and dressings is essential.

As discussed earlier, MRSA is an emerging problem and difficult to treat infection. Both bactericidal and bacteriostatic agents have been effective in the treatment of MRSA. A number of antibiotics, both oral and intravenous, are recommended in treating soft tissue and bone infected with MRSA and are outlined in Table 22.1. It has also been suggested that minocycline is an effective therapeutic option and provides rapid improvement and resolution of MRSA infection following prolonged and unsuccessful therapy with doxycy-

Table 22.1 Antibiotics recommended in treating soft tissue and bone infected with MRSA

Antibiotic	Route of administration	Main benefits	Main problems
Erythromycin (macrolide)	PO (main) and IV	Widespread experience of use	Comparatively poor oral absorption, GI side effects
Clindamycin (macrolide)	PO (main) and IV	Excellent bone penetration	Risk of *Clostridium difficile* diarrhoea
Linezolid (bacteriostatic)	PO (main) and IV	Excellent bioavailability and tissue penetration. Well tolerated; resistance rare	Reversible myelosuppression on prolonged courses; expensive
Daptomycin	IV	Once-daily administration Resistance rare	Skeletal muscle toxicity. Creatine kinase monitoring required
Vancomycin (glycopeptide)	IV	Widespread experience of use. Studies on bone penetration is less conclusive	Nephrotoxicity – monitoring required Increasing resistance concerns
Teicoplanin (glycopeptide)	IV	Less nephrotoxic than vancomycin Once-daily administration	Monitoring required Concerns regarding resistance
Doxycycline (tetracycline)	PO	Once-daily administration	Nausea ± vomiting, oesophageal irritation
Minocycline (tetracycline)	PO (main) and IV	Good safety profile and efficacy against MRSA; inexpensive	
Tigecycline (bacteriostatic)	IV	Use in polymicrobial infection	GI side effects
Rifampicin (bactericidal)	PO (main) and IV	Excellent tissue and bone penetration	Must be used in combination Extensive interactions Liver function monitoring
Fusidic acid	PO (main) and IV	Excellent tissue and bone penetration	Must be used in combination

PO per oral, *IV* intravenous, *GI* gastrointestinal, *MRSA* methicillin-resistant *staphylococcus aureus*
Adapted from Thompson and Townsend [22], with permission from Elsevier

cline, in cases of doxycycline-related MRSA resistance [21]. Choice of antibiotics under these circumstances should be guided by local standards of microbiological guidance and recommendations.

An important consideration in SSc-related digital ulceration is the presence of calcinosis that may contribute to the initiation and chronicity of ulceration and infection. Mannose-binding lectin levels and markers of oxidative stress, the advanced glycation/lipoperoxidation end products with their respective receptor, have been found to be upregulated in SSc patients with calcinosis [23, 24]. Recent mass spectrometric analysis on protein composition of calcinotic deposits from a small cohort of patients with SSc revealed a subset of immune-related components with neutrophils, immunoglobulins and complement system, thus supporting that immunoinflammatory response may underlie the aetiopathogenesis of dystrophic calcinosis [25].

There is evidence to suggest that tetracyclines including minocycline may have anti-inflammatory effects with suppression of key cytokines including tumour necrosis factor-alpha (TNF-α) and interleukins (IL-6 and IL-1β). Other potential mechanisms include downregulation of collagenolytic enzymes including matrix metalloproteinases, elastase and cathepsins with augmentation of antioxidant effects [26, 27]. In support of this, minocycline was reported to be effective in the treatment of calcinosis in a small case series of nine patients [28], and while its use has not been formally evaluated in a larger study, minocycline may be considered in selected patients with ulcers associated with calcinosis.

Observational Data from Royal Free Hospital (2014–2015)

Table 22.2 summarises recent data on our experience on the management of SSc-related infected digital ulcers with antibiotics in an unselected cohort of patients followed up in a specialist nurse-led digital ulcer clinic over a 12-month period. Consistent with the published literature, *Staph aureus* remains the most frequently isolated pathogen in our cohort. A majority of these pathogens were either MRSA or MSSA despite the routine practice of topical decolonisation of our patients. This highlights the complexity and challenge in the management of soft tissue infection in SSc given the chronicity of the disease, frequent hospitalisations with recurrent antibiotic use and associated use of immunosuppressive agents in this disease. The other pathogens encountered were *Pseudomonas aeruginosa*, *Enterobacter cloacae* and *Serratia marcescens*. On the other hand, normal skin flora was demonstrated in 25%, and the significance of this needs to be considered in the appropriate clinical context.

All patients had initial treatment with the penicillin group (flucloxacillin and co-amoxiclav). Subsequent courses of antibiotics were either macrolide (erythromycin or clarithromycin) or tetracycline synthetic (doxycycline). The patients received the antibiotics over 1–4 weeks. Prolonged antibiotic treatment was given to three patients who had digital ulcers complicated by osteomyelitis. All three patients received doxycycline; one patient received teicoplanin before switching to doxycycline. Patient 12 received prolonged 3-month course of doxycycline even though no osteomyelitis was detected and swab culture only demonstrated normal skin flora. The rationale for extended therapy was based on the anecdotal evidence of doxycycline on chronic inflammation associated with poor ulcer healing. Similarly, minocycline and pamidronate were continued for Patient 11 with underlying calcinosis complicating the ulcer. In addition to antibiotics, all 12 patients received concomitant treatment for Raynaud's and digital ulcers with prostacyclin analogue, vasodilators, endothelin receptor antagonist (bosentan) or PDE5 inhibitor (sildenafil), antiplatelets alone or in combination. All 12 patients showed good clinical response and improvement of their ulcers with negative wound swabs at the end of the observation period. An illustrative case with patient 2 is shown in Fig. 22.6.

Table 22.2 Observational data on antibiotics use in infected digital ulcers in 12 SSc patients at the Royal Free Hospital from 2014 to 2015

Patient	Antibiotics	Antibiotics duration	Swab culture and sensitivity	Therapies	Complications
1	Fluclox	4 weeks	*P. aeruginosa*	Ilo, sil, los	No OM
2	Fluclox, doxy	1 week, 12 weeks	MSSA (S: fluclox), MRSA (S: teic). Repeat swab (NG)	Ilo, sil, los, nif, clo	OM
3	Fluclox, doxy	4 weeks (Doxy)	*P. aeruginosa* (S: cipro, taz). Repeat swab (NG)	Sil, ena, asp	OM
4	Fluclox	1 week, 3 weeks	MSSA (S: fluclox)	Ilo, sil, IVIG, asp, los	No OM
5	Fluclox	2 weeks	Normal skin flora	Ilo, asp, fluox, dil, monopril	
6	Fluclox, claryth (total of 4 courses)	1–2 weeks each	MRSA (S: mupirocin)	Ilo, sil, asp, los, GTN patch	No OM
7	Aug; day 11 ceft (allergy), switched to teic and genta; doxy	2 weeks (augm), 3 days (teic and genta), 4 weeks (doxy)	MSSA (S: fluclox, eryth, claryth)	Ilo, sil, los, asp	OM
8	Aug, fluclox, doxy	4 weeks (fluclox), 4 weeks (doxy)	MSSA (S: fluclox, eryth, claryth)	Ilo	NA
9	Fluclox	2 weeks	*E. cloacae* (S: cipro) Possibility of colonising flora	Ilo, los, clo	NA
10	Fluclox, eryth	1 week each	*S. marcescens* (R: amp, aug, cephal) Possibility of colonising flora	Ilo, sil, amlo, ram, bosentan	NA
11	Fluclox, claryth	2 weeks each	MRSA (S: cipro, clinda, eryth, fucidin, teic)	Minocycline, pamidronate	Calcinosis
12	Fluclox, doxy	5 weeks, 12 weeks	Normal skin flora	Ilo	No OM

Fluclox flucloxacillin, *doxy* doxycycline, *claryth* clarithromycin, *eryth* erythromycin, *aug* aumentin, *teic* teicoplanin, *genta* gentamicin, *ceft* ceftriaxone, *cipro* ciprofloxacin, *taz* tazocin, *amp* ampicillin, *cephal* cephalexin, *clinda* clindamycin, *ilo* iloprost, *sil* sildanefil, *los* losartan, *nif* nifedipine, *clo* clopidogrel, *asp* aspirin, *ena* enalapril, *dil* diltiazem, *fluox* fluoxetine, *amlo* amlodipine, *ram* ramipril, *IVIG* intravenous immunoglobulin, *GTN* glyceryl trinitrate, *P. aeruginosa Pseudomonas aeruginosa*, *E. cloacae Enterobacter cloacae*, *S. marcescens Serratia marcescens*, *NG* no growth, *MSSA* methicillin-sensitive *Staphylococcus aureus*, *MRSA* methicillin-resistant *Staphylococcus aureus*, *OM* osteomyelitis, *S* sensitive, *R* resistant, *NA* not applicable

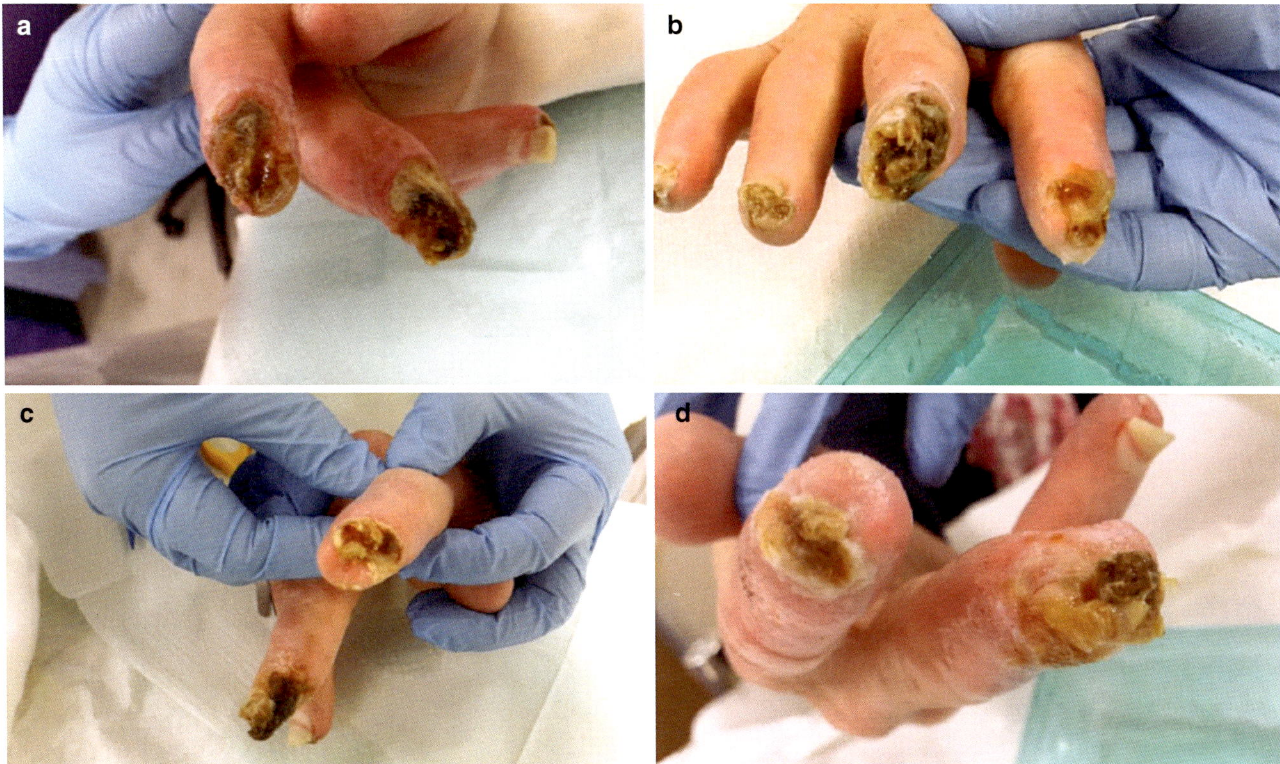

Fig. 22.6 The serial photographs ((**a**) baseline, (**b**) week 2, (**c**) week 6, (**d**) week 10)) demonstrate the temporal course of treatment response with prolonged course of doxycycline in a SSc patient with severe chronic non-healing digital ulcers predominantly right index and middle fingers complicated with MRSA osteomyelitis. Multidisciplinary approach with expert advice from microbiologist and close monitoring and regular wound care in a specialist nurse-led digital ulcer clinic was critical in managing this complex case

Conclusion

Infection should be considered in all DU, and management involves local and systemic therapy together with general management of SSc vasculopathy. Early and prompt recognition based on clinical signs and symptoms is critical. Patient education and awareness of this complication ideally within a dedicated SSc digital vascular clinic is pivotal for the prevention of digital ulcers and management of these patients. Early treatment with appropriate antibiotics and local wound care are crucial to prevent complications such as osteomyelitis and gangrene. Empirical choice of antibiotics and definitive treatments should be guided according to local practice. A multidisciplinary approach across all levels of medical and surgical teams is essential to guide diagnostic and therapeutic management.

Acknowledgment We would like to acknowledge Ms. Annalyn Nunag, our specialist nurse for her contribution towards collection of data from patients with digital ulceration treated with antibiotics.

References

1. Denton CP, et al. Demographic, clinical and antibody characteristics of patients with digital ulcers in systemic sclerosis: data from the DUO Registry. Ann Rheum Dis. 2012;71:718–21.
2. Matucci-Cerinic M, et al. Elucidating the burden of recurrent and chronic digital ulcers in systemic sclerosis: long-term results from the DUO Registry. Ann Rheum Dis. 2016;75(10):1770–6.
3. Bootun R. Effects of immunosuppressive therapy on wound healing. Int Wound J. 2013;10:98–104.
4. Bosanquet DC, Harding KG. Wound duration and healing rates: cause or effect? Wound Repair Regen. 2014;22:143–50.
5. Xu D, et al. Clinical characteristics of systemic sclerosis patients with digital ulcers in China. Clin Exp Rheumatol. 2013;31(Suppl 76):S46–9.
6. Ingraham K, Steen V. Morbidity of digital tip ulceration in scleroderma (abstract). Arthritis Rheum. 2006;54(supplement 9):578.
7. Allanore Y, et al. Clinical characteristics and predictors of gangrene in patients with systemic sclerosis and digital ulcers in the Digital Ulcer Outcome Registry: a prospective, observational cohort. Ann Rheum Dis. 2016;75(9):1736–40.
8. Fiori G, Galluccio F, Braschi F, Amanzi L, Miniati I, Conforti ML, et al. Vitamin E gel reduces time of healing of digital ulcers in systemic sclerosis. Clin Exp Rheumatol. 2009;27:51–4.
9. Nihtyanova SI, Brough GM, Black CM, Denton CP. Clinical burden of digital vasculopathy in limited and diffuse cutaneous systemic sclerosis. Ann Rheum Dis. 2008;67(1):120–3.
10. Cutolo M, Herrick AL, Distler O, Becker MO, Beltran E, Carpentier P, et al. Nailfold videocapillaroscopic features and other clinical risk factors for digital ulcers in systemic sclerosis: a multicenter, prospective cohort study. Arthritis Rheumatol. 2016;68(10):2527–39.
11. Denton CP, et al. BSR and BHPR guideline for the treatment of systemic sclerosis. Rheumatology (Oxford). 2016;55(10):1906–10.
12. Hughes M, et al. Consensus best practice pathway of the UK Scleroderma Study Group: digital vasculopathy in systemic sclerosis. Rheumatology (Oxford). 2015;54(11):2015–24.
13. Klein S, et al. Evidence-based topical management of chronic wounds according to the T.I.M.E. principle. J Dtsch Dermatol Ges. 2013;11(9):819–29.
14. Gürgen M. Excess use of antibiotics in patients with non-healing ulcers. EMWA J. 2014;14(1):17.
15. Sherber NS, Wigley FM. Evaluation and management of skin disease. Scleroderma: from pathogenesis to comprehensive management. New York: Springer; 2016. p. 483–4.
16. Gualtierotti R, Adorni G, Lubatti C, Zeni S, Meroni PL, Ingegnoli F. Digital ulcer management in patients with systemic sclerosis. OA Arthritis. 2014;2(1):2.
17. Giuggioli D, Manfredi A, Colaci M, Lumetti F, Ferri C. Scleroderma digital ulcers complicated by infection with fecal pathogens. Arthritis Care Res (Hoboken). 2012;64(2):295–7.
18. Giuggioli D, Manfredi A, Colaci M, Lumetti F, Ferri C. Osteomyelitis complicating scleroderma digital ulcers. Clin Rheumatol. 2013;32(5):623–7.
19. Moran GJ, Krishnadasan A, Gorwitz RJ, Fosheim GE, McDougal LK, Carey RB, et al. Methicillin-resistant S. aureus infections among patients in the emergency department. N Engl J Med. 2006;355(7):666–74.
20. Steen V, Denton CP, Pope JE, Matucci-Cerinic M. Digital ulcers: overt vascular disease in systemic sclerosis. Rheumatology (Oxford). 2009;48 Suppl:iii19–24.
21. Cunha BA. Minocycline is a reliable and effective oral option to treat meticillin-resistant Staphylococcus aureus skin and soft-tissue infections, including doxycycline treatment failures. Int J Antimicrob Agents. 2014;43(4):386–7.
22. Thompson S, Townsend R. Pharmacological agents for soft tissue and bone infected with MRSA: which agent and for how long? Injury. 2011;42(Suppl 5):S7–10.
23. Osthoff M, Ngian GS, Dean MM, et al. Potential role of the lectin pathway of complement in the pathogenesis and disease manifestations of systemic sclerosis: a case inverted question mark control and cohort study. Arthritis Res Ther. 2014;16:480.
24. Davies CA, Herrick AL, Cordingley L, et al. Expression of advanced glycation end products and their receptor in skin from patients with systemic sclerosis with and without calcinosis. Rheumatology (Oxford, England). 2009;48:876–82.
25. Gallas A, Hunter CA, Blanford CF, Lockyer NP, Herrick AL, Winpenny REP. Protein composition of systemic sclerosis-related calcinotic deposits [abstract]. Rheumatology (Oxford, England). 2017;56(Suppl 2):35.
26. Nüesch E, Rutjes AW, Trelle S, Reichenbach S, Jüni P. Doxycycline for osteoarthritis of the knee or hip. Cochrane Database Syst Rev. 2009;4:CD007323.
27. Di Caprio R, Lembo S, Di Costanzo L, Balato A, Monfrecola G. Anti-inflammatory properties of low and high doxycycline doses: an in vitro study. Mediat Inflamm. 2015;2015:329418.
28. Robertson LP, Marshall RW, Hickling P. Treatment of cutaneous calcinosis in limited systemic sclerosis with minocycline. Ann Rheum Dis. 2003;62(3):267–9.

Alternative Therapeutic Approaches in Skin Ulcers Due to Systemic Sclerosis

Nabil George, Todd Kanzara, and Kuntal Chakravarty

Alternative Approaches

Among the main principles of medical treatment, it has become evident that the use of alternative non-pharmaceutical therapies should play a more significant role in management. We present and discuss the various modalities and their mechanisms in this chapter aiming to highlight their efficacy and current evidence base in the treatment of digital ulcerations in scleroderma.

Hyperbaric Oxygen Therapy

The concept of hyperbaric oxygen therapy (HBOT) aims to raise the partial pressure of oxygen in plasma alongside saturating haemoglobin. By confining the patient within a compression chamber and raising atmospheric pressures to 2–2.5 atmospheric absolute units (ATA), a partial pressure of oxygen (PO_2) at or greater than 100 kPa [1, 2] can be established.

Plasma becomes highly oxygenated, and oxygen diffusion into tissues increases, thereby addressing the cellular hypoxia. Furthermore, the effects of HBOT have been shown to reduce postischaemic oedema, ameliorating tissue perfusion and the microcirculation [3]. Physiologically, the effect of raising the partial pressure of oxygen induces vasoconstriction though with compensatory higher oxygenation [4, 5]. Additionally, the delivery of high concentration of oxygen tends to increase the formation of free radicals, such as reactive oxygen species (ROS) and reactive nitrogen species (RNS) that in turn upregulates antioxidants [6]. As shown in the diagram below (Fig. 23.1), the overall therapeutic effects of HBOT can be explained by the anti-inflammatory and pro-regenerative mechanisms mediated via cellular signalling pathways [1].

Currently, the National Health Service of England has commissioned the use of HBOT for use in decompression illness, gas embolism and acute carbon monoxide poisoning [2]. However, the potential for its use in other disease states has also been extensively investigated [5, 7]. A Cochrane review regarding chronic diabetic ulcers illustrated an improvement in wound healing with supplementary HBOT, at least in the short term [8]. Table 23.1 shows HBOT applied in DU of scleroderma and its outcome. The studies shown identified patients with intractable peripheral ulcers associated with scleroderma. In all cases where HBOT was considered, patients' healing potential was assessed in terms of perfusion indices using transcutaneous oximetry. A reading greater than 300 mmHg under hyperbaric oxygen delivery

N. George
Medicine/Surgery, North Middlesex University Hospital, London, UK

T. Kanzara
Otolaryngology, Southend Hospital, Southend, Essex, UK

K. Chakravarty (✉)
Rheumatology, Royal Free Hospital NHS Foundation Trust, London, UK

© Springer Nature Switzerland AG 2019
M. Matucci-Cerinic, C. P. Denton (eds.), *Atlas of Ulcers in Systemic Sclerosis*, https://doi.org/10.1007/978-3-319-98477-3_23

satisfied the criteria for HBOT. As results showed, the outcomes were variable at 6 months post-HBOT with complete healing of some ulcers but not others, though consistently tissue perfusion had improved.

Such case reports shed light on the potential of HBOT in treating ulcers of scleroderma. The technicalities of such modality of treatment involve patients committing significant time in the chamber as well as being able to tolerate the confined space. Logistically, hyperbaric chambers are still not widely available; with various chambers of different treatment capabilities scattered across the United Kingdom and Northern Ireland [11] and over 500 across North America

[12]. Additionally, the side effects of hyperbaric treatment include barotrauma of cavities, such as the ears, sinuses, teeth, eyes, gastrointestinal tract and lungs [13]. Careful monitoring of patients and pre-procedure assessments to identify any risk of barotrauma as well as appropriate reversal of atmospheric pressures require qualified and trained staff to manage the process.

In summary, HBOT has the potential to become a vital adjunct in treating digital ulcers associated with scleroderma. However, more studies and research is required, especially randomised controlled trials, as we have only seen sparse evidence published.

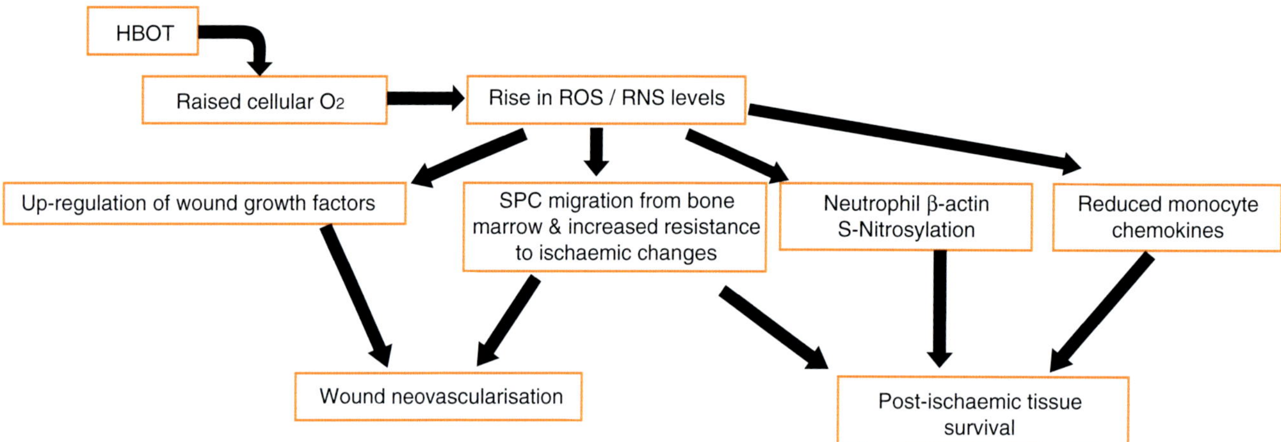

Fig. 23.1 Signalling pathways involved in tissue neovascularisation and tissue viability as induced by HBOT. At the centre of these pathways are ROS/RNS that act as signalling molecules, leading to various signalling cascades and promoting growth factors, stem cells recruitment and reduction in inflammatory mediators. SDF-1 stromal-derived factor-1, TGFβ1 transforming growth factor β1, VEGF vascular endothelial growth factor, SPC stem/progenitor cells, HIF-1/2 hypoxia inducible factor 1/2, HO-1 haem oxygenase-1, HSP heat shock proteins. (Modified from Thom [1])

Table 23.1 HBOT used for DU of scleroderma [9, 10]

Study		Patient	Methods	Outcomes
Markus et al. (2006) [9]	Case 1.	Bilateral medial malleoli ulcers in a patient with scl-70 antibodies positive scleroderma	HBOT at 2.4 ATA for 90 minutes per session, 5 days a week for 6 weeks	6 months post-HBOT: Complete healing with no recurrence
	Case 2.	Bilateral symmetrical ulcers of the third digits in a patient with overlap syndrome [systemic lupus erythematosus and limited scleroderma]	HBOT at 2.4 ATA for 90 minutes per session, 5 days a week for 6 weeks	6 months post-HBOT: Complete healing of right-sided ulcer Left sided digit remained ulcerated Overall perfusion improvement
Gerodimos et al. (2013) [10]	Case 1.	Ulcers at the left medial malleolus and right first toe in a patient with limited cutaneous scleroderma	HBOT at 2.4 ATA for 90 minutes per session for 34 sessions + regular debridement	Complete healing of the left ankle ulcer Right toe ulcer incompletely healed; though tissue perfusion improved (avoided amputation)

Botox

The botulinum toxin (Botox) is a neurotoxin derived from the gram-positive anaerobic bacterium *Clostridium botulinum*. Historically it has been described as the 'sausage poison' due to its association with an episode of mass poisoning following a feast on contaminated sausage and ham (not due to its morphology) [14]. Ever since, it has been developed to treat many conditions, as listed in Table 23.2.

Of the seven toxins produced by *Clostridium botulinum* (types A, B, C1, D, E, F, G), the neurotoxins A (or Botox-A), B and E are the most potent to humans with a potential to cause fatal botulism, particularly the former. The main targets of the botulinum toxin are acetylcholine systems at the neuromuscular junctions (NMJ), autonomic ganglia, postganglionic parasympathetic nerve endings and postganglionic sympathetic nerve endings. The toxin polypeptide itself comprises a heavy and a light chain. The combined mechanisms of the toxins include blocking neurotransmitter release at cholinergic nerve terminals [15–20], resulting in depressed endplate potentials at the NMJ and subsequent muscle paralysis [21]. At other sites of action, cholinergic mechanisms are also inhibited, such as at eccrine epithelia driven by acetylcholine (explaining its use in hyperhidrosis) and at smooth muscle structures [15]. One study [22] addressed the effects of Botox-A on different classes of cotransmitters at autonomic neurovasculature. Their findings implicated Botox-A in the partial inhibition of noradrenergic systems of vasoconstriction as well as eliminating cholinergic presynaptic inhibition of vasodilator neurones, conferring a state of vasodilatation independent of nitric oxide-mediated vasodilation. Animal studies have also shown that surgical flaps treated with Botox-A exhibited an increase in survival rate due to improved circulation and increased expression of vascular endothelial growth factor (VEGF) [23–26].

Further, recent studies illustrated the role of Botox-A, which also protected against endothelial damage in vitro by reducing the oxidative damage elicited during ischaemia-reperfusion injury [27]. In the study, episodes of ischaemia were induced as intermittent hypoxia to tissue, in an attempt to mimic ischaemia-reperfusion injury, the putative causal mechanism of Raynaud's phenomenon (RP). Altogether, these properties of Botox have made it a potential candidate in the management of digital ischaemia seen in Raynaud's phenomenon and associated ulceration. Subjectively and objectively, symptoms of RP such as pain, numbness, digital stiffness and perfusion as well as ulcer healing seem to improve by administration of Botox-A [28–34]. From local experience at the Royal Free London NHS Foundation Trust, an established scleroderma centre in London, Botox has been observed to provide symptomatic relief, mostly for ulcers occurring at or around the proximal and distal interphalangeal joints of digits (Fig. 23.2). The drawbacks of using Botox-A, however, include lack of standardised injection protocols and the potential side effects of botulinum at the target site. Local muscle weakness, albeit transient, has been reported [30]. Nonetheless, randomised controlled trials with Botox-A for RP and specifically addressing ulcerations are needed to substantiate the long-term effects and efficacy of such treatment.

Table 23.2 The established role of Botox in other conditions [15–19]

Domain						
Neuromuscular	Idiopathic focal dystonia	Craniocervical spasms and dystonias	Facial dystonias	Tardive dystonia	Chronic migraines	Primary hyperhidrosis
Pelvic floor	Detrusor-related overactive bladder					
Ocular	Primary/secondary eso/exotropia	Nonconcomitant misalignment	Paralytic strabismus	Restrictive or myogenic strabismus		
Cosmetic/ dermatologic	Glabellar lines	Facial and neck wrinkles, creases and lines				

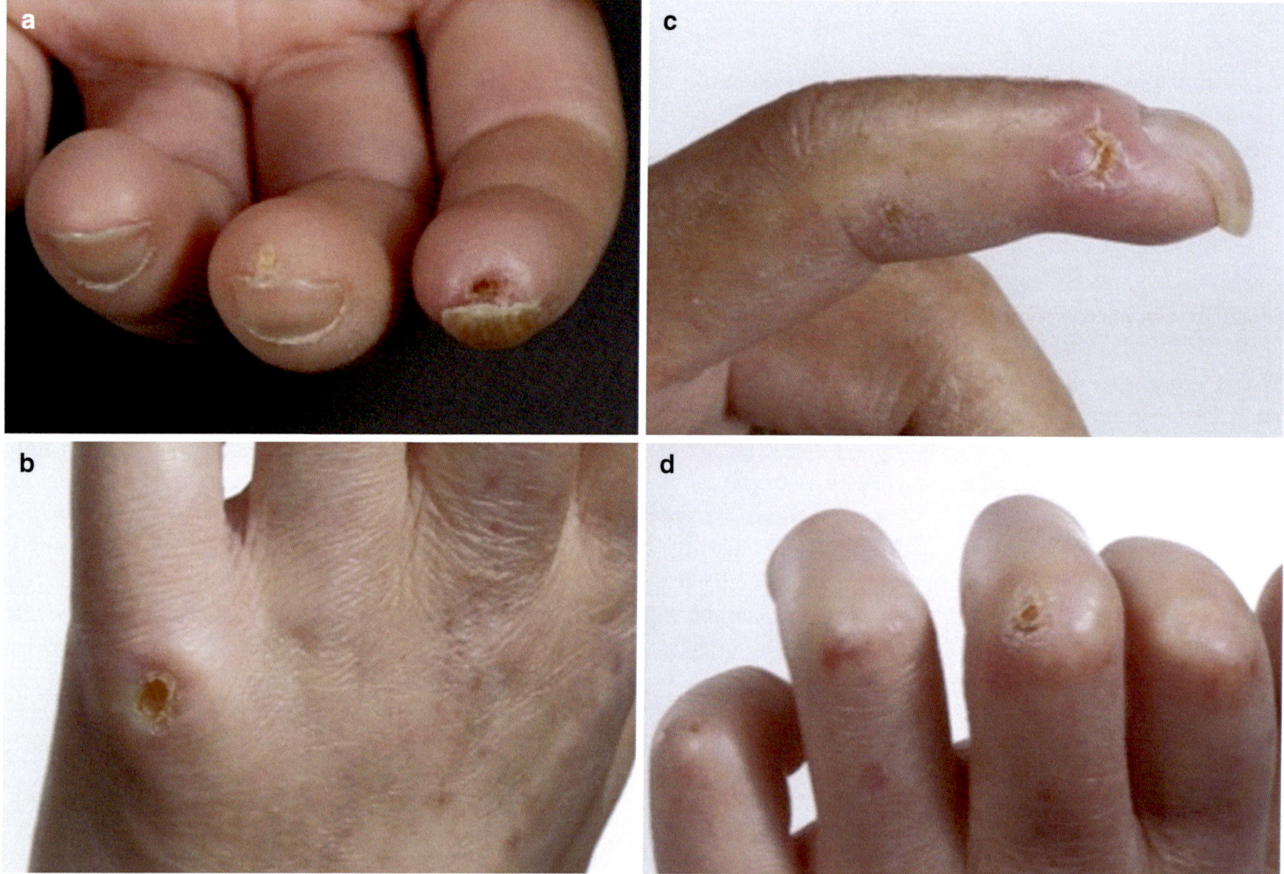

Fig. 23.2 Collection of images taken from patients with scleroderma with associated digital ulcerations due to trauma. From local clinical experience, ulcers occurring at the pulps (**a**) and the metacarpophalangeal (MCP) (**b**) region have not yielded much success when treated with Botox. However, symptomatic relief may be obtained when treating ulcers occurring around or at the distal (**c**) and proximal (**d**) interphalangeal joints. (Images from Salford Royal NHS Foundation Trust hospital, England, UK)

Vitamin E

Though technically an umbrella term for the various isomers of tocopherols and tocotrienols, vitamin E (the nutritional term) has become synonymous with the biologically active form, α-tocopherol. As a lipophilic molecule, it enters from the diet in chylomicrons and is carried in plasma as very low-density lipoproteins (VLDL). This essential vitamin plays a significant role in scavenging lipid peroxyl radicals terminating chain reactions of lipid peroxidation. Oxygen free radicals initiate the chain peroxidation of lipids, be it at the terminals of phospholipid membranes or low-density lipoproteins. α-Tocopherol evidently plays an important role in erythrocyte membrane stability by breaking this chain reaction. Upon scavenging free radicals, the oxidised form of vitamin E requires ascorbic acid (vitamin C) to regenerate and regain potency [35]. Evaluation of vitamin E has implicated it in maintaining endothelial integrity, inhibiting inflammatory adhesion molecules and pro-inflammatory cytokine release, as well as vasodilation and reducing plate-let aggregation via prostaglandin pathways [36–40]. The following figure depicts the mechanisms of action elicited by α-tocopherol that may help protect the endothelium and cellular membranes (Fig. 23.3).

Patients with scleroderma exhibit low levels of vitamin E [41]. Clinical experience and case reports have shown the potential of this antioxidant in promoting beneficial skin changes, whether administered systemically or topically [42, 43]. Fiori and colleagues enrolled a group of 27 patients with known scleroderma-associated digital ulcers and studied the effects of a locally formulated vitamin E gel on topical application (Table 23.3).

The results showed that administration of vitamin E achieved more rapid wound healing, with better pain control, in turn reducing costs of any supplementary medications. However, the study did not address the long-term effects of such management. Further research with a larger sample size and prospective long-term follow-up is necessary to comprehensively ascertain the benefits of vitamin E as an alternative therapy for digital ulcers in scleroderma.

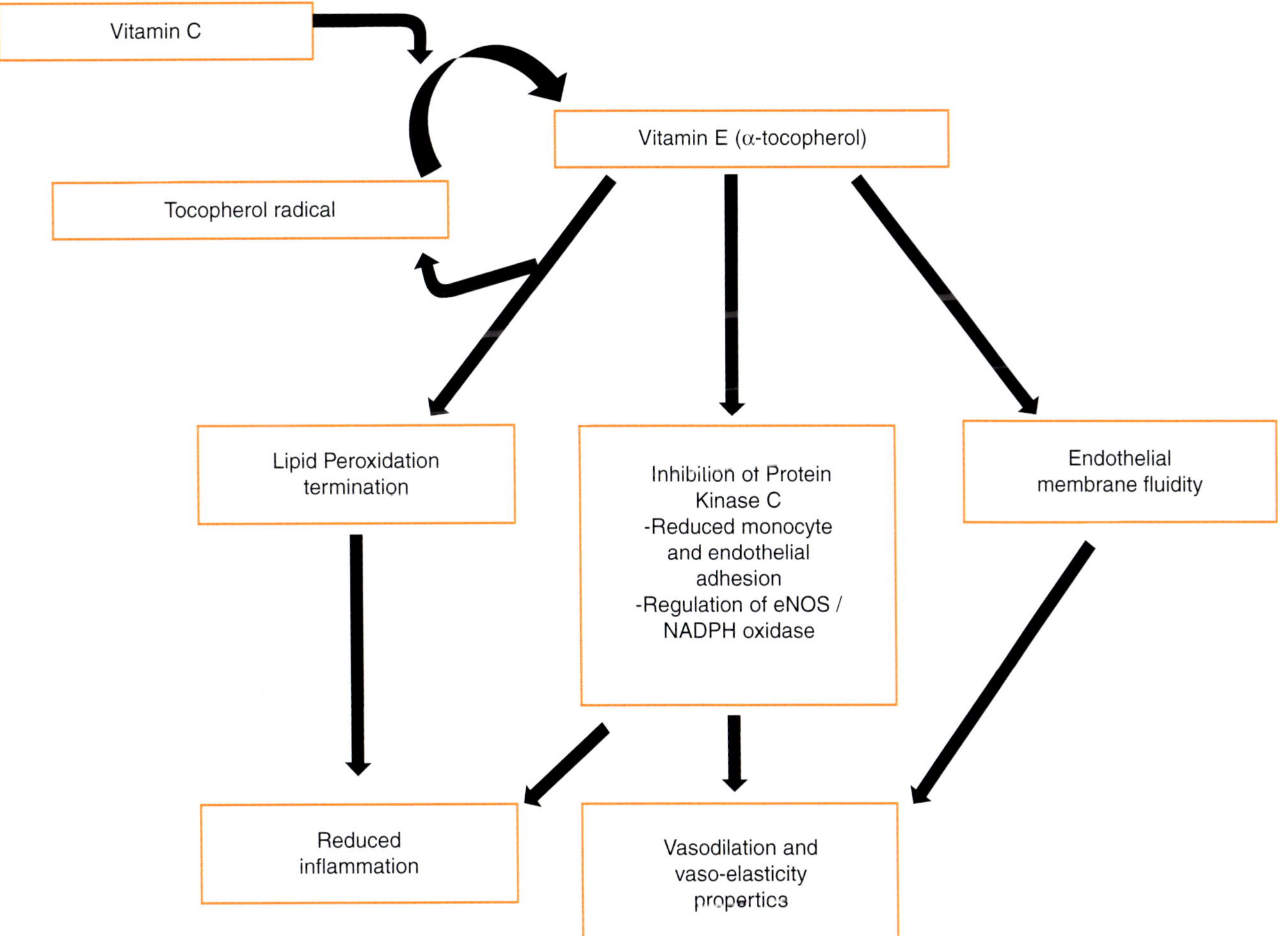

Fig. 23.3 Overview of the proposed wound healing and endothelial functions of vitamin E. Its actions involve maintaining cellular membrane stability as well as reducing inflammation while preventing damage to the elasticity of the endothelium. Recycling of vitamin E requires adequate presence of ascorbic acid (vitamin C). *eNOS* endothelial nitric oxide synthase, *NADPH* nicotinamide adenine dinucleotide phosphate

Table 23.3 Effect of vitamin E on digital ulcers of scleroderma

Study	Numbers	Methods	Outcomes	Potential
Fiori et al. (2009) [44]	27 patients with scleroderma digital ulcers	15 on experimental arm – topical vitamin E gel alongside wound care protocol	Mean time to healing: 7 weeks faster wound healing than controls	Faster healing, reduction in pain, reduction in consumption of other medications (including analgesics)
		vs. 12 on wound care protocol only	Reduction of pain at 18 sessions vs. 26 sessions for controls	

Topical Nitric Oxide Agents

Nitric oxide-generating agents can act as potent vasodilators via the metabolite nitrogen monoxide – or nitric oxide (NO). This is achieved by the formation of *S-nitrosothiols* intermediates as effective donors of NO [45]. NO binds the haem group of guanylate cyclase, activating this enzyme and releasing cyclic guanosine monophosphate (cGMP). The increasing number of cGMP lowers intracellular calcium and at the level of the endothelium relaxes smooth muscle cells. Moreover, the role of NO extends beyond its vasodilatory effects. Other functions include inhibition of platelet aggregation, killing of pathogens, bladder control and mediation of neurologic pathways [46]. Production of NO endogenously is derived from the nitric oxide synthase enzymes (NOS), comprising three recognised isoforms (Table 23.4).

Several literature reports have described increased levels of NO [47–52] in patients with scleroderma, while others have described the contrary [53]. The pattern, however, seems to show a tendency towards increased NO with higher levels of iNOS. Certainly, iNOS expression seems to correlate with worsening grades of disease progression at the digits [51, 52].

Regarding digital ulceration, however, Tucker and colleagues trialled topical sodium nitrite containing gels and tested these on the forearms and digits of patients with severe RP. The vasodilatory effects of NO were elicited in both patients with RP and healthy controls, though more so at the forearms than at the fingers [54]. They suggested a potential role for the use of this agent in the acute onset of RP. Further trials, using a customised formulation of a topical nitrate agent (namely MQX 503), also showed improvement in RP subjectively in terms of RP episodes and duration, pain, stiffness and hand disability, with better blood flow at the digits [55, 56]. Application of a preparation of glyceryl trinitrate (GTN) at the digits was also objectively shown to improve perfusion confirmed by laser Doppler ultrasonography [57].

Despite the raised NO levels that may be observed in scleroderma patients, it seems exogenous NO application may benefit these patients with RP symptoms and its sequelae. Conversely, the above-mentioned trials only investigated short-term effects of topical nitrite agents. Reported side effects of topical applications included headaches, dizziness, light headedness and local paraesthesia/skin irritation. Randomised controlled studies looking at long-term effects, dosages and standardisation of a topical regime are necessary. Nonetheless, this modality seems to offer a potential avenue in tackling RP and possibly preventing associated ulceration of the digits.

Table 23.4 The various types of NOS and their expression and effects physiologically [45, 46]

Isoform	Sites	Expression	Effects
Neuronal NOS (nNOS)	Neuronal	Constitutive, but levels inducible	Response to excitatory amino acids Neurotransmission/neuromodulation Synaptic plasticity (including long-term memory)
Inducible NOS (iNOS)	Inflammation (organs, endothelium or immune cells) Lung epithelium	Inducible	Free radical damage to pathogens Excess implicated in disease states
Endothelial NOS (eNOS)	Endothelium Some neuronal tissue	Constitutive, but levels inducible	Vasodilation Inhibition of platelet aggregation

External Compressions

Mechanical force to improve tissue perfusion is a simple yet effective modality. Applying external pneumatic pressure to limbs can improve blood flow, be it by continuous or intermittent compressions [58–60]. Pneumatic pressure creates a favourable arteriovenous gradient that allows perfusion of capillaries, vasodilation due to effects of sheer stress and loss of venous pressure leading to an inhibition of the autoregulation of the vasculature [61].

Many case series have identified intermittent pneumatic compressions (IPC) as having beneficial therapeutic outcomes in managing critical limb ischaemia. Limb salvage, wound healing, relief of pain at rest, increased blood flow to the affected limb, improved limb mobility, avoidance of limb amputation and an improved quality of life were among the positive outcomes reported in such studies [62–65]. A similar potential was observed in the context of scleroderma ulcers. Filho and co-workers looked at the effects of IPC in 17 patients with ulcers associated with scleroderma. Using IPC allowed for frequent healing of ulcers in the fingers and toes [66]. Confirmation of such healing in scleroderma was observed in a study where 5 h a day of IPC achieved healing of digital ulcers after 21 weeks, with a reduction in pain after commencing therapy [58].

As of yet, no large prospective and randomised controlled trials have been published regarding external pneumatic compressions. Nonetheless, the concept of compressions to alleviate distal ischaemia holds much promise. Many pneumatic devices have been marketed for other purposes, for example, for deep vein thromboprophylaxis [67]. Should enough evidence arise that favours their use in ulcers of scleroderma, then a rapid expansion in provision is conceivable.

Ultrasound Therapy

Ultrasonography has become a mainstay across various medical and surgical specialties, including therapeutic applications (such as physical therapy, lithotripsy, tissue ablation, bone fracture healing, transdermal drug delivery enhancement, thrombus dissolution and others) [68]. There has also been an increasing interest in the use of ultrasound in the treatment of chronic wounds.

One study looked at the effects of using non-contact, low frequency ultrasound therapy on venous ulcers [69]. In the randomised and controlled trial, it was observed that supplementing standard wound care with ultrasound therapy provided significant relief in pain after 4 weeks. Furthermore, ulcer area showed a significant reduction for patients receiving ultrasound adjunct compared to standard wound care alone, with twice the number of ulcers achieving complete healing after 7 weeks into treatment compared to the control arm. In another retrospective study looking at chronic wounds below the knee of various aetiologies, non-contact ultrasound therapy delivered by means of a saline mist intermediate also achieved more healing of wounds with a higher rate of healing compared to controls [70]. The mechanisms by which ultrasound seems to supplement better healing can be attributed to its debridement effects. It has been shown to destroy bacterial biofilms at wound sites through transient cavitation and bubble dynamics. Further, it promotes neovascularisation and favourable granulation tissue modification [71–74]. The Food and Drug Administration have recently approved this technique of non-contact low frequency ultrasound delivered with saline mist for 'wound healing through wound cleansing and maintenance debridement by the removal of yellow slough, fibrin, tissue exudates and bacteria' [75].

A case report of a 68-year-old male with a painful ulcer on his left second finger associated with limited cutaneous sclerosis highlighted the benefits of ultrasound therapy. Unable to tolerate regular debridement due to pain, the authors opted for ultrasound therapy along with standard daily dressings. After 6 weeks of 5 min application of ultrasonography, three times a week, the patient reported being pain-free from the ulcer and complete closure of the wound site was seen at 10 weeks [76]. This case report highlights the importance of trialling alternative therapies and can be a foundation stone for further research into digital ulcers. Prospective follow-up studies are required to determine the long-term effects of this modality of treatment. Certainly, the use of ultrasound requires competency and is highly operator-dependent. As with many treatment modalities involving chronic lesions, adherence to a strict and well-designed management protocol is crucial.

Iontophoresis

Iontophoresis is the process of delivering electric currents at microampere (μA) amplitude to aid and enhance the transfer of ionised compounds, such as medicines or chemicals, into the skin. Figure 23.4 illustrates this concept in a simplistic manner.

The idea is to be able to tolerate committing the affected skin area into a solution that aids in the ionisation of the drug to be delivered and close the electrical circuit for the system to function. Closure of the circuit could be done either by using one limb (or the affected area) in the iontophoresis device while on the same limb attaching the return cathode, or by using the contralateral limb also submersed in a solution (such as saline) as the downstream electrode.

Some uses of iontophoresis include treatment of hyperhidrosis (particularly of the palms and soles), where patients are required to undergo two to four sessions a week using tap water as the ionising solution only, though glycopyrronium bromide (an antimuscarinic agent) may be used with caution [77]. Delivery of vasodilatory agents with iontophoresis has also been studied. Circulatory enhancement, as observed using laser Doppler, was achieved when using iontophoresis to deliver acetylcholine (Ach) and sodium nitroprusside (NaNP) in patients with scleroderma [78, 79]. A later study examined the effect of iontophoresis in healthy subjects and the use of vasodilatory Ach and NaNP on a single finger and compared that blood flow to the adjacent finger. Their results confirmed an improved perfusion of the affected digit only [80]. A couple of years later, another study examined eight patients with scleroderma, but no ulcerations, and the response to finger-only iontophoresis at a current of 200 μA using Ach and NaNP solutions. The study found an improvement in blood flow in the fingers, with no systemic side effects [81].

The evidence is there that perfusion is ameliorated when using iontophoresis to deliver Ach and NaNP. However, results confirming whether this would prevent or help in the management of scleroderma ulcers are yet to be published.

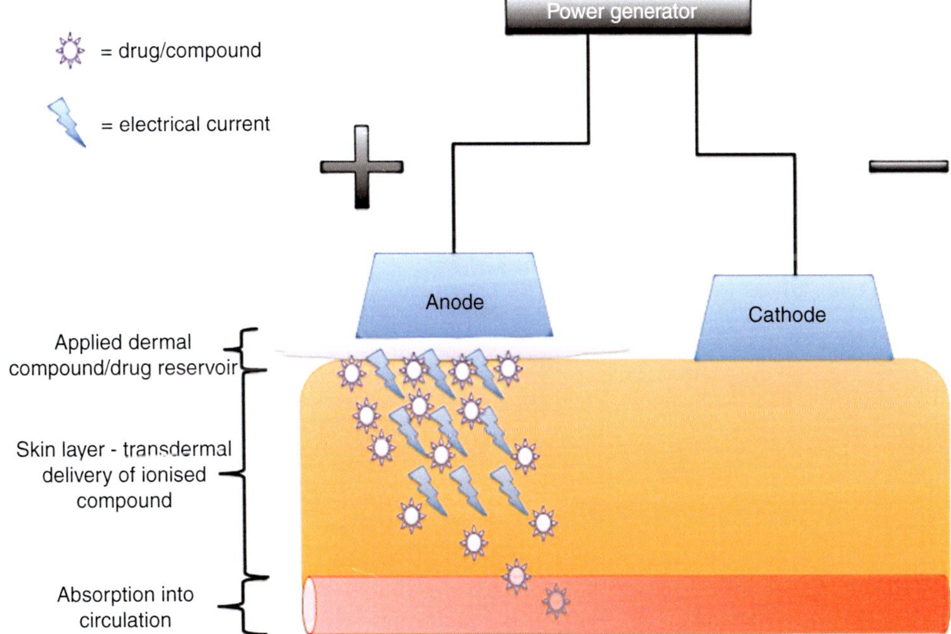

Fig. 23.4 Illustration of the mechanism of iontophoresis: a closed circuit current is required to ensure flow of ionised matter across the target area

Maggot Debridement Therapy (MDT)

Biodebridement, biosurgery, wound myiasis, larval therapy or maggot debridement therapy (MDT) refer to the use of living larvae of the greenbottle fly, *Lucilia sericata*, for the treatment of wounds. Historically, ancient tribal paintings from the Maya of Central America as well as from Australia's aboriginals depict the use of larvae for medicinal purposes. However, following the introduction of antibiotics, the popularity of larval therapy suffered [82].

Though an unpleasant thought for some, MDT is becoming more widely looked into as it has shown therapeutic benefits for pressure sores, decubitus ulcers, diabetic ulcers, neurovascular and vascular ulcers, osteomyelitis, necrotising fasciitis, postsurgical wound infections and burns [83]. The means by which maggots promote wound debridement include mechanical and enzymatic mechanisms. The maggot's mouth acts as a hook that latches onto necrotic tissue and along with their rough body surface allow for mechanical debridement as they crawl. Additionally, the excretions and secretions derived from maggots include enzymes and compounds (such as allantoin, sulfhydryl radicals, calcium cysteine, glutathione, collagenases and serine proteases, among others) that digest necrotic tissue and bacterial biofilms. Maggots have also been shown to ingest and kill bacteria in their guts as well as producing ammonia and altering environmental pH, inhibiting further bacterial growth [84]. Other maggot secretions have been shown to reduce complement proteins as well as enhancing growth factors from macrophages [82]. The use of MDT in chronic ulcers and wounds confirmed that healing time was shortened and improved the healing rate, which can potentially reduce the use of antibiotics while stimulating earlier onset tissue regeneration [84, 85]. Though no study has yet shown the use of MDT in the ulcers associated with scleroderma, this could be a promising new avenue for research.

Herbal Remedies

One cannot mention alternative medicine without delving into the realms of herbal remedies. To date, no herbal remedy has been identified or researched that may help in the treatment of scleroderma-associated ulcers, as per the authors' literature review. One study based in China looked into the cellular and molecular benefits of using Yiqihuoxue formula (Yqx), a traditional Chinese medication whose two main components are derived from the *Astragalus membranaceus* and *Salvia miltiorrhiza* plants [86]. *Astragalus membranaceus* is a perennial plant, native to the North and East of China, Mongolia and Korea. Its root is extracted and dried then used as the medicinal entity [87]. *Salvia miltiorrhiza*

(red sage/Chinese sage) is a deciduous perennial plant, indigenous to Japan and commonly found in grassy forests and along streams in the West and Southwest of China. Its root is the main medicinal component [88]. The study identified a role for Yqx as being anti-fibrotic when applied to skin cells harvested from bleomycin-induced mice models (daily bleomycin subcutaneous injections for 3 weeks leading to skin fibrosis) as well as cultured fibroblasts from the skin of patients with scleroderma. It was postulated that the active ingredient of *Salvia miltiorrhiza* – salvianolic acid B (SAB) – acted against the cytokine transformation growth factor beta (TGF-β) signalling pathway involved in collagen production by fibroblasts, a process that is abnormally augmented in scleroderma [89, 90]. The immunomodulatory effects of *Astragalus membranaceus* were highlighted as its main contributing effect [86].

Another plant that has been studied is the *Capparis spinosa* – a green spiny shrub that naturally grows along the Mediterranean basin as well as the North-West of China. Its methanol extract has been shown to act as an antioxidant [91]. When applied to fibroblasts derived from scleroderma lesions, there was significant protection from free radical damage as well as exhibiting fibrotic-modulatory effects [92].

The studies discussed above only addressed the microbiologic effects of the herbal medications. Though potentially they exhibit anti-fibrotic effects, their application at a clinical level is yet to be determined. Further research in the uses of such remedies in patients with scleroderma ulcers is required.

Conclusion

Our experience suggests that alternative therapies may complement mainstream treatment in carefully selected cases. As we have seen, there are many potential alternative therapies that are being researched and applied at a preliminary clinical level. Research into the efficacy of most of these therapies is in its embryonic stages with some holding much promise. However, they are far from supplanting established treatments. Large-scale clinical trials with robust study methodologies are required to prove efficacy of most of the alternative treatments. We have seen hyperbaric oxygen therapy and topical vitamin E gels showing much potential, though only backed by case reports. There remains a lack of evidence addressing the long-term benefits and side effects of the therapies discussed. As such, alternative therapies may only provide a provisional complementary aid until further trials and studies prove otherwise.

Early disease recognition, basic wound care and preventative lifestyle measures are the cornerstone of managing digital ulcers. The importance of patient education and multidisciplinary team work cannot be overstated.

References

1. Thom SR. Oxidative stress is fundamental to hyperbaric oxygen therapy. J Appl Physiol. 2009;106:988–95.
2. NHS Commissioning board. Clinical commissioning policy: the use of hyperbaric oxygen therapy; 2013.
3. Nylander G, Lewis D, Nordstrom H, Larsson J. Reduction of post-ischemic edema with hyperbaric oxygen. Plast Reconstr Surg. 1985;76(4):596–603.
4. Duling BR. Microvascular responses to alterations in oxygen tension. Circ Res. 1972 Oct;31:481–9.
5. Juha HA, Niinikoski MD. Clinical hyperbaric oxygen therapy, wound perfusion, and transcutaneous oximetry. Wold Journal of Surgery. 2004;28(3):307–11.
6. Halliwell B, Gutteridge JMC. Free radicals in biology and medicine. 3rd ed. Oxford: Oxford University Press; 2000.
7. de Andrade SM, Santos ICRV. Hyperbaric oxygen therapy for wound care. Revista Gaucha de Enfermagem. 2016;37(2): e59257.
8. Krane P, Bennett MH, Martyn-St James M, Schnabel A, Debus SE. Hyperbaric oxygen therapy for chronic wounds (Review): The Cochrane Collaboration; 2012.
9. Markus YM, Bell MJ, Evans AW. Ischemic scleroderma wounds successfully treated with hyperbaric oxygen therapy. J Rheumatol. 2006;33(8):1694–6.
10. Gerodimos C, Stefanidou S, Kotsiou M, Melekos T, Mesimeris T. Hyperbaric oxygen treatment of intractable ulcers in a systemic sclerosis patient. Aristotle Univ Med J. 2013;40(3):19–22.
11. UKDiving.co.uk. Hyperbaric Chamber Locations Across The UK. [Online].; July 2015 [cited 16 February 2017]. Available from: http://www.ukdiving.co.uk/information/hyperbaric.htm.
12. Worldwide Hyperbaric Chamber Locator, Contact London Recompression & Hyperbaric facilities - The London Diving Chamber. All Regions >> North America. [Online]. February 2017. [cited 16 February 2017]. Available from: http://www.londondivingchamber.co.uk/index.php?id=contact&page=11®ion=8&country=64
13. Bove AA. Merck Manual. [Online]; 2013 [cited 2015 March 16. Available from: http://www.merckmanuals.com/home/injuries_and_poisoning/diving_and_compressed_air_injuries/barotrauma.html
14. Erbguth FJ. Historical notes on botulism, Clostridium botulinum, botulinum toxin, and the idea of the therapeutic use of the toxin. Mov Dis. 2004;19(Suppl 8):S2–6.
15. Nigam PK, Nigam A. Botulinum Toxin. Indian J Dermatol. 2010;55(1):8–14.
16. National Institute for Health and Care Excellence. Botulinum toxin type A for the prevention of headaches in adults with chronic migraine [Guidance]. 2012.
17. National Institute for Health and Care Excellence. Idiopathic overactive bladder syndrome: botulinum toxin A [Guidance]. 2012.
18. U.S. Food and Drug Administration. Information for Healthcare Professionals: OnabotulinumtoxinA (marketed as Botox/Botox Cosmetic), AbobotulinumtoxinA (marketed as Dysport) and RimabotulinumtoxinB (marketed as Myobloc) [Report]. 2013.
19. National Institute for Health and Care Excellence. Endoscopic thoracic sympathectomy for primary hyperhidrosis of the upper limb [Guidance]. 2014.
20. Singh BR. Intimate details of the most poisonous poison. Nat Struct Biol. 2000;7(8):617–9.
21. Pestronk A. Neuromuscular Disease Center. [Online]. 2014 [cited 2015 April 19. Available from: http://neuromuscular.wustl.edu/nother/bot.htm
22. Morris JL, Jobling P, Gibbins IL. Differential inhibition by botulinum neurotoxin A of cotransmitters released from autonomic vasodilator neurons. Am J Physiol Heart Circu Physiol. 2001;281(5):H2124–32.
23. Kim YS, Roh TS, Lee WJ, Yoo WM, Tark KC. The effect of botulinum toxin A on skin flap survival in rats. Wound Repair Regen. 2009;17(3):411–7.
24. Schweizer F, Schweizer R, Zhang S, Kamat P, Contaldo C, Rieben R, et al. Botulinum toxin A and B raise blood flow and increase survival of critically ischemic skin flaps. J Surg Res. 2013;184(2):1205–13.
25. Kim TK, Oh EJ, Chung JY, Park JW, Cho BC, Chung HY. The effects of botulinum toxin A on the survival of a random cutaneous flap. J Plast Reconstr Aesthet Surg. 2009 July;62(7):906–13.
26. Park TH, Rah DK, Chong Y, Kim JK. The effects of botulinum toxin a on survival of rat TRAM flap with vertical midline scar. Ann Plast Surg. 2015 January;74(1):100–6.
27. Uchiyama A, Yamada K, Perera B, Ogino S, Yokoyama Y, Takeuchi Y, et al. Protective effect of botulinum toxin A after cutaneous ischemia-reperfusion injury. Sci Rep. 2015;13(5):9072 (1–6).
28. Neumeister MW, Chambers CB, Herron MS, Webb K, Wietfeldt J, Gillespie JN, et al. Botox therapy for ischemic digits. Plast Reconstr Surg. 2009;124(1):191–201.
29. Sycha T, Graninger M, Auff E, Schnider P. Botulinum toxin in the treatment of Raynaud's phenomenon: a pilot study. Eur J Clin Investig. 2004;34(4):312–3.
30. Van Beek AL, Lim PK, Gear AJL, Pritzker MR. Management of vasospastic disorders with botulinum toxin A. Plast Reconstr Surg. 2007 January;119(1):217–26.
31. Fregene A, Ditmars D, Siddiqui A. Botulinum toxin type A: a treatment option for digital ischemia in patients with Raynaud's phenomenon. J Hand Surg. 2009;34(3):446–52.
32. Smith L, Polsky D, Franks AG. Botulinum toxin-A for the treatment of Raynaud syndrome. Arch Dermatol. 2012;148(4):426–8.
33. Neumeister MW. Botulinum toxin type A in the treatment of Raynaud's phenomenon. J Hand Surg. 2010;35(12):2085–92.
34. Serri J, Legre R, Veit V, Guardia C, Gay AM. Botulinum toxin type A contribution in the treatment of Raynaud's phenomenon due to systemic sclerosis. Ann Chir Plast Esthet. 2013;58(6):658–62.
35. Halliwell B, Gutteridge JMC. Free radicals in biology and medicine. 3rd ed. Oxford: Oxford University Press; 2000.
36. Singh U, Jialal I. Anti-inflammatory effects of alpha-tocopherol. Ann N Y Acad Sci. 2004;1031:195–203.
37. Singh U, Devaraj S, Jialal I. Vitamin E, oxidative stress and inflammation. Annu Rev Nutr. 2005;25:151–74.
38. Burton GW, Traber MG. Vitamin E: antioxidant activity, biokinetics, and bioavailability. Annu Rev Nutr. 1990;10:357–82.
39. Freedman JE, Keaney JFJ. Vitamin E inhibition of platelet aggregation is independent of antioxidant activity. J Nutr. 2001;131(2):374–77S.
40. Wu D, Liu L, Meydani M, Meydani SN. Vitamin E increases production of vasodilator prostanoids in human aortic endothelial cells through opposing effects on cyclooxygenase-2 and phospholipase A2. J Nutr. 2005;135(8):1847–53.
41. Lundberg AC, Akesson A, Akesson B. Dietary intake and nutritional status in patients with systemic sclerosis. Ann Rheum Dis. 1992;51(10):1143–8.
42. Burgess JF, Pritchard JE. Tocopherol (vitamin E) therapy in sclerosis of the legs with ulcer. Can Med Assoc J. 1948;59(3):242–7.
43. Panin G, Strumia R, Ursini F. Topical alpha-tocopherol acetate in the bulk phase. Eight years of experience in skin treatment. Ann N Y Acad Sci. 2006;1031(1):443–7.
44. Fiori G, Galluccio F, Braschi F, Amanzi L, Miniati I, Conforti ML, et al. Vitamin E gel reduces time of healing of digital ulcers in systemic sclerosis. Clin Exp Rheumatol. 2009;27:S51–4.
45. Ignarro LJ, Cirino G, Casini A, Napoli C. Nitric oxide as a signaling molecule in the vascular system: an overview. J Cardiovasc Pharmacol. 1999;34(6):879–86.

46. Halliwell B, Gutteridge JMC. Free radicals in biology and medicine. Oxford, Oxford University Press; 2000.
47. Cotton SA, Herrick AL, Jayson MIV, Freemont AJ. Endothelial expression of nitric oxide synthases and nitrotyrosine in systemic sclerosis skin. J Pathol. 1999;189(2):273–8.
48. Andersen GN, Caidahl K, Kazzam E, Petersson AS, Waldenstrom A, Mincheva-Nilsson L, et al. Correlation between increased nitric oxide production and markers of endothelial activation in systemic sclerosis: findings with the soluble adhesion molecules E-selectin, intercellular adhesion molecule 1, and vascular cell adhesion molecule 1. Arthritis Rheum. 2000;43(5):1085–93.
49. Yamamoto T, Katayama I, Nishioka K. Nitric oxide production and inducible nitric oxide synthase expression in systemic sclerosis. J Rheumatol. 1998;25(2):314–7.
50. Takagi K, Kawaguchi Y, Hara M, Sugiura T, Hargai M, Kamatani N. Serum nitric oxide (NO) levels in systemic sclerosis patients: correlation between NO levels and clinical features. Clin Exp Immunol. 2003;134(3):538–44.
51. Sud A, Khullar M, Wanchu A, Bambery P. Increased nitric oxide production in patients with systemic sclerosis. Nitric Oxide. 2000;4(6):615–9.
52. Matucci-Cerinic M, Kahaleh MB. Beauty and the beast. The nitric oxide paradox in systemic sclerosis. Rheumatology (Oxford). 2002;41(8):843–7.
53. Allanore Y, Borderie D, Hilliquin P, Hernvann A, Levacher M, Lemarechal H, et al. Low levels of nitric oxide (NO) in systemic sclerosis: inducible NO synthase production is decreased in cultured peripheral blood monocyte/macrophage cells. Rheumatology (Oxford). 2001;40(10):1089–96.
54. Tucker AT, Pearson RM, Cooke ED, Benjamin N. Effect of nitric-oxide-generating system on microcirculatory blood flow in skin of patients with severe Raynaud's syndrome: a randomised trial. Lancet. 1999;354(9191):1670–5.
55. Chung L, Shapiro L, Fiorentino D, Baron M, Shanahan J, Sule S, et al. MQX-503, a novel formulation of nitroglycerin, improves the severity of Raynaud's phenomenon. Arthritis Rheum. 2009;60(3):870–7.
56. Hummers LK, Dugowson CE, Dechow FJ, Wise RA, Gregory J, Michalek J, et al. A multi-centre, blinded, randomised, placebo-controlled, laboratory-based study of MQX-503, a novel topical gel formulation of nitroglycerine, in patients with Raynaud phenomenon. Ann Rheum Dis. 2013 December;72(12):1962–7.
57. Anderson ME, Moore TL, Hollis S, Jayson MIV, King TA, Herrick AL. Digital vascular response to topical glyceryl trinitrate, as measured by laser Doppler imaging, in primary Raynaud's phenomenon. Rheumatology (Oxford). 2002;41(3):324–8.
58. Pfizenmaier DH, Kavros SJ, Liedl DA, Cooper LT. Use of intermittent pneumatic compression for treatment of upper extremity vascular ulcers. Angiology. 2005;56(4):417–22.
59. Rosales-Velderrain A, Padilla M, Choe CH, Hargens AR. Increased microvascular flow and foot sensation with mild continuous external compression. Physiol Rep. 2013;1(7):e00157.
60. Labropoulos N, Leon LR, Bhatti A, Melton S, Kang SS, Mansou AM, et al. Hemodynamic effects of intermittent pneumatic compression in patients with critical limb ischemia. J Vasc Surg. 2005;42(4):710–6.
61. Delis KT. The case for intermittent pneumatic compression of the lower extremity as a novel treatment in arterial claudication. Perspect Vasc Surg Endovasc Ther. 2005;17(1):29–42.
62. Chang ST, Hsu JT, Chu CM, Pan KL, Jang SJ, Lin PC, et al. Using intermittent pneumatic compression therapy to improve quality of life for symptomatic patients with Infrapopliteal diffuse peripheral obstructive disease. Circ J. 2012;76(4):971–6.
63. Sultan S, Hamada N, Soylu E, Fahy A, Hynes N, Tawfick W. Sequential compression biomechanical device in patients with critical limb ischemia and nonreconstructible peripheral vascular disease. J Vasc Surg. 2011;54(2):440–6.
64. van Bemmelen PS, Gitlitz DB, Faruqi RM, Weiss-Olmanni J, Brunetti VA, Giron F, et al. Limb salvage using high-pressure intermittent compression arterial assist device in cases unsuitable for surgical revascularization. Arch Surg (Chicago III: 1960). 2001;136(11):1280–5.
65. Kavros SJ, Delis KT, Turner NS, Voll AE, Liedl DA, Gloviczki P, et al. Improving limb salvage in critical ischemia with intermittent pneumatic compression: a controlled study with 18-month follow-up. J Vasc Surg. 2008;47(3):543–9.
66. Filho JP, Sampaio-Barros PD, Parente JB, Menezes FH, Potério GB, Samara AM, et al. Rhythmic external compression of the limbs: a method for healing cutaneous ulcers in systemic sclerosis. J Rheumatol. 1998;25(8):1540–3.
67. National Institute for Health and Care Excellence. NICE National Institute for Health and Care Excellence. [Online]. 2010 [cited 2015 May 3. Available from: https://www.nice.org.uk/guidance/cg92/chapter/Key-priorities-for-implementation#reducing-the-risk-of-vte
68. Miller D, Smith N, Bailey M, Czarnota G, Hynynen K, Makin I, et al. Overview of therapeutic ultrasound applications and safety considerations. J Ultrasound Med. 2012;31(4):623–34.
69. Gibbons GW, Orgill DP, Serena TE, Novoung A, O'Connell JB, Li WW, et al. A prospective, randomized, controlled trial comparing the effects of noncontact, low-frequency ultrasound to standard care in healing venous leg ulcers. Ostomy Wound management. 2015;61(1):16–29.
70. Kavros SJ, Liedl DA, Boon AJ, Miller JL, Hobbs JA, Andrews KL. Expedited wound healing with noncontact, low-frequency ultrasound therapy in chronic wounds: a retrospective analysis. Advances in skin and wound care. 2008;21(9):416–23.
71. Lai J, Pittelkow MR. Physiological effects of ultrasound mist on fibroblasts. Int J Dermatol. 2007;46(6):587–93.
72. Thawer HA, Houghton PE. Effects of ultrasound delivered through a mist of saline to wounds in mice with diabetes mellitus. J Wound Care. 2004;13(5):171–6.
73. Stanisic MM, Provo BJ, Larson DL, Kloth LC. Wound Debridement with 25 kHz Ultrasound. Advances in Skin and wound care. 2005;18(9):484–90.
74. Maan ZN, Januszyk M, Rennert RC, Duscher D, Rodrigues M, Fujiwara T, et al. Expedited Wound Healing with Noncontact, Low-Frequency Ultrasound Therapy in Chronic Wounds: A Retrospective Analysis. Plastic and reconstructive surgery. 2014;134(3):402e–11e.
75. Department of Health and Human Services. Food and Drug Administration. MIST Therapy System 510(K) Premarket Notification; David L. Bremseth, Pharm D. Vice President, Clinical and Regulatory affairs. Celleration, Inc. 10250 Valley View Road, Suite 137, Eden Prairie, Minnesota 55344. 2005 May 17.
76. Fleming CP. Sound evidence: acoustic pressure wound therapy in the treatment of a vasculopathy-associated digital ulcer: a case study. Ostomy Wound management. 2008;54(4):62–5.
77. National Institute for Health and Care Excellence. NICE; National Institute for Health and Care Excellence. [Online].; 2013 [cited 2015 May 5. Available from: http://cks.nice.org.uk/hyperhidrosis" \l "!scenario.
78. Anderson ME, Hollis S, Moore T, Jayson MIV, Herrick AL. Non-invasive assessment of vascular reactivity in forearm skin of patients with primary Raynaud's phenomenon and systemic sclerosis. Br J Rheumatol. 1996;35:1281–8.
79. Anderson ME, Campbell F, Hollis S, Moore T, MIV J, Herrick AL. Non-invasive assessment of digital vascular reactivity in patients with primary Raynaud's phenomenon and systemic sclerosis. Clinical and experimental rheumatology. 1999;17(1):49–54.
80. Murray AK, Herrick AL, Gorodkin RE, Moore TL, King TA. Possible therapeutic use of vasodilator iontophoresis. Microvasc Res. 2005 January;69(1–2):89–94.

81. Murray AK, Moore TL, King TA, Herrick AL. Vasodilator iontophoresis a possible new therapy for digital ischaemia in systemic sclerosis? Rheumatology (Oxford). 2008 January;47(1):76–9.

82. Gottrup F, Jorgensen B. Maggot Debridement: An Alternative Method for Debridement. Eplasty Journal of Plastic surgery. 2011;11(e33):290–302.

83. Whitaker IS, Welck M, Whitaker MJ, Conroy FJ. From the bible to biosurgery: Lucilia sericata--plastic surgeon's assistant in the 21st century. Plast Reconstr Surg. 2006;117(5):1670–1.

84. Sherman RA. Mechanisms of maggot-induced wound healing: what do we know, and where do we go from Here? Evid Based Complement Alternat Med. 2014;2014:1–13.

85. Sun X, Jiang K, Chen J, Wu L, Lu H, Wang A, et al. A systematic review of maggot debridement therapy for chronically infected wounds and ulcers. Int J Infect Dis. 2014;25:32–7.

86. Wu T, Chu H, Tu W, Song M, Chen D, Yuan J, et al. Dissection of the mechanism of traditional Chinese medical prescription-Yiqihuoxue formula as an effective anti-fibrotic treatment for systemic sclerosis. BMC Complement Altern Med. 2014;14(224)

87. University of Maryland Medical Center. University of Maryland Medical Center. [Online]. 2013 [cited 2015 May 4]. Available from: http://umm.edu/health/medical/altmed/herb/astragalus

88. Wang BQ. Salvia Miltiorrhiza: chemical and pharmacological review of a medicinal plant. Journal of Medicinal plants research. 2010;4(25):2813–20.

89. Sonnylal S, Denton CP, Zheng B, Keene DR, He R, Adams HP, et al. Postnatal induction of transforming growth factor beta signaling in fibroblasts of mice recapitulates clinical, histologic, and biochemical features of scleroderma. Arthritis Rheum. 2007;56(1):334–44.

90. Kawakami T, Ihn H, Xu W, Smith E, LeRoy C, Trojanowska M. Increased expression of TGF-beta receptors by scleroderma fibroblasts: evidence for contribution of autocrine TGF-beta signaling to scleroderma phenotype. J Invest Dermatol. 1998;110(1):47–51.

91. Germano MP, De Pasquale R, D'Angelo V, Catania S, Silvari V, Costa C. Evaluation of extracts and isolated fraction from Capparis spinosa L. buds as an antioxidant source. J Agric Food Chem. 2002;50(5):1168–71.

92. Yl C, Li X, Zheng M. Capparis spinosa protects against oxidative stress in systemic sclerosis dermal fibroblasts. Arch Dermatol Res. 2010;302(5):349–55.

Part IX

Future Strategies: Regenerative Medicine

Nicoletta Del Papa, Eleonora Zaccara, Gabriele Di Luca,
and Wanda Maglione

Introduction

Wound repair is a complex biological process based on different and overlapped stages, namely, hemostasis, inflammation, cell proliferation, and tissue regeneration [1]. After an injury, multiple biological pathways are immediately activated and synchronized to maintain the integrity of normal tissues. However, healing of wounds is significantly compromised in a number of medical conditions, such as ischemia, diabetes, chronic renal failure, infection, and radiation exposure, which subsequently lead to loss of body parts such as extremities, an impaired quality of life, and even mortality due to wound-related infective complications. The mechanisms of inadequate healing include prolonged inflammation, decreased cellular infiltration, modified extracellular matrix (ECM) formation, reduced growth factors, and impaired vascularization [2, 3]. The dysregulation of all these cellular and molecular signals is even considered an important mechanism supporting digital ulcers (DUs) in systemic sclerosis (SSc). Furthermore, in SSc, the progressive rarefaction of capillaries, thickening of the vessel wall, and luminal narrowing, even promoted by perivascular fibrotic tissue, are responsible for persistent tissue hypoxia and oxidative stress [4]. Moreover, a defect in the angiogenic reparative machine, based on the niche microenvironment and progenitor cell involvement, has been hinted as an additional pathogenic mechanism for DU onset in the course of SSc [5].

Although therapeutic advances in SSc have been made through a better biological understanding and availability of candidate therapies, DUs and their complications still impact significantly on patients' quality of life and hand function.

Despite advances in wound closure techniques and devices, there is still a critical need for new methods of enhancing the healing process to achieve optimal outcomes.

Stem Cells in Skin Ulcer Healing

The attempt to find new treatments for SSc DUs leads researchers to investigate the use of stem cells for potential ulcer healing applications. Recently, stem cell therapies have emerged as a new approach for regeneration and repair of damaged organs and tissues in various diseases [6–8].

The major advantage of the stem cell approach is the availability of a great number of cells that are self-renewing and able to differentiate into various cell types. Among stem cells, embryonic stem cells and induced pluripotent stem cells have enormous potentials [9, 10]; however their therapeutic use is limited by several limitations including ethical considerations, genetic manipulation, and unknown cell regulation mechanisms. In recent years, adult mesenchymal stem cells (MSCs) have been used in many animal and human studies as an attractive candidate for cell-based therapies. Their use does not give rise to any ethical problem, and from the clinical perspective, their low immunogenicity allows a safe therapeutic application in allogeneic and even xenogeneic settings [11, 12]. MSCs isolated from bone marrow (BM) stroma are one of the representatives and mostly used adult stem cells and have the potential for in vitro differentiation [13]. Many studies have demonstrated that intravenous or intradermal administration of MSCs enhanced cutaneous wound healing, such as acute wounds, diabetic ulcers, radiation ulcers, and ulcers in the course of collagen diseases, in animals and humans [14–21].

In a pilot study, Nevskaya et al. showed that local implantation of BM-CD34+ in SSc ischemic skin ulcers in hands induced a rapid and evident beneficial effect on vascular symptoms resulting in ulcer healing and amelioration of Raynaud's phenomenon [22]. Similarly, other authors showed that statin may have beneficial effects on vascular manifestations of SSc, through improvement in endothelial function, suppression of the inflammatory response, and mobilization of endothelial progenitor stem cells [23, 24]. Particularly, Abou-Raya et al. [25] published the first

N. Del Papa (✉) · E. Zaccara · G. Di Luca · W. Maglione
Department of Rheumatology, ASST Gaetano Pini, Milan, Italy
e-mail: nicoletta.delpapa@asst-pini-cto.it

© Springer Nature Switzerland AG 2019
M. Matucci-Cerinic, C. P. Denton (eds.), *Atlas of Ulcers in Systemic Sclerosis*, https://doi.org/10.1007/978-3-319-98477-3_24

randomized, double-blind, placebo-controlled clinical trial evaluating the effect of atorvastatin on vascular manifestations of SSc. They observed significant reductions in the overall number of DUs and in the mean number of new DUs per patient in the statin group [25].

Adipose Tissue in Ulcer Healing: Translational Relevance

Although BM-MSCs are available, potential problems might be represented by the low number of harvested cells, by the invasive procedure, and by the potential donor site morbidity. In contrast, adipose tissue is more accessible and has a higher yield of MSCs, and adipose-derived mesenchymal stem cells (ADSCs) share many properties with their bone marrow counterpart [12] in terms of morphology, differentiation potential, cell surface markers, and transcriptomic and proteomic profile [13, 26–29]. Thus they are studied as one of the leading sources for regenerative medicine research.

Liposuction along with surgical excision of fat tissue has facilitated the extraction of adipose tissue for many years. Independent studies have determined that liposuction aspiration alone does not significantly alter the viability of fat cells [30]. A further adaptation of this procedure, by regulating the centrifugation speed, induced an optimal cell recovery consisting of a highly heterogeneous cell suspension defined as stromal vascular fraction (SVF).

SVF contains a small percentage of pre-adipocytes or adipocyte progenitors (adipose-derived stem cells, ADSCs) along with endothelial cells, fibroblasts, pericytes, and different blood cells [31, 32].

ADSCs

ADSCs display properties similar to those observed in BM-MSCs in terms of cell surface markers and differentiation into multiple cell lines (i.e., osteogenic, chondrogenic, and adipogenic cell lineages in vitro). Similar to BM-MSCs, ADSCs have been shown to be immunoprivileged since they do not express major histocompatibility complex and inhibit proliferation of activated peripheral blood mononuclear cells, suggesting a role for modulating the immune system in inflammatory disorders or allogeneic transplantation [12, 33].

Due to these characteristics, ADSCs appear to be an ideal population of stem cells for practical regenerative medicine, given that they are plentiful, of autologous tissue origin, and non-immunogenic and are more easily available. Based on this background knowledge, they have rapidly advanced into clinical trials for treatment of a broad range of conditions.

With regard to wound healing, preclinical and, more recently, clinical trials have shown that ADSCs are effective in the treatment of acute and chronic skin wounds [34–36]. However, the exact mechanisms by which ADSCs promote tissue repair are still elusive and not well understood. It is probable that ADSCs can initiate and/or favor tissue repair and regeneration by a number of nonexclusive mechanisms. First, in a site of injured tissue, ADSCs may work as "building blocks" by directly migrating and differentiating into resident cell types [36]. Ebrahimian et al. skillfully demonstrated in mouse wound models that healing processes were related to differentiation of green fluorescent protein-positive ADSCs into keratinocytes and endothelial cells [37]. Neovascularization is thought to be a fundamental phase in the wound healing process. Several in vitro studies have documented the ability of expanded ADSCs to undergo endothelial differentiation [38–41]. Particularly, the addition of VEGF to culture conditions increased the expression of endothelial markers and the development of endothelial structures by ADSCs [33]. These in vitro findings have been further supported by in vivo studies showing that the administration of ADSCs accelerated wound healing by increasing vascular structures and skin perfusion [42–44].

However, the contribution of ADSCs to tissue repair is much wider when one considers the enormous secretome reservoir of these stem cells [45–47]. ADSCs secrete many different growth factors such as insulin-like growth factor (IGF), hepatocyte growth factor (HGF), and vascular endothelial growth factor (VEGF) [45–47]. Different studies have shown that these growth factors are effective in wound healing animal models [36, 48] since the use of ADSC-conditioned medium by itself could enhance wound healing outcomes [47–49]. More recently, new prospects have emerged from the observation that ADSCs reside in a hypoxic microenvironment [50]. Based on this consideration, several studies have shown the effects of hypoxia on functionality of ADSCs, including proliferation, differentiation, survival rate, and cytokine or growth factor secretions. In reality, hypoxia exposure does not modify ADSC morphology and surface marker expression, but enhances their proliferation rate and preserves their stemness as shown by the increased expression of levels of stemness genes [50]. With regard to ADSC differentiation into the three cell lineages, chondrocytes, osteocytes, and adipocytes, data from hypoxic conditions are contrasting and not conclusive, since the different percentages of oxygen tension in the experimental conditions can diversely affect (either reduce or enhance) the differentiation. Interestingly, it has been demonstrated that hypoxia improves ADSC angiogenic potential via upregulation of anti-apoptotic and angiogenic factors (e.g., VEGF and angiogenin) [50]. Moreover, in response to hypoxia, ADSCs stimulate angiogenesis more strongly than

BM-MSCs [51, 52] as shown by the higher upregulation of genes for pro-angiogenic factors and downregulation of anti-angiogenic genes in ADSCs. The paracrine pro-angiogenic effects of ADSCs have been demonstrated in in vitro experimental conditions where the addition of conditioned medium (CM) of hypoxic-treated ADSCs induced endothelial proliferation and tube formation [50]. The neo-vessel formation was also confirmed in vivo, after topical application of CM from hypoxia-cultured human ADSCs in murine models of wound healing [53]. Besides paracrine signaling of angiogenesis, hypoxia stimulates the direct differentiation of ADSCs into endothelial-like cells expressing typical endothelial markers (CD31, VE-cadherin, Tie2, angiopoietin receptor, and von Willebrand factor) [54]. Finally, hypoxia regulates the expression of SDF-1 and its receptors (CXCR4 principally) on ADSC surface, which promotes migration, homing, and engraftment of transplanted ADSCs in damaged tissues [50, 52]. The fact that ADSC-induced neoangiogenesis may be enhanced in hypoxic experimental conditions is an additional favorable aspect in the perspective of using ADSCs in an in vivo hypoxic wound environment.

Other SVF Cell Populations

There is still a lack of information concerning the characterization of the cell subpopulations constituting the SVF. Beyond the presence of the well-studied ADSCs, the SVF population (the freshly uncultured cell population) derived from adipose tissue include an unknown number of cells: hematopoietic, endothelial progenitors, immune cells, fibroblasts, pericytes, mature endothelial cells, immune cells, and other uncharacterized cells [33, 55]. The high variations in the percentage of detection for certain cell surface markers could be explained in the different gating strategies applied during the flow cytometric studies and the cellular separation procedures. Finally, it is not possible to exclude that donor variability could influence the final composition of SVF. All these considerations are important both to clarify the biological potentialities of SVF preparations and to understand, bearing in mind the therapeutic applications, whether SVF composition is qualitatively and/or quantitatively different in healthy versus disease subjects.

Despite the wide interest in ADSCs, at present it is known that SVF contains only a small percentage of ADSCs, estimated at 2–10% [55]. Li et al. reported three additional subpopulations of interest that can be isolated and cultured from SVF. The first is CD31+/34-, which is classified as "mature endothelial," with the endothelial marker CD31, lacking the progenitor marker CD34. The second is subpopulation classified as "endothelial progenitors," CD31+/34+. The third subpopulation represents a pericyte group and is characterized by surface markers CD146+/90+/31−/34- [56]. These cells reside adjacent to the blood vessel walls and are known to be important contributors in the endothelial repair processes.

The term "endothelial progenitor cells" (EPCs) is fundamentally used to refer to populations of cells that are capable of differentiation into mature endothelial cells (ECs), with physiological roles in angiogenesis (the sprouting of new blood vessels from existing ones) and vasculogenesis (de novo formation of vascular networks) [57]. Recent research identifies two major categories of endothelial precursors, hematopoietic EPCs and nonhematopoietic EPCs, largely different in their ontological origins and surface markers, both potentially important as cell source for vascular regenerative therapies.

The density of pericytes in the SVF is unknown, ranging from 3 to 5% [58]. Pericytes are mural cells of the microcirculation that have been shown to play key roles in regulating microvascular morphogenesis, stability, and permeability. During angiogenesis, pericytes migrate to newly vascularized tissues regulating endothelial cell growth [59]. Of note, recent work has revealed that pericytes share several characteristics with ADSCs, but very little is known about their real potentialities in the adipose environment and their relationship with pluripotent cell counterparts.

It is known that a large subpopulation of SVF consists of monocytes, macrophages, and T-cells [58]. Macrophages present in the SVF predominantly express M2 markers, representing, in the spectrum of all macrophage activation states, the reparative arm characterized by its involvement in tissue remodeling and immune regulation. Their presence usually contrasts or balances the inflammatory macrophages (termed M1), characterized by the production of high levels of pro-inflammatory cytokines [58]. However, the macrophage composition in SVF needs further detailed studies.

The real number of T-cells present in SVF is still unknown. Adipose tissue-derived Treg cells are distinct from their counterparts in lymphoid organs based on their transcriptional profile, T-cell receptor repertoire, and cytokine and chemokine receptor expression pattern [60]. Interestingly, Tregs in SVF express a much higher level of IL-10 in comparison with lymph node Tregs, further supporting a higher anti-inflammatory potential for adipose-derived Tregs [60].

At the moment, the most important rationale in clinical use and research interest in SVF originates from the awareness of the presence of ADSCs. The non-MSC component of the SVF is composed of heterogenous cell populations still waiting to be characterized. Some of these cells show stemness characteristics, some express common surface markers, and others have different functional abilities, although human adipose tissue is generally seen as a source of cells with angiogenic potential.

Adipose Tissue in Scleroderma Ulcer Healing: Clinical Relevance

Overview on Surgery Techniques

The fat grafting technique, also known as lipofilling, was first described by Coleman [61]. It is the most common procedure used in plastic surgery to restore many types of aesthetic or pathological defects of soft tissues. First used to obtain a filler effect, interest in the use of adipose tissue has increased due to the evidence of its regenerative capabilities and biological effects. Over time, multiple variations of this first technique have been developed to obtain better performance. Autologous fat grafting (AFG) is a minimally invasive procedure with limited patient discomfort consisting of three stages. Aspirated or suctioned fat is processed by centrifuging to obtain a "purified" sample. By centrifugation, the fat is then separated in the oil, fluid, and blood supernatants. As a result, a concentrated fat sample that contains not only the fat cells or adipocytes but also the stem cells and a variety of growth factors is obtained. Some surgeons add a further step and isolate the stem cell population from the fatty tissue.

Currently, there is no agreement among authors about the best method of processing fat grafts. In addition, there is no conclusive proof that using the stem cell population alone is of any additional benefit compared with the SVF preparations. Finally, recent research suggests that most of the regenerative ADSC effects might be related to their paracrine functions as shown by the benefit induced by ADSC extracellular vesicles and secretion factors in neurodegenerative diseases, ischemic damages, and wound healing [48, 58].

AFG Applications to Skin Features of Scleroderma Spectrum Diseases

In the last few years, AFG and its subsequently evolved procedures have been applied to localized scleroderma cutaneous lesions, firstly in linear scleroderma and in different types of morphea [reviewed in 62]. In most of these cases, a significant increase of skin elasticity and thickening was reported, with both aesthetic and functional improvement of the treated skin areas, while no serious side effects were observed during and after these procedures. Prompted by these results, AFG has been successfully used in the treatment of systemic sclerosis (SSc) perioral changes, responsible for functional limitations and aesthetical impairments [63–65]. The same procedure has been used in a few studies showing similar good clinical results without any significant complication. The anti-fibrotic effects of AFG have been further demonstrated by Granel et al. [66] in an open-label study aimed at evaluating the safety, tolerability, and potential efficacy of AFG procedure in SSc hand disability. The authors obtained autologous SVF from lipoaspirates, using an automated filtration processing system, and subsequently injected SVF into the subcutaneous tissue of each finger. They observed a significant improvement of all the parameters used for evaluating hand skin elasticity and function from 2 months [66]. Altogether these results confirm the efficacy and safety of all types of AFG procedures in the treatment of skin fibrotic lesions related to scleroderma, regardless of the type of fat preparation and/or purification. However, the present data do not allow us to attribute the reported clinical benefit common to all the studies to a specific subpopulation of cells or a specific mechanism. Del Papa et al. clearly provided evidence that AFG is able to induce neoangiogenesis in the lip skin as suggested by the significant improvement induced by lipofilling in microvascular patterns at labial capillaroscopy [63]. Moreover, the AFG in the perioral area produced a neoproliferation of dermal capillaries and reduced the fibrotic changes with a partial restoration of the dermal structure, supporting the advanced concept of the regenerative capacity of adipose tissue, probably via a pro-angiogenic process [63].

AFG Applications in Scleroderma Digital Ulcers

Scleroderma DUs are primarily the result of an obstructive vasculopathy of the fingers and toes, characterized by progressive vessel intima thickening and final lumen occlusion. In poorly oxygenated tissues, tissue regeneration is arrested in an inflammatory phase. The increase in inflammatory cells, associated with vascular insufficiency, leads to an abnormal production of inflammatory cytokines, loss of important growth factors, and an increase in secretion of matrix metalloproteinases. Additional complicating factors are represented by infections, epidermal thinning in patients with longstanding disease, and skin being tightly stretched over joints, with associated contractures. Therefore, the progression of the proper sequence of events responsible for SSc ulcer healing is impaired, and the response to conventional therapies is compromised. In this scenario, the attempt to find new treatments for SSc DUs has led researchers to investigate the use of stem cells for potential ulcer healing applications.

As described above, all the findings regarding the use of AFG in the treatment of SSc skin lesions support the hypotheses that the observed clinical benefits induced by AFG are mainly due to a vascular response. This issue was actually first confirmed by Bank et al. [67] who observed an unexpected reduction in the DU number after AFG in 11 patients with unresponsive Raynaud's phenomenon [RP] secondary to connective tissue disease (nine SSc and two mixed connective tissue disease). Using Coleman's technique, they injected the SVF along palmar, dorsal, and digital hand vessels without causing major complications, such as severe infection, loss of digits, or vascular or tendon injury. Although the extremity perfusion improvement was not statistically significant, they observed a significant reduction of number, duration, and severity of cold attacks and a DU improvement in some patients. Granel et al. observed similar results by injecting autologous SVF into the subcutaneous tissue of SSc fingers. They showed a significant improvement of Raynaud's condition scale and HD and a reduction trend of the DU number [66]. Moreover they noticed a significant rapid hand pain reduction by VAS scale from month 2 to month 6, but it was not confirmed at year 1. The modified Rodnan skin score (mRSS) at the hands improved significantly only at year 1 suggesting a possible continuous and progressive effect on skin fibrosis [66]. These data are expected to be confirmed in an ongoing controlled clinical trial [68].

Focusing on SSc ulcers, two studies were aimed to verify the AFG efficacy on ulcer healing [69, 70]. Del Bene et al. [69] treated nine SSc patients by AFG for a total of 15 ulcers, and the follow-up timeframe was of 3 months. They performed AFG according to Coleman's technique from 2 to 8 months after the ulcer onset. They injected 2–3 ml of the SVF obtained by centrifugation at the border of the larger ulcers or at the finger base of the smaller digital ulcers. They observed complete healing in ten DUs and size reduction >50% in two, within 8–12 weeks. They referred an improvement of pain in almost all patients/ulcers treated, associated with a reduction in analgesic use [69].

Del Papa et al. [70] proposed AFG treatment to 15 patients with similar and long-lasting SSc DUs on fingertips. The grafting procedure consisted of an injection of 0.5–1 ml of adipose SVF at the basis of the corresponding finger by sequential introduction of small aliquots in different directions from the injection site in order to spread the implanted adipose fraction as widely as possible around the finger base. Adipose tissue was obtained by Coleman's technique at the abdominal site, followed by a centrifugation at $920 \times g$ for 3 min in sterile conditions. As observed in the other studies, no adverse event was recorded. The primary end point was the time to heal the cardinal ulcer, while reduction of pain intensity [VAS scale] and of analgesic consumption represented secondary end points. A rather fast complete epithelialization of the DUs was reached in all of the enrolled patients [mean time to healing 4.23 weeks] associated with a significant reduction in pain intensity after a few weeks. The clinical benefit was further supported by a significant increase of the number of capillaries at 3 and 6 months at nailfold videocapillaroscopy and a significant after treatment reduction of digit artery resistivity measured by high-resolution echocolor Doppler [70].

In conclusion all these studies demonstrated that adipose tissue-based therapy is safe and efficient in ameliorating the local microvascular features associated with SSc vascular complications, including long-lasting DUs. Despite the limitations of these studies, including the short-term observation, the limited number of patients, and the open-label design, the promising results obtained should be regarded as a starting point for future clinical trials and applications.

Conclusions and Future Prospectives

Despite advances in DU-advanced topical medications and closure devices, at present there is no consensus regarding treatment of DUs in scleroderma. In particular, no drug has given evidence to reverse the microvasculopathy associated with scleroderma tissue damage. In this discouraging scenario, stem cell therapies have emerged as therapeutic alternatives for repair of damaged tissues. Due to their capacity to self-renew, proliferate, and differentiate in multi-lineage cells, stem cells, in particular those derived from adult tissues like the bone marrow and fat, may well place such cells with great potential in regenerative medicine. Interest in the use of adipose tissue is ever increasing due to the ease of access, abundant supply, and lack of ethical concerns. Despite the growing interest in autologous fat grafting applications in different degenerative disorders such as neurological diseases, diabetes, heart failure, and wound healing, there is no agreement on the best technique to perform AFG. No definite indications are known about the proper selection of donor sites, methods of harvest, process, and placement of fat grafts. With regard to the treatment of SSc DUs, it should be noted that different types of ulcers might have different healing outcomes when using fat graft as a therapy. Indeed experimental data suggest that the microenvironment can regulate ADSC function when in contact [71]. Moreover the injection of adipose-derived cells in SSc DUs could induce more or less positive results based on the acute ischemic or chronic fibrotic subset of treated ulcers. Such a difference might obviously dictate different therapeutic rationales in the use of AFG in the treatment of SSc skin complications.

Many basic scientific questions remain to be addressed. Although the mechanisms by which ADSCs and other SVF components, together with their secretory factors, have been well studied, the possibility that these cells can be useful in ulcer healing still remains to be clarified in depth. In addition, it has not yet been fully elucidated whether adipose-derived cell populations from SSc patients share the same therapeutic potential as cells derived from normal donors. In the autologous set, comparison between SSc and healthy fat donors is a topic of important debate. Recently our group showed that ADSCs from patients with SSc exhibit the same phenotypic pattern as well as the same proliferative, differentiation potentials and immunosuppressive properties as those from normal controls [72]. In addition, we observed that both SSc and normal ADSCs were able to support both normal and SSc endothelial cells to perform tube formation in normoxic condition. The latter capability appeared to be enhanced under hypoxic condition and, in a comparable way, in all types of ADSC-endothelial cell co-cultures including those where SSc-EC were tested. This is in contrast to what has been reported in studies concerning BM-MSCs from patients with SSc, which have been shown to be somehow defective in their proliferative potential, as well as to express a partially different phenotype [72].

On the whole, these data suggest that ADSCs from patients with SSc maintain normal phenotype and unchanged proliferation capacity. Their unaltered immunosuppressive and neoangiogenetic potentials strongly support the use of these cells in future cell-based therapeutic trials in SSc.

References

1. Gurtner GC, Werner S, Barrandon Y, Longaker MT. Wound repair and regeneration. Nature. 2008;453(7193):314–21.
2. Guo S, DiPietro LA. Factors affecting wound healing. J Dent Res. 2010;89:219–29.
3. Menke NB, Ward KR, Witten TM, Bonchev DG, Diegelmann RF. Impaired wound healing. Clin Dermatol. 2007;25:19–25.
4. Gabrielli A, Avvedimento EV, Krieg T. Scleroderma. N Engl J Med. 2009;360(19):1989–2003.
5. Distler JH, Gay S, Distler O. Angiogenesis and vasculogenesis in systemic sclerosis. Rheumatology. 2006;45(Suppl 3):iii26–7.
6. Mimeault M, Hauke R, Batra S. Stem cells: a revolution in therapeutics-recent advances in stem cell biology and their therapeutic applications in regenerative medicine and cancer therapies. Clin Pharmacol Therap. 2007;82:252–64.
7. Körbling M, Estrov Z. Adult stem cells for tissue repair—a new therapeutic concept? N Engl J Med. 2003;349:570–82.
8. Parker AM, Katz AJ. Adipose-derived stem cells for the regeneration of damaged tissues. Expert Opinion on Biological Ther. 2006;6:567–78.
9. Korin N, Levenberg S. Engineering human embryonic stem cell differentiation. Biotechnol Genet Eng Rev. 2007;24:243–61.
10. Park I-H, Arora N, Huo H, Maherali N, Ahfeldt T, Shimamura A, et al. Disease-specific induced pluripotent stem cells. Cell. 2008;134:877–86.
11. Caplan AI. Adult mesenchymal stem cells: when, where, and how. Stem Cells Int. 2015;2015:628767.
12. Strioga M, Viswanathan S, Darinskas A, Slaby O, Michalek J. Same or not the same? Comparison of adipose tissue-derived versus bone marrow-derived mesenchymal stem and stromal cells. Stem Cell Dev. 2012;21(14):2724–52.
13. Pittenger MF, Mackay AM, Beck SC, Jaiswal RK, Douglas R, Mosca JD, et al. Multilineage potential of adult human mesenchymal stem cells. Science. 1999;284(5411):143–7.
14. Motegi SI, Ishikawa O. Mesenchymal stem cells: the roles and functions in cutaneous wound healing and tumor growth. J Dermatol Sci. 2017;86(2):83–9.
15. Lu D, Chen B, Liang Z, Deng W, Jiang Y, Li S, et al. Comparison of bone marrow mesenchymal stem cells with bone marrow-derived mononuclear cells for treatment of diabetic critical limb ischemia and foot ulcer: a double-blind, randomized, controlled trial. Diabetes Res Clin Pract. 2011;92:26–36.
16. Procházka V, Gumulec J, Jaluvka F, Salounová D, Jonszta T, Czerny D, et al. Cell therapy, a new standard in management of chronic critical limb ischemia and foot ulcer. Cell Transplant. 2010;19:1413–24.
17. Kirana S, Stratmann B, Lammers D, Negrean M, Stirban A, Minartz P, et al. Wound therapy with autologous bone marrow stem cells in diabetic patients with ischaemia-induced tissue ulcers affecting the lower limbs. Int J Clin Pract. 2007;61:690–4.
18. Hanson SE, Kleinbeck KR, Cantu D, Kim J, Bentz ML, Faucher LD, et al. Local delivery of allogeneic bone marrow and adipose tissue-derived mesenchymal stromal cells for cutaneous wound healing in a porcine model. J Tissue Eng Regen Med. 2016;10(2):E90–100.
19. Ichioka S, Yokogawa H, Sekiya N, Kouraba S, Minamimura A, Ohura N, et al. Determinants of wound healing in bone marrow-impregnated collagen matrix treatment: impact of microcirculatory response to surgical debridement. Wound Repair Regen. 2009;17:492–7.
20. Ichioka S, Kouraba S, Sekiya N, Ohura N, Nakatsuka T. Bone marrow-impregnated collagen matrix for wound healing: experimental evaluation in a microcirculatory model of angiogenesis, and clinical experience. Br J Plast Surg. 2005;58(8):1124–30.
21. Mizuno H, Miyamoto M, Shimamoto M, Koike S, Hyakusoku H, Kuroyanagi Y. Therapeutic angiogenesis by autologous bone marrow cell implantation together with allogeneic cultured dermal substitute for intractable ulcers in critical limb ischaemia. J Plast Reconstr Aesthet Surg. 2010;63(11):1875–82.
22. Nevskaya T, Ananieva L, Bykovskaia S, Eremin I, Karandashov E, Khrennikov J, et al. Autologous progenitor cell implantation as a novel therapeutic intervention for ischaemic digits in systemic sclerosis. Rheumatology. 2009;48(1):61–4.
23. Kuwana M. Potential benefit of statins for vascular disease in systemic sclerosis. Curr Opin Rheumatol. 2006;18:594–600.
24. Del Papa N, Cortiana M, Vitali C, Silvestris I, Maglione W, Comina DP, et al. Simvastatin reduces endothelial activation and damage but is partially ineffective in inducing endothelial repair in systemic sclerosis. J Rheumatol. 2008;35(7):1323–8.
25. Abou-Raya A, Abou-Raya S, Helmii M. Statins: potentially useful in therapy of systemic sclerosis-related Raynaud's phenomenon and digital ulcers. J Rheumatol. 2008;35:1801–8.
26. Gronthos S, Franklin DM, Leddy HA, Robey PG, Storms RW, Gimble JM. Surface protein characterization of human adipose tissue-derived stromal cells. J Cell Physiol. 2001;189:54–63.
27. Musina R, Bekchanova E, Sukhikh G. Comparison of mesenchymal stem cells obtained from different human tissues. Bull Exp Biol Med. 2005;139:504–9.
28. Katz AJ, Tholpady A, Tholpady SS, Shang H, Ogle RC. Cell surface and transcriptional characterization of human adipose derived adherent stromal (hADAS) cells. Stem Cells. 2005;23:412–23.
29. Liu TM, Martina M, Hutmacher DW, Hui JHP, Lee EH, Lim B. Identification of common pathways mediating differentiation of bone marrow-and adipose tissue-derived human mesenchymal stem cells into three mesenchymal lineages. Stem Cells. 2007;25:750–60.
30. Shim YH, Zhang RH. Literature review to optimize the autologous fat transplantation procedure and recent technologies to improve graft viability and overall outcome: a systematic and retrospective analytic approach. Aesthet Plast Surg. 2017;41(4):815–31.
31. Yoshimura K, Shigeura T, Matsumoto D, Sato T, Takaki Y, Aiba-Kojima E, et al. Characterization of freshly isolated and cultured cells derived from the fatty and fluid portions of liposuction aspirates. J Cell Physiol. 2006;208:64–76.
32. Eto H, Suga H, Matsumoto D, Inoue K, Aoi N, Kato H, et al. Characterization of structure and cellular components of aspirated and excised adipose tissue. Plast Reconstr Surg. 2009;124:1087–97.
33. Gimble JM, Katz AJ, Bunnell BA. Adipose-derived stem cells for regenerative medicine. Circ Res. 2007;100(9):1249–60.
34. Wong VW, Gurtner GC, Longaker MT. Wound healing: a paradigm for regeneration. Mayo Clin Proc. 2013;88(9):1022–31.

35. Shingyochi Y, Orbay H, Mizuno H. Adipose-derived stem cells for wound repair and regeneration. Expert Opin Biol Ther. 2015;15(9):1285–92.
36. Hassan WU, Greiser U, Wang W. Role of adipose-derived stem cells in wound healing. Wound Repair Regen. 2014;22(3):313–25.
37. Ebrahimian TG, Pouzoulet F, Squiban C, Buard V, André M, Cousin B, et al. Cell therapy based on adipose tissue-derived stromal cells promotes physiological and pathological wound healing. Arterioscler Thromb Vasc Biol. 2009;29(4):503–10.
38. Cao Y, Sun Z, Liao L, Meng Y, Han Q, Zhao RC. Human adipose tissue-derived stem cells differentiate into endothelial cells in vitro and improve postnatal neovascularization in vivo. Biochem Biophys Res Commun. 2005;332:370–9.
39. Planat-Benard V, Silvestre JS, Cousin B, Andre M, Nibbelink M, Tamarat R, et al. Plasticity of human adipose lineage cells toward endothelial cells: physiological and therapeutic perspectives. Circulation. 2004;109:656–63.
40. Rehman J, Traktuev D, Li J, Merfeld-Clauss S, Temm-Grove CJ, et al. Secretion of angiogenic and antiapoptotic factors by human adipose stromal cells. Circulation. 2004;109:1292–8.
41. Fraser JK, Schreiber R, Strem B, Zhu M, Alfonso Z, Wulur I, et al. Plasticity of human adipose stem cells toward endothelial cells and cardiomyocytes. Nat Clin Pract Cardiovasc Med. 2006;3(Suppl 1):S33–7.
42. Kim EK, Li G, Lee TJ, Hong JP. The effect of human adipose-derived stem cells on healing of ischemic wounds in a diabetic nude mouse model. Plast Reconstr Surg. 2011;128(2):387–94.
43. Atalay S, Coruh A, Deniz K. Stromal vascular fraction improves deep partial thickness burn wound healing. Burns. 2014;40(7):1375–83.
44. Rodriguez J, Boucher F, Lequeux C, Josset-Lamaugarny A, Rouyer O, Ardisson O, et al. Intradermal injection of human adipose-derived stem cells accelerates skin wound healing in nude mice. Stem Cell Res Ther. 2015;6:241.
45. Lee SM, Lee SC, Kim SJ. Contribution of human adipose tissue-derived stem cells and the secretome to the skin allograft survival in mice. J Surg Res. 2014;188:280–9.
46. Hsiao ST-F, Asgari A, Lokmic Z, Sinclair R, Dusting GJ, Lim SY, et al. Comparative analysis of paracrine factor expression in human adult mesenchymal stem cells derived from bone marrow, adipose, and dermal tissue. Stem Cells Dev. 2012;21:2189–203.
47. Park BS, Jang KA, Sung JH, Park JS, Kwon YH, Kim KJ, et al. Adipose-derived stem cells and their secretory factors as a promising therapy for skin aging. Dermatol Surg. 2008;34:1323–6.
48. Cerqueira MT, Pirraco RP, Marques AP. Stem cells in skin wound healing: are we there yet? Adv Wound Care (New Rochelle). 2016;5(4):164–75.
49. Cross KJ, Mustoe TA. Growth factors in wound healing. Surg Clin North Am. 2003;83:531.
50. Choi JR, Yong KW, Wan Safwani WK. Effect of hypoxia on human adipose-derived mesenchymal stem cells and its potential clinical applications. Cell Mol Life Sci. 2017;74(14):2587–600.
51. Kim Y, Kim H, Cho H, Bae Y, Suh K, Jung J. Direct comparison of human mesenchymal stem cells derived from adipose tissues and bone marrow in mediating neovascularization in response to vascular ischemia. Cell Physiol Biochem. 2007;20(6):867–76.
52. Rubina K, Kalinina N, Efimenko A, Lopatina T, Melikhova V, Tsokolaeva Z, et al. Adipose stromal cells stimulate angiogenesis via promoting progenitor cell differentiation, secretion of angiogenic factors, and enhancing vessel maturation. Tissue Eng Part A. 2009;15(8):2039–50.
53. Hsiao ST, Lokmic Z, Peshavariya H, Abberton KM, Dusting GJ, Lim SY, et al. Hypoxic conditioning enhances the angiogenic paracrine activity of human adipose-derived stem cells. Stem Cells Dev. 2013;22(10):1614–23.
54. Bekhite MM, Finkensieper A, Rebhan J, Huse S, Schultze-Mosgau S, Figulla HR, et al. Hypoxia, leptin, and vascular endothelial growth factor stimulate vascular endothelial cell differentiation of human adipose tissue-derived stem cells. Stem Cells Dev. 2014;23(4):333–51.
55. Bourin P, Bunnell BA, Casteilla L, Dominici M, Katz AJ, March KL, et al. Stromal cells from the adipose tissue-derived stromal vascular fraction and culture expanded adipose tissue-derived stromal/stem cells: a joint statement of the International Federation for Adipose Therapeutics and Science (IFATS) and the International Society for Cellular Therapy (ISCT). Cytotherapy. 2013;15(6):641–8.
56. Li H, Zimmerlin L, Marra KG, Donnenberg VS, Donnenberg AD, Rubin JP. Adipogenic potential of adipose stem cell subpopulations. Plast Reconstr Surg. 2011;128(3):663–72.
57. Sukmawati D, Tanaka R. Introduction to next generation of endothelial progenitor cell therapy: a promise in vascular medicine. Am J Transl Res. 2015;7:411–21.
58. Dykstra JA, Facile T, Patrick RJ, Francis KR, Milanovich S, Weimer JM, et al. Concise review: fat and furious: harnessing the full potential of adipose-derived stromal vascular fraction. Stem Cells Transl Med. 2017;6(4):1096–108.
59. Dar A, Itskovitz-Eldor J. Therapeutic potential of perivascular cells from human pluripotent stem cells. J Tissue Eng Regen Med. 2015;9(9):977–87.
60. Cipolletta D. Adipose tissue-resident regulatory T cells: phenotypic specialization, functions and therapeutic potential. Immunology. 2014;142(4):517–25.
61. Coleman SR. Structural fat grafting: more than a permanent filler. Plast Reconstr Surg. 2006;118(3 Suppl):108S–20S.
62. Del Papa N, Zaccara E, Andracco R, Maglione W, Vitali C. Adipose-derived cell transplantation in systemic sclerosis: state of the art and future perspectives. J Scleroderma Relat Disord. 2017;2:33–41.
63. Del Papa N, Caviggioli F, Sambataro D, Zaccara E, Vinci V, Di Luca G, et al. Autologous fat grafting in the treatment of fibrotic perioral changes in patients with systemic sclerosis. Cell Transplant. 2015;24:63–72.
64. Onesti MG, Fioramonti P, Carella S, Fino P, Marchese C, Scuderi N. Improvement of mouth function disability in systemic sclerosis patients over one year in a trial of fat transplantation versus adipose-derived stromal cells. Stem Cells Int. 2016;2016:2416192.
65. Sautereau N, Daumas A, Truillet R, Jouve E, Magalon J, Veran J, et al. Efficacy of autologous microfat graft on facial handicap in systemic sclerosis patients. Plast Reconstr Surg Glob Open. 2016;4(3):e660.
66. Granel B, Daumas A, Jouve E, Harlé JR, Nguyen PS, Chabannon C, et al. Safety, tolerability and potential efficacy of injection of autologous adipose derived stromal vascular fraction in the fingers of patients with systemic sclerosis: an open-label phase I trial. Ann Rheum Dis. 2015;74(12):2175–82.
67. Bank J, Fuller SM, Henry GI, Zachary LS. Fat grafting to the hand in patients with Raynaud phenomenon: a novel therapeutic modality. Plast Reconstr Surg. 2014;133(5):1109–18.
68. ClinicalTrials.gov: NCT02558543.
69. Del Bene M, Pozzi MR, Rovati L, Mazzola I, Erba G, Bonomi S. Autologous fat grafting for scleroderma-induced digital ulcers. An effective technique in patients with systemic sclerosis. Handchir Mikrochir Plast Chir. 2014;46:242–7.
70. Del Papa N, Di Luca G, Sambataro D, Zaccara E, Maglione W, Gabrielli A, et al. Regional implantation of autologous adipose tissue-derived cells induces a prompt healing of long-lasting indolent digital ulcers in patients with sys-temic sclerosis. Cell Transplant. 2015;24(11):2297–305.
71. Koenen P, Spanholtz TA, Maegele M, Stürmer E, Brockamp T, Neugebauer E, et al. Acute and chronic wound fluids inversely influence adipose-derived stem cell function: molecular insights into impaired wound healing. Int Wound J. 2015;12(1):10–6.
72. Capelli C, Zaccara E, Cipriani P, Di Benedetto P, Maglione W, Andracco R, et al. Phenotypical and functional characteristics of "in vitro" expanded adipose-derived mesenchymal stromal cells from patients with systemic sclerosis. Cell Transplant. 2017;26(5):841–54.

Part X

Atlas

Marco Matucci-Cerinic, Christopher P. Denton,
Tiziana Pucci, Francesca Braschi, Claudia Fantauzzo,
and Lucia Paganelli

Digital Ulcers

Loss of epidermal covering with a break in the basement membrane (which separates dermis from epidermis). It appears clinically as visible blood vessels, fibrin, granulation tissue and/or underlying deeper structures (e.g., muscle, ligament, fat) or as it would appear on debridement.

(J Scleroderma Relat Disord 2017; 2:115–120)

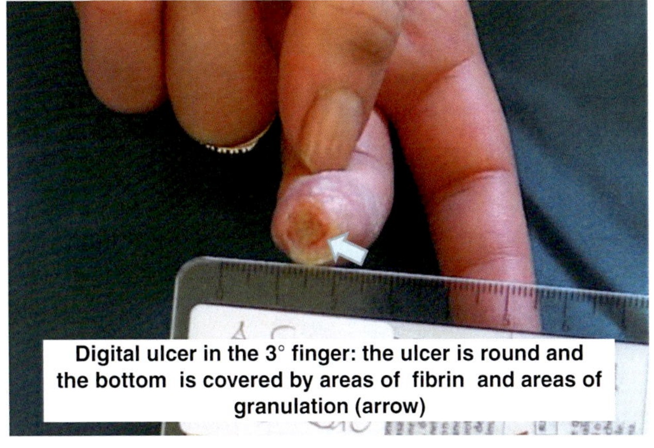

Digital ulcer in the 3° finger: the ulcer is round and the bottom is covered by areas of fibrin and areas of granulation (arrow)

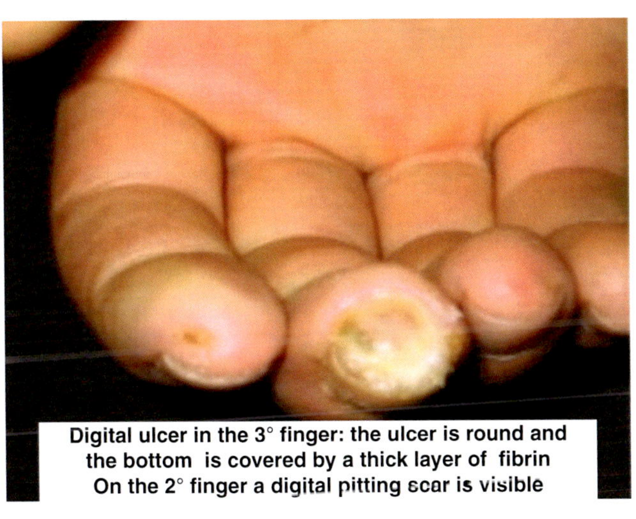

Digital ulcer in the 3° finger: the ulcer is round and the bottom is covered by a thick layer of fibrin
On the 2° finger a digital pitting scar is visible

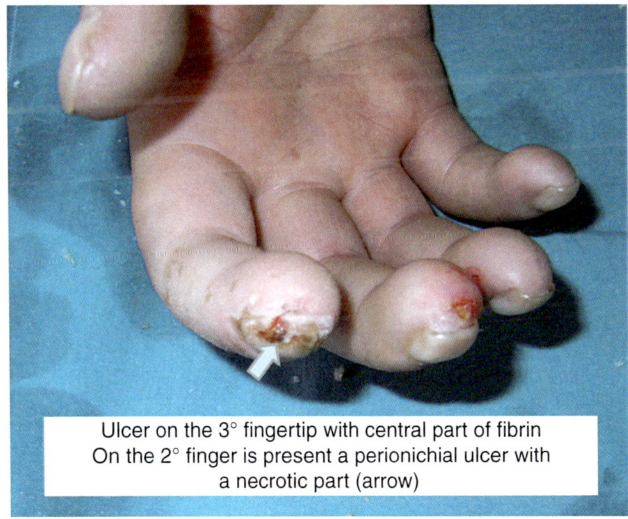

Ulcer on the 3° fingertip with central part of fibrin
On the 2° finger is present a perionichial ulcer with a necrotic part (arrow)

M. Matucci-Cerinic (✉)
Department of Experimental and Clinical Medicine, University of Florence, Florence, Italy

Department of Geriatric Medicine, Division of Rheumatology, AOUC, Florence, Italy
e-mail: marco.matuccicerinic@unifi.it

C. P. Denton
Division of Medicine, University College London, Centre for Rheumatology, Royal Free Hospital, London, UK

T. Pucci · F. Braschi · C. Fantauzzo · L. Paganelli ·
Department of Experimental and Clinical Medicine, University of Florence, Florence, Italy

Department of Geriatric Medicine, Division of Rheumatology, AOUC, Florence, Italy

Health Professional Department, AOUC, Florence, Italy

© Springer Nature Switzerland AG 2019
M. Matucci-Cerinic, C. P. Denton (eds.), *Atlas of Ulcers in Systemic Sclerosis*, https://doi.org/10.1007/978-3-319-98477-3_25

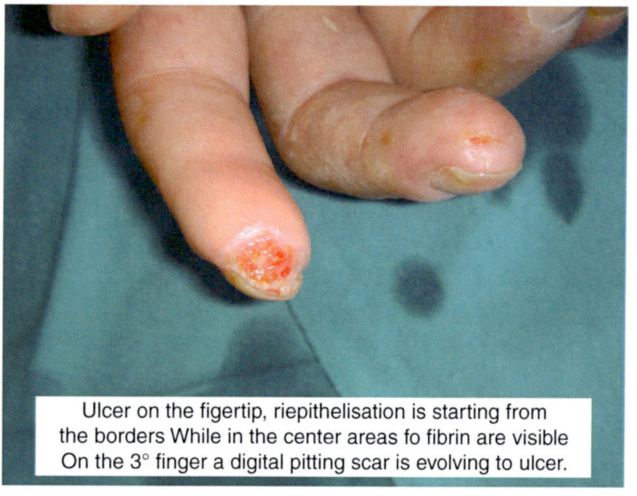

Ulcer on the figertip, riepithelisation is starting from the borders While in the center areas fo fibrin are visible On the 3° finger a digital pitting scar is evolving to ulcer.

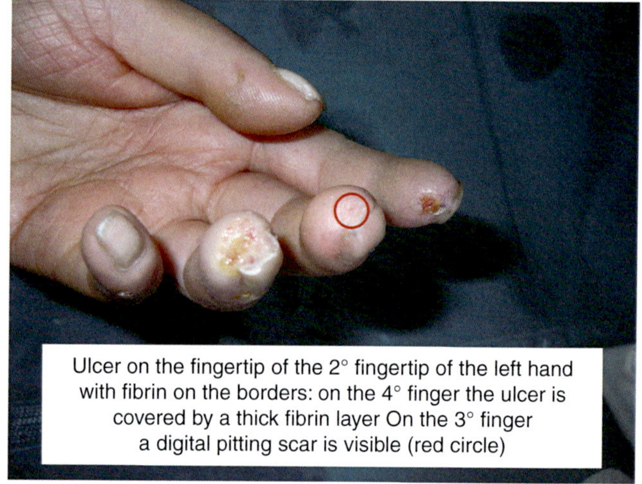

Ulcer on the fingertip of the 2° fingertip of the left hand with fibrin on the borders: on the 4° finger the ulcer is covered by a thick fibrin layer On the 3° finger a digital pitting scar is visible (red circle)

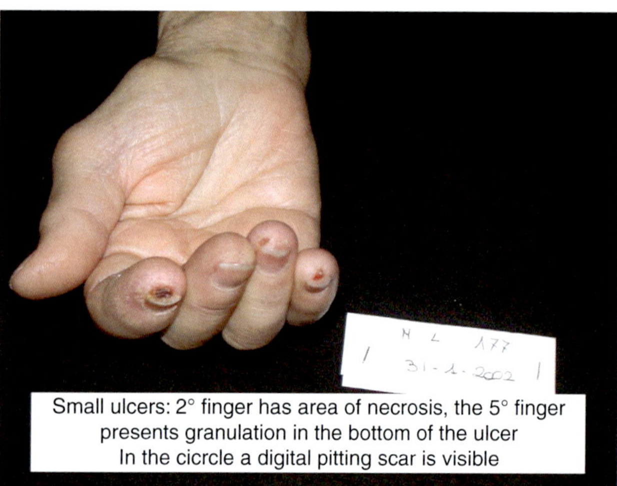

Small ulcers: 2° finger has area of necrosis, the 5° finger presents granulation in the bottom of the ulcer In the cicrcle a digital pitting scar is visible

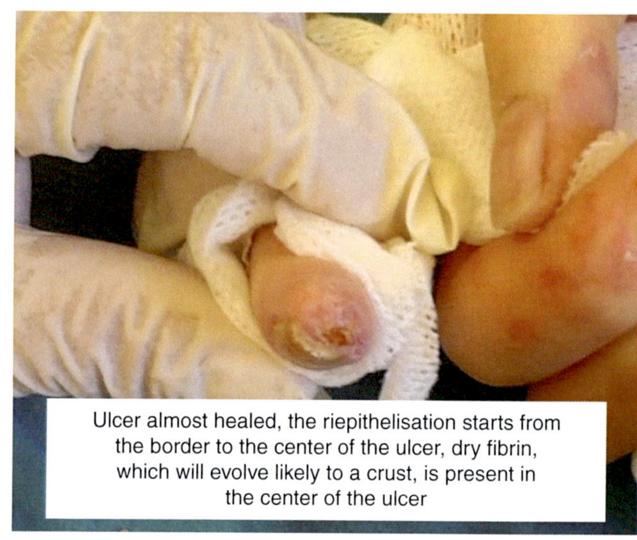

Ulcer almost healed, the riepithelisation starts from the border to the center of the ulcer, dry fibrin, which will evolve likely to a crust, is present in the center of the ulcer

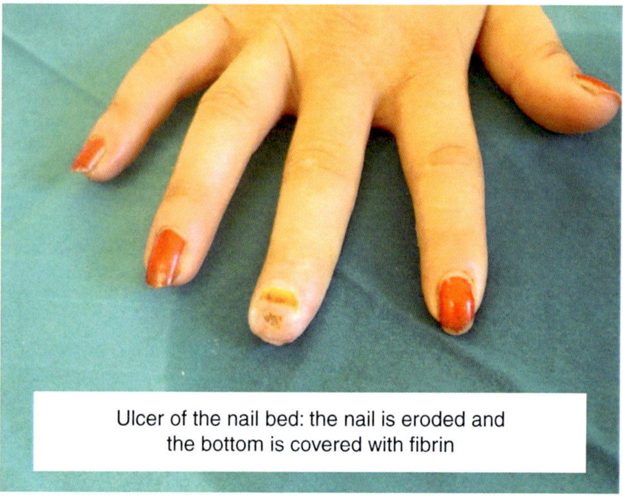

Ulcer of the nail bed: the nail is eroded and the bottom is covered with fibrin

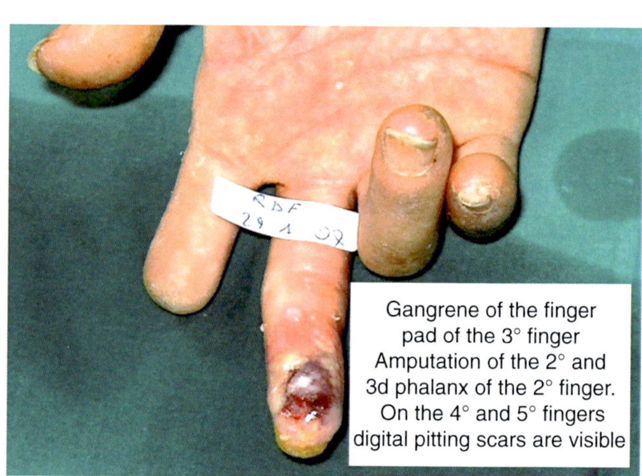

Gangrene of the finger pad of the 3° finger Amputation of the 2° and 3d phalanx of the 2° finger. On the 4° and 5° fingers digital pitting scars are visible

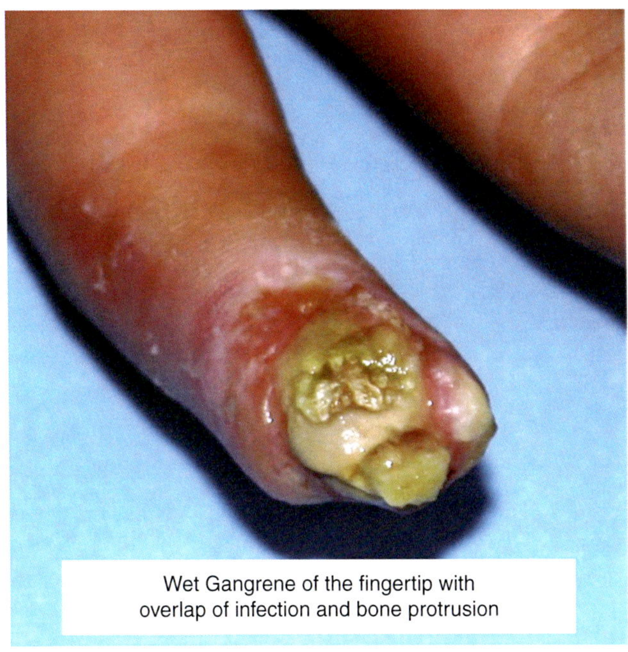

Wet Gangrene of the fingertip with
overlap of infection and bone protrusion

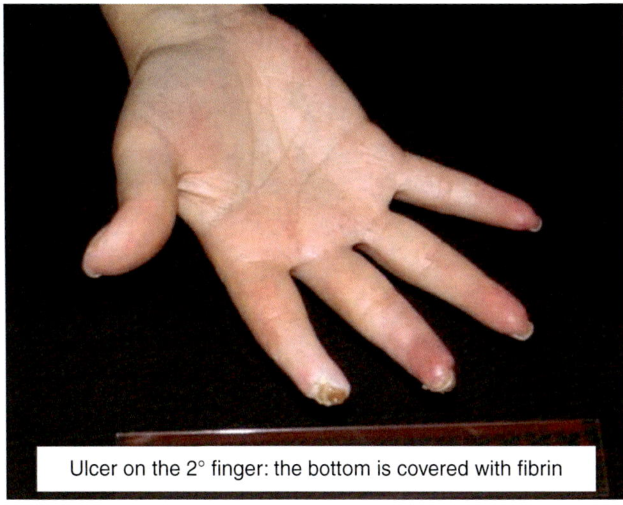

Ulcer on the 2° finger: the bottom is covered with fibrin

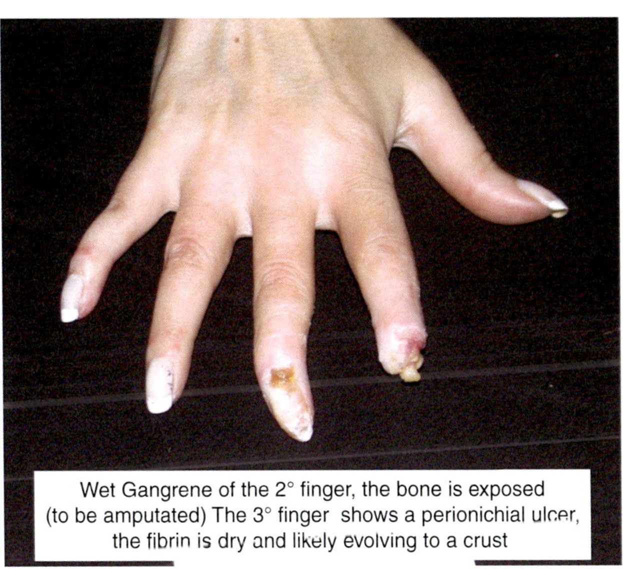

Wet Gangrene of the 2° finger, the bone is exposed
(to be amputated) The 3° finger shows a perionichial ulcer,
the fibrin is dry and likely evolving to a crust

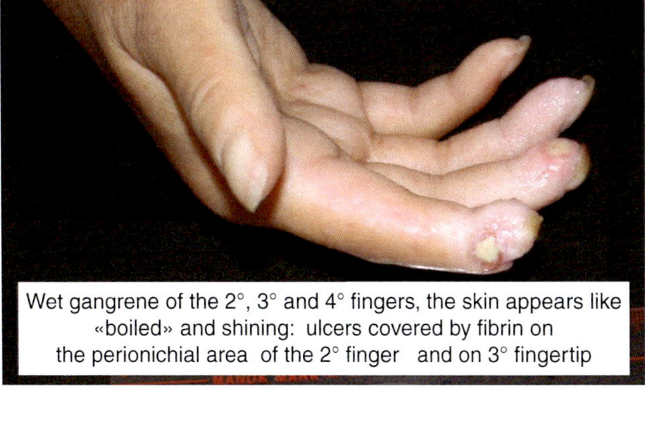

Wet gangrene of the 2°, 3° and 4° fingers, the skin appears like
«boiled» and shining: ulcers covered by fibrin on
the perionichial area of the 2° finger   and on 3° fingertip

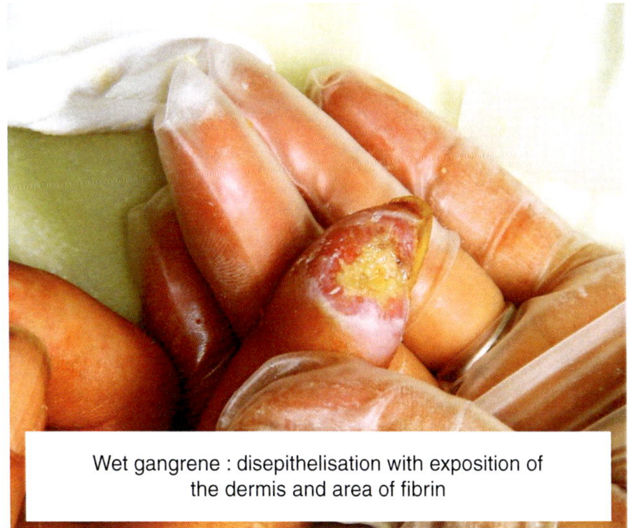

Wet gangrene : disepithelisation with exposition of
the dermis and area of fibrin

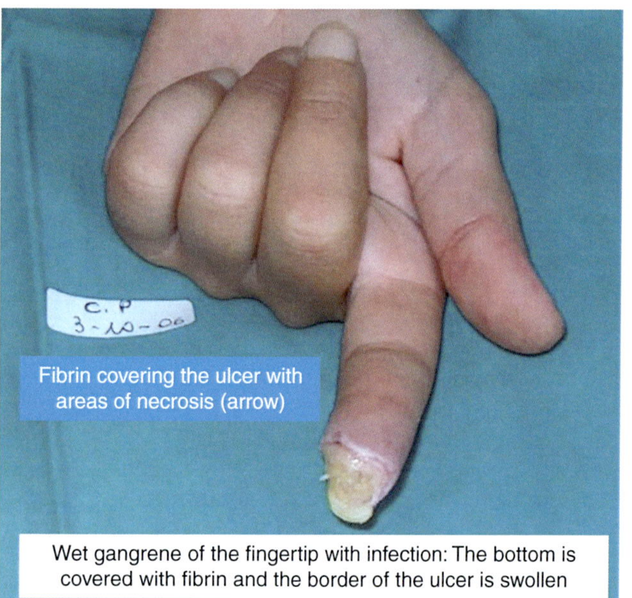

Wet gangrene of the fingertip with infection: The bottom is covered with fibrin and the border of the ulcer is swollen

Calcinosis

Detected either clinically or radiographically. Calcinosis is defined as palpable, dermal and/or subcutaneous or intramuscular calcific deposits. It is usually located in digits or over large proximal joints or extensor surfaces of distal extremities

(Ann Rheum Dis. 2013;72:1747)

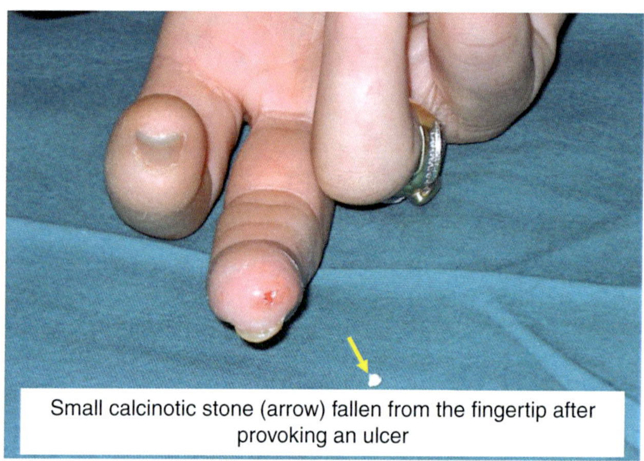

Small calcinotic stone (arrow) fallen from the fingertip after provoking an ulcer

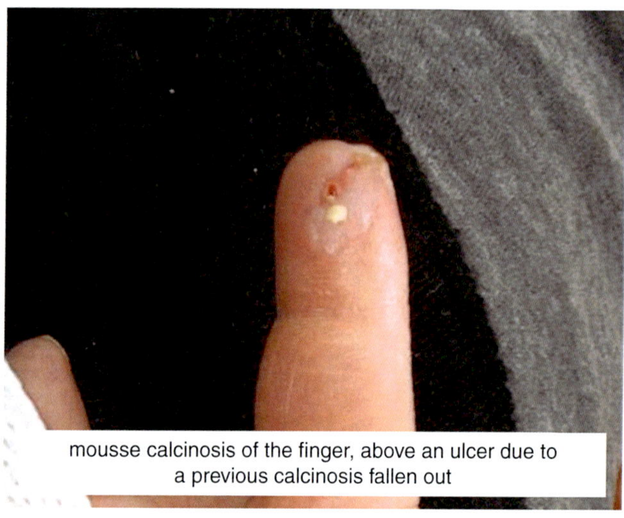

mousse calcinosis of the finger, above an ulcer due to a previous calcinosis fallen out

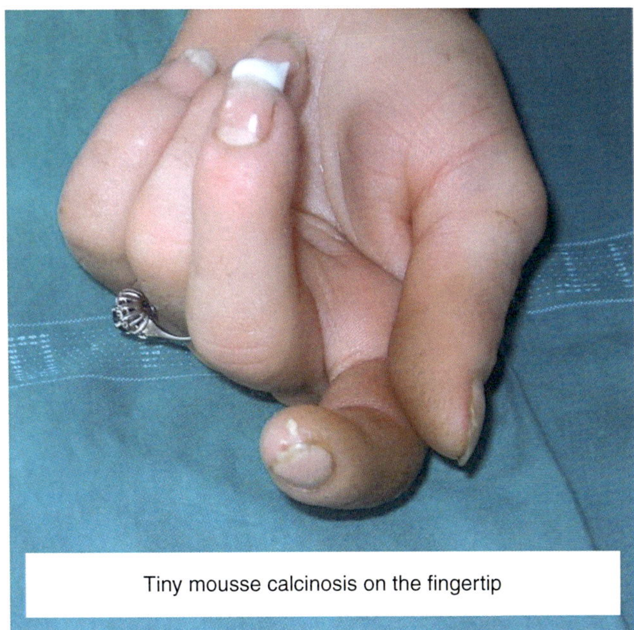

Tiny mousse calcinosis on the fingertip

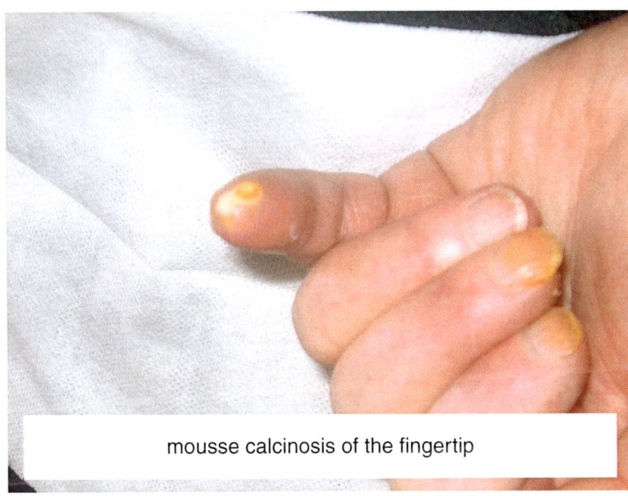

mousse calcinosis of the fingertip

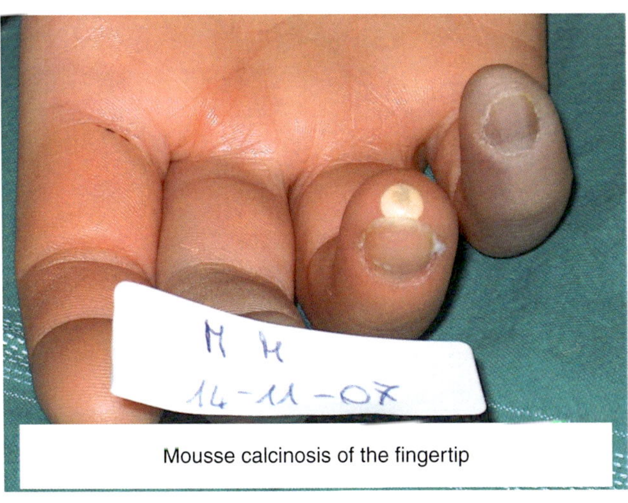

Mousse calcinosis of the fingertip

Digital Pitting Scars

small-sized hyperkeratosis sometimes overlying a cutaneous depression

> Digital pitting scars are depressed areas at the tips *and other areas on the finger* as a result of chronic ischemia, rather than trauma or exogenous causes

> (Ann Rheum Dis 2013;72:1747)

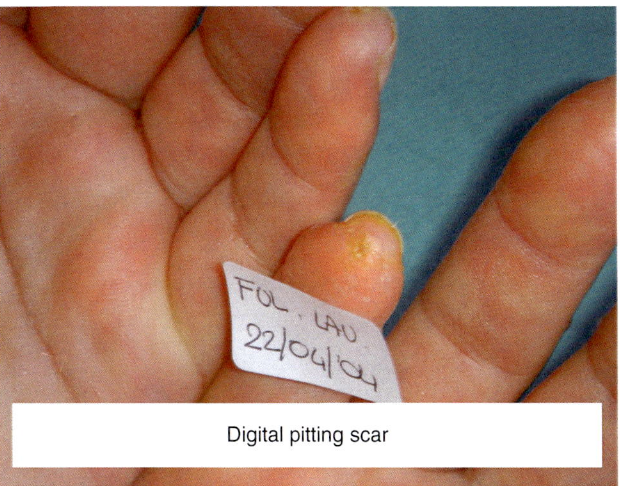

Digital pitting scar

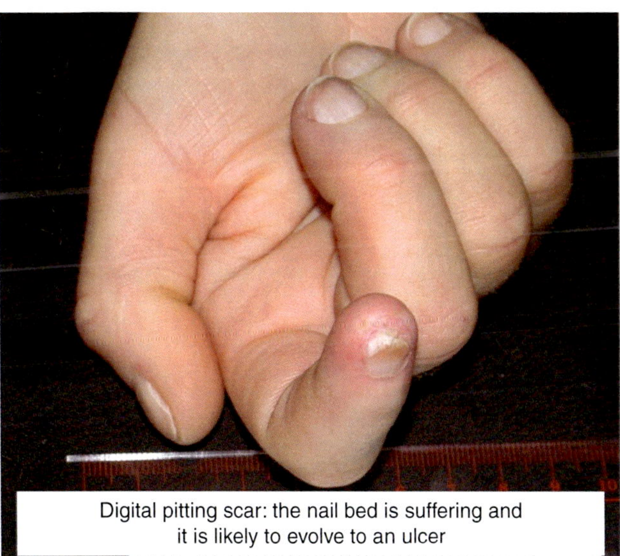

Digital pitting scar: the nail bed is suffering and it is likely to evolve to an ulcer

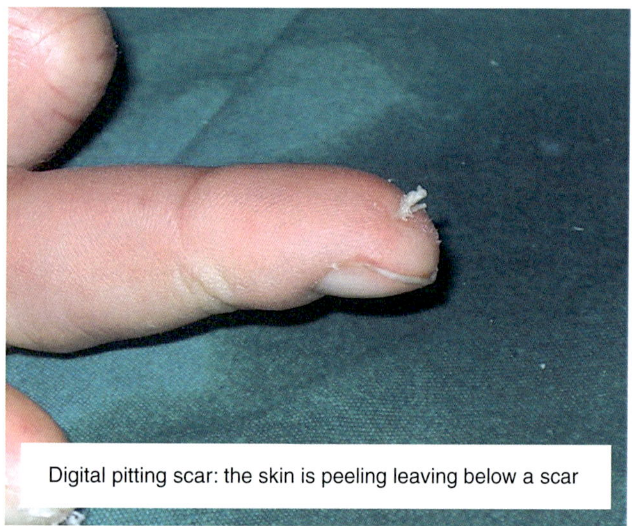

Digital pitting scar: the skin is peeling leaving below a scar

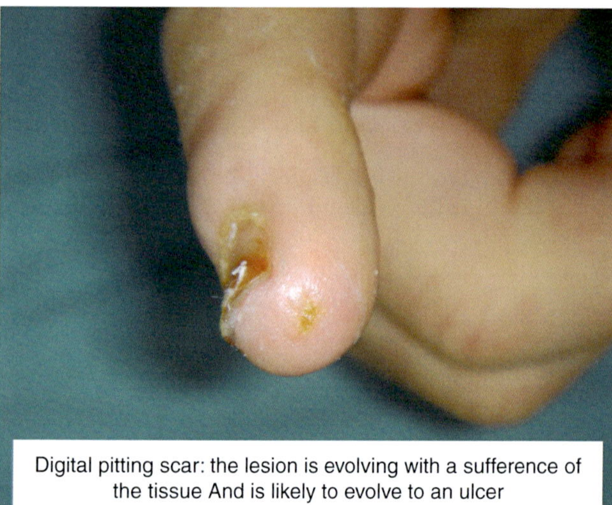

Digital pitting scar: the lesion is evolving with a sufference of
the tissue And is likely to evolve to an ulcer
if not adequately managed

Necrosis

Pathologic death of tissue resulting from irreversible damage.

End result of infarction of a superficial area, often associated with secondary infection.

It may be classified in wet (frequently linked to infection) or dry necrosis.

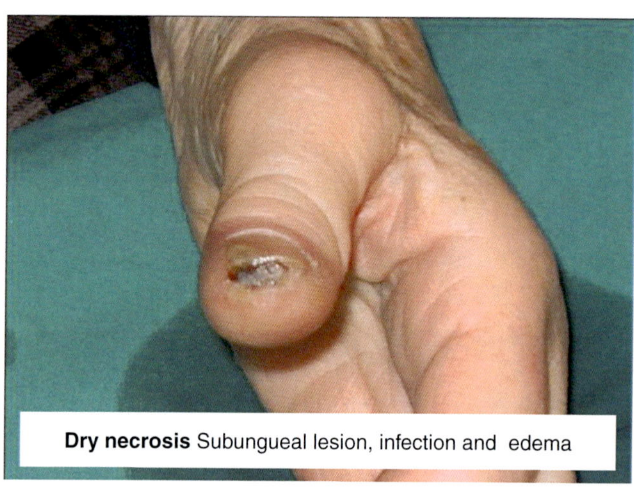

Dry necrosis Subungueal lesion, infection and edema

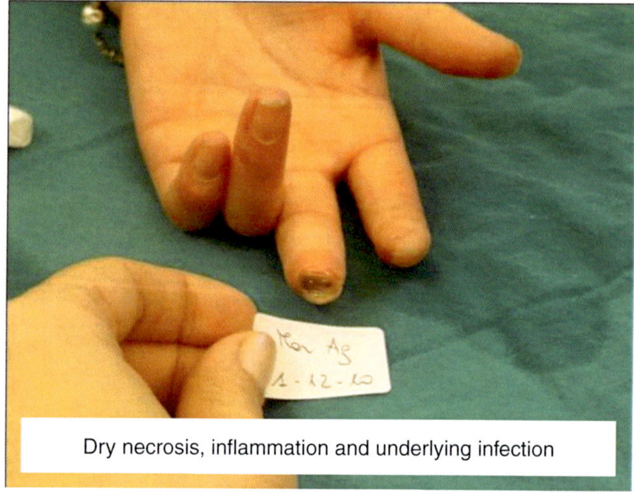

Dry necrosis, inflammation and underlying infection

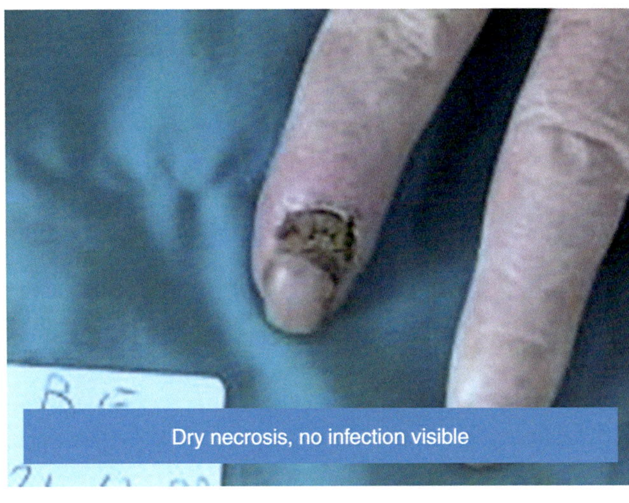

Dry necrosis, no infection visible

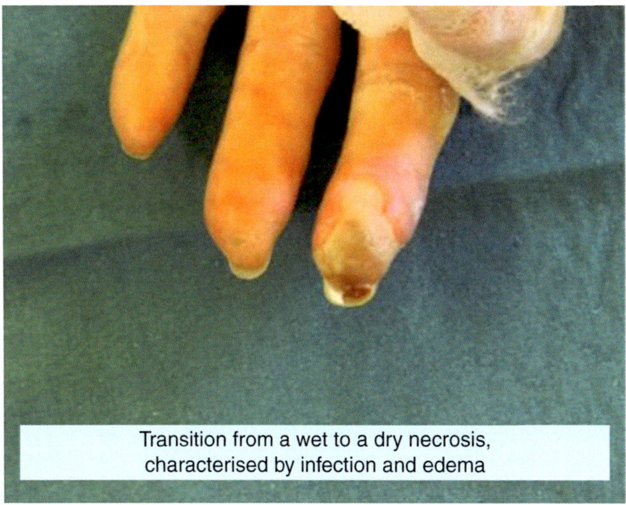

Transition from a wet to a dry necrosis, characterised by infection and edema

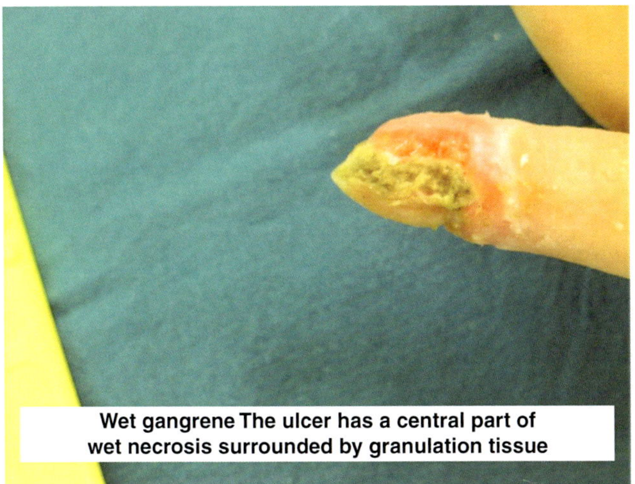

Wet gangrene The ulcer has a central part of wet necrosis surrounded by granulation tissue

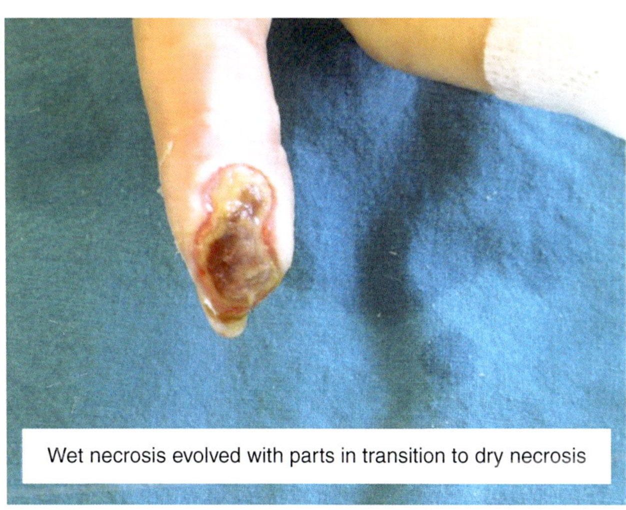

Wet necrosis evolved with parts in transition to dry necrosis

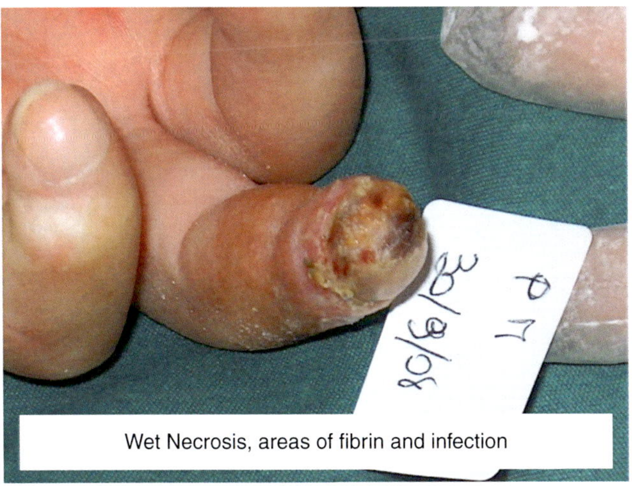

Wet Necrosis, areas of fibrin and infection

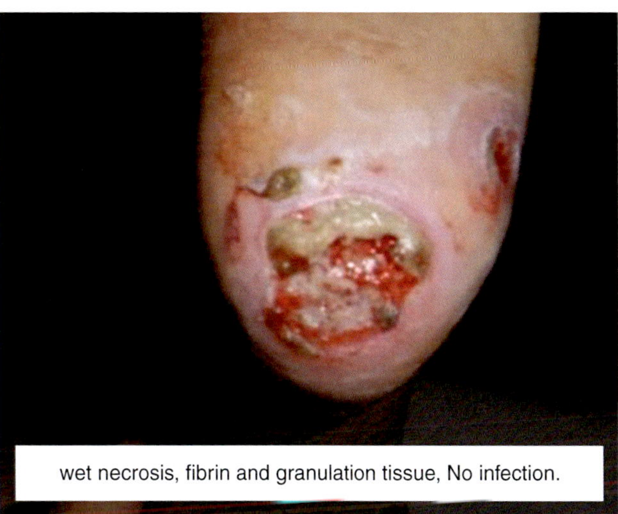

wet necrosis, fibrin and granulation tissue, No infection.

Eschar

A thick, coagulated crust expression of *superficial necrosis*.
May overlie an area of ulceration.

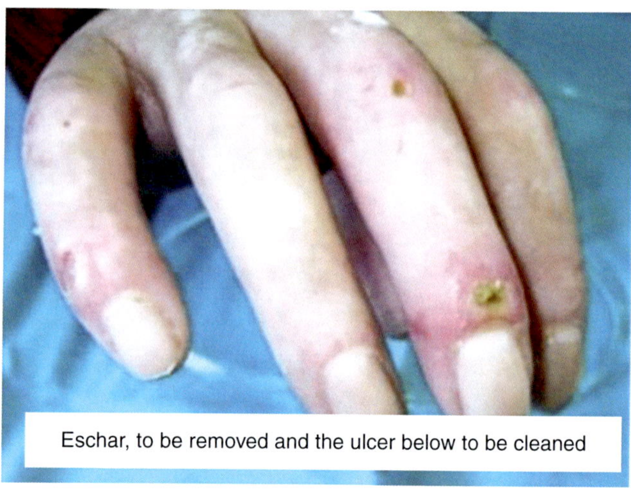

Eschar, to be removed and the ulcer below to be cleaned

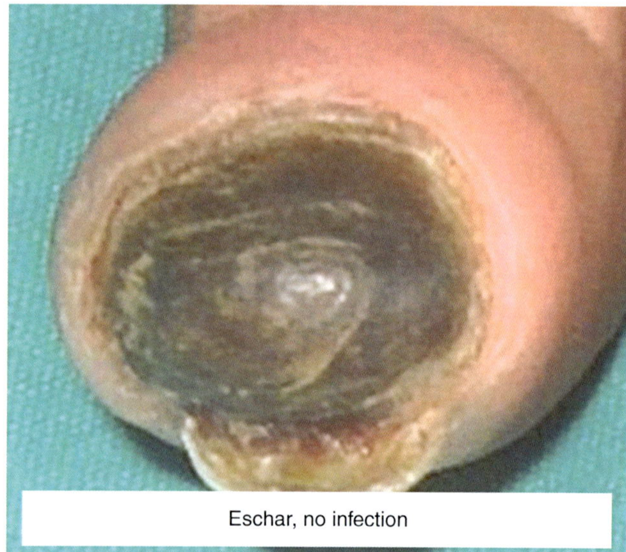

Eschar, no infection

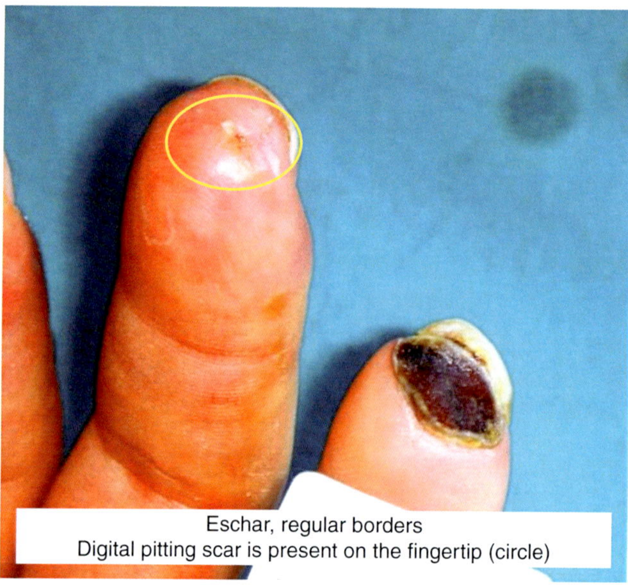

Eschar, regular borders
Digital pitting scar is present on the fingertip (circle)

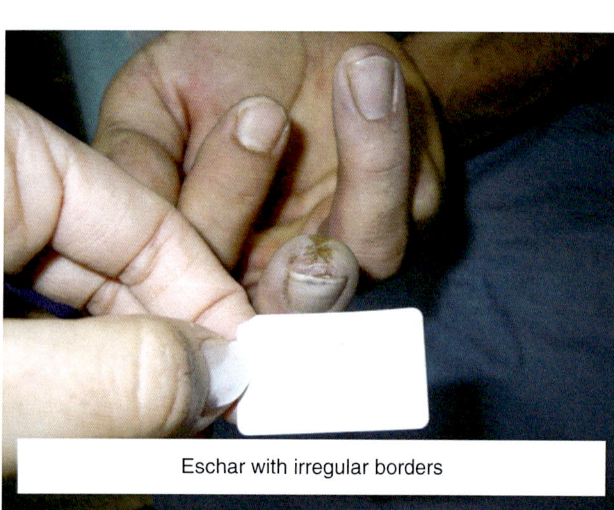

Eschar with irregular borders

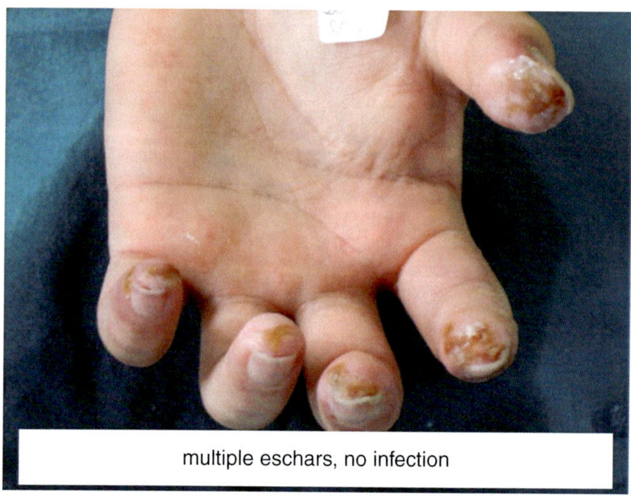

multiple eschars, no infection

Gangrene

Deep tissue necrosis due to obstruction or loss of blood supply; it may be localised to a small area or involve an entire finger, and may be wet or dry according to evolution, reflecting the degree of adjacent tissue perfusion, time course of necrosis and presence or type of associated secondary infection.

It usually evolves from a wet phase to a dry phase.

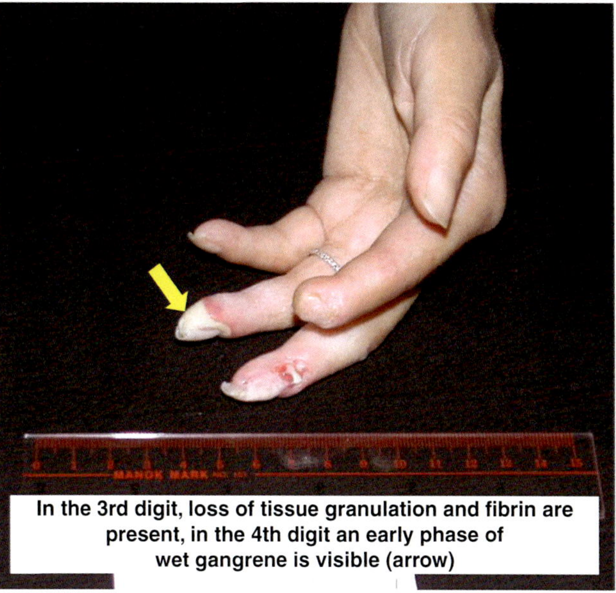

In the 3rd digit, loss of tissue granulation and fibrin are present, in the 4th digit an early phase of wet gangrene is visible (arrow)

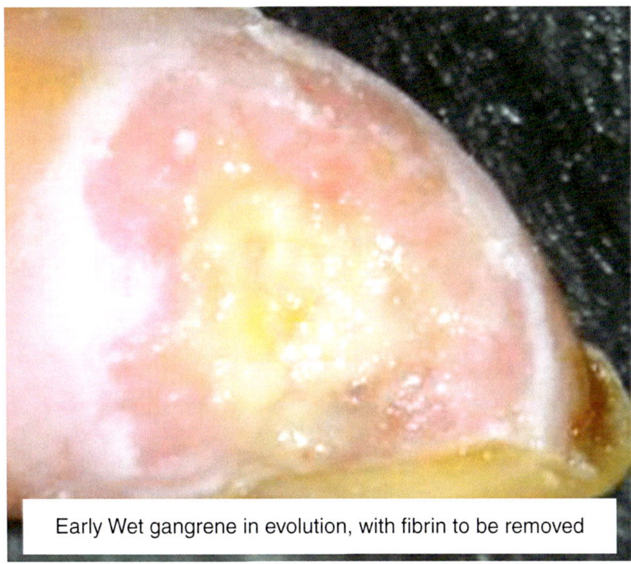

Early Wet gangrene in evolution, with fibrin to be removed

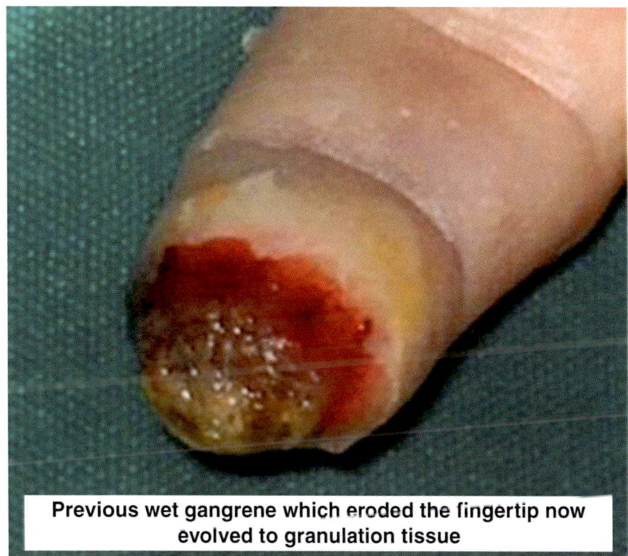

Previous wet gangrene which eroded the fingertip now evolved to granulation tissue

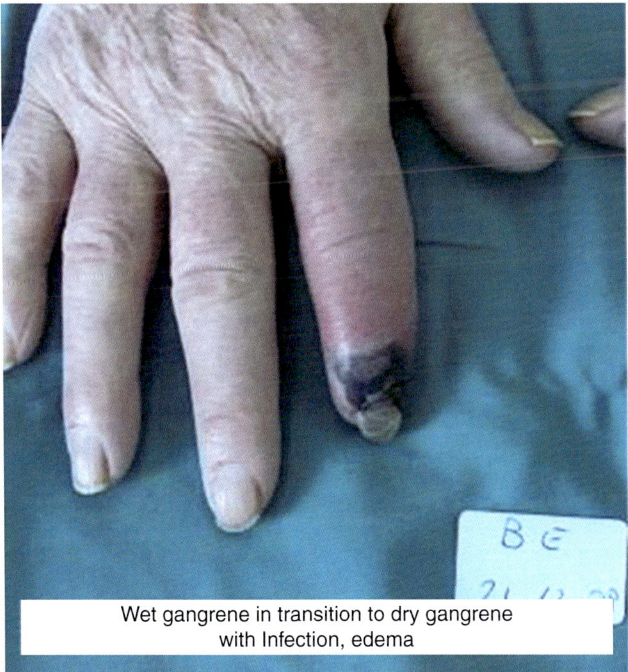

Wet gangrene in transition to dry gangrene with Infection, edema

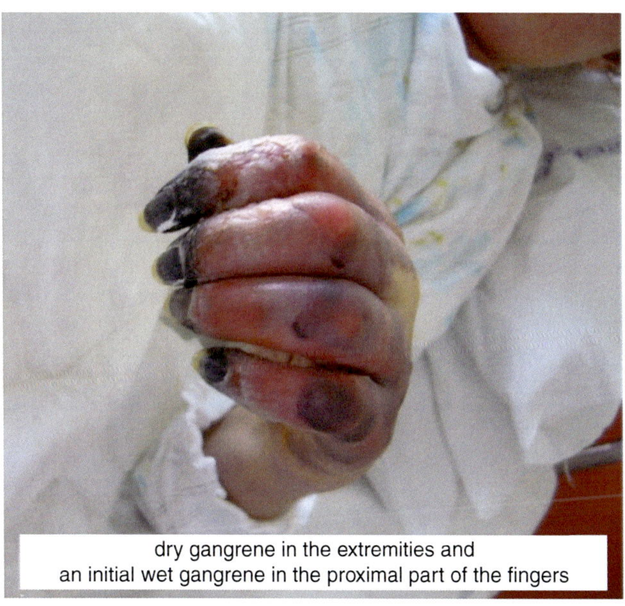

dry gangrene in the extremities and an initial wet gangrene in the proximal part of the fingers

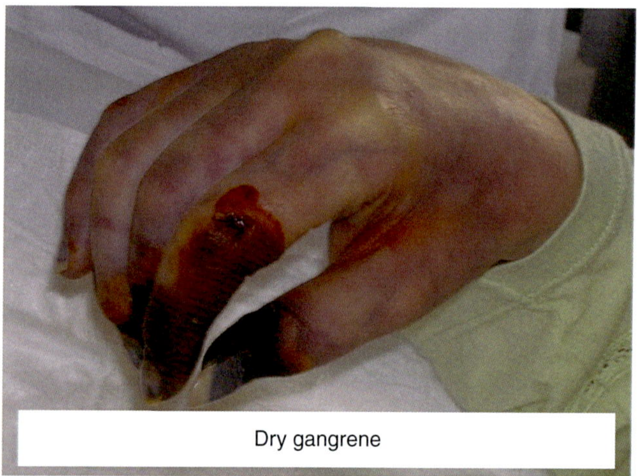

Dry gangrene

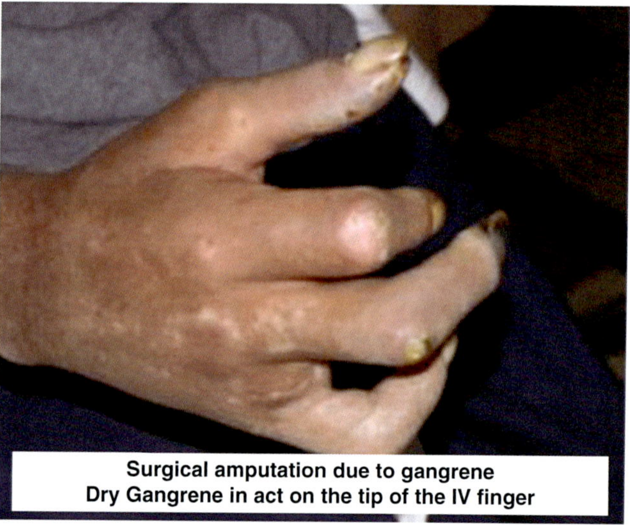

Surgical amputation due to gangrene
Dry Gangrene in act on the tip of the IV finger

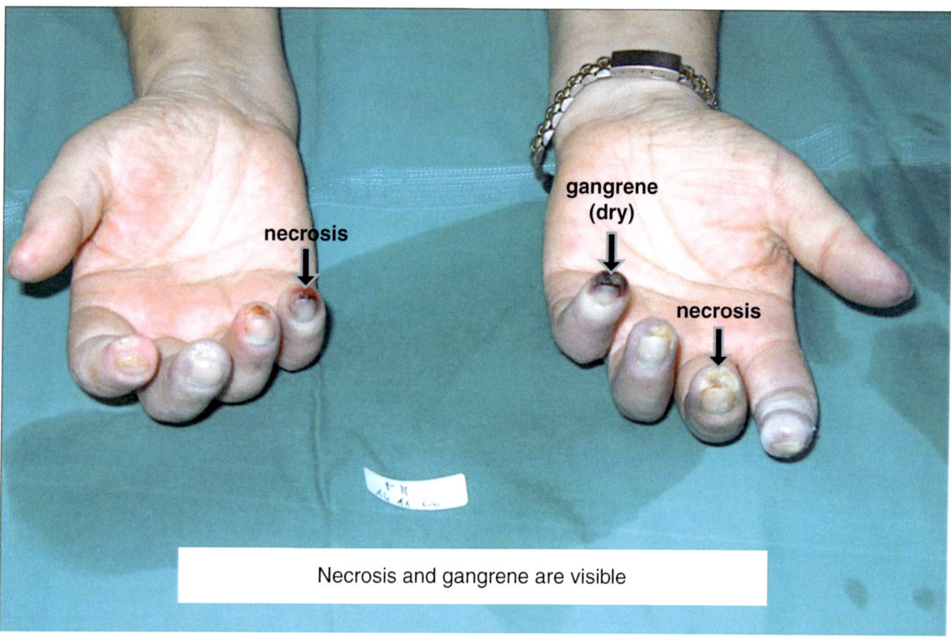

Necrosis and gangrene are visible

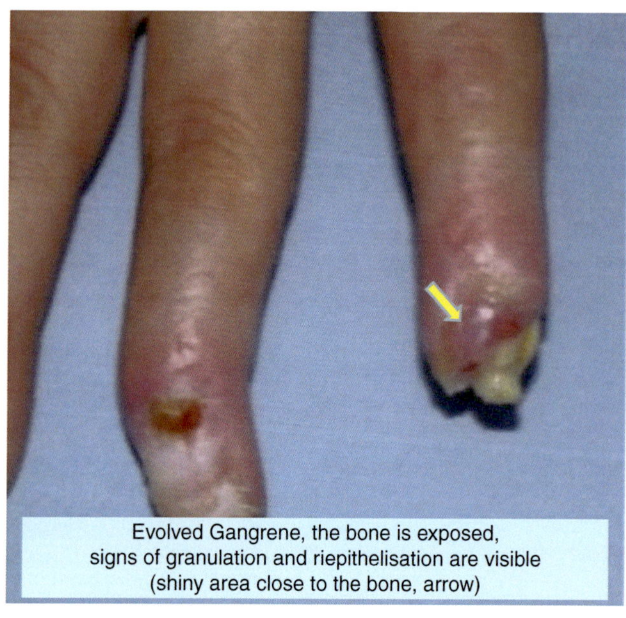

Evolved Gangrene, the bone is exposed,
signs of granulation and riepithelisation are visible
(shiny area close to the bone, arrow)

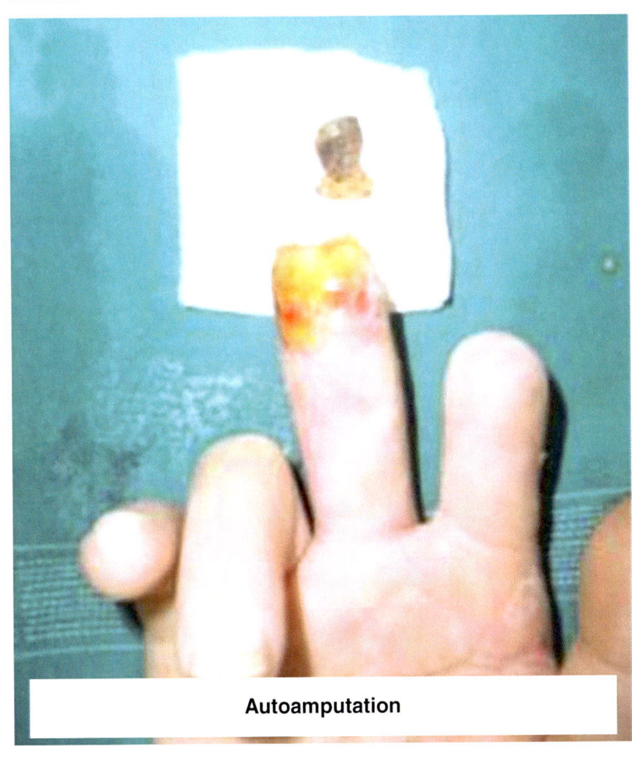

Autoamputation

Re-epithelialization

Formation of epithelium over a denuded surface.
This may cover partially or completely the ulcer.
It is always preceded by granulation which leads to progressive healing of the ulcer.

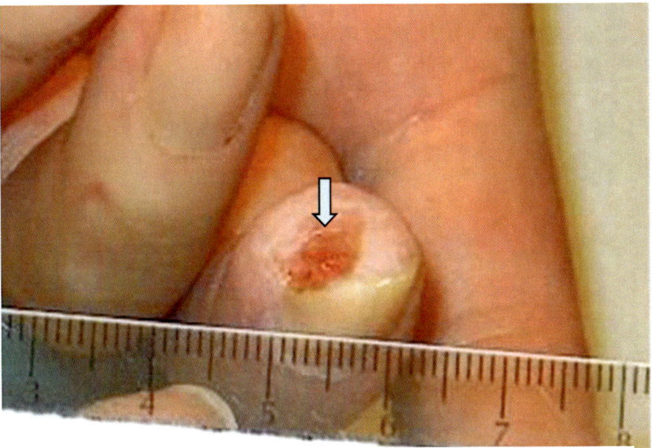

The red area on the ulcer border (arrow) fresh granulating tissue in the bottom of the ulcer.

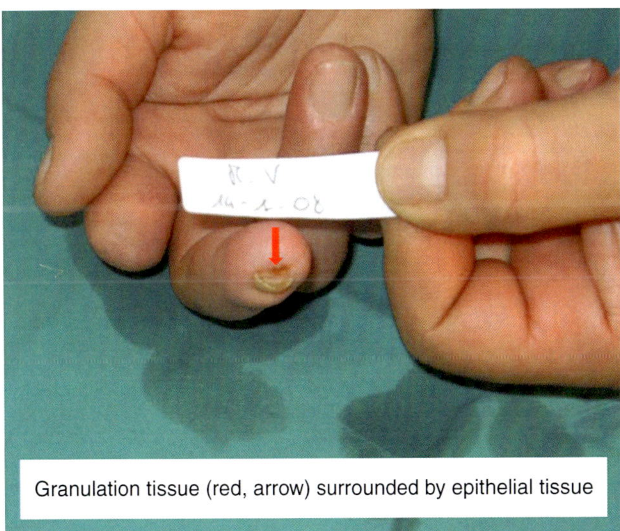

Granulation tissue (red, arrow) surrounded by epithelial tissue

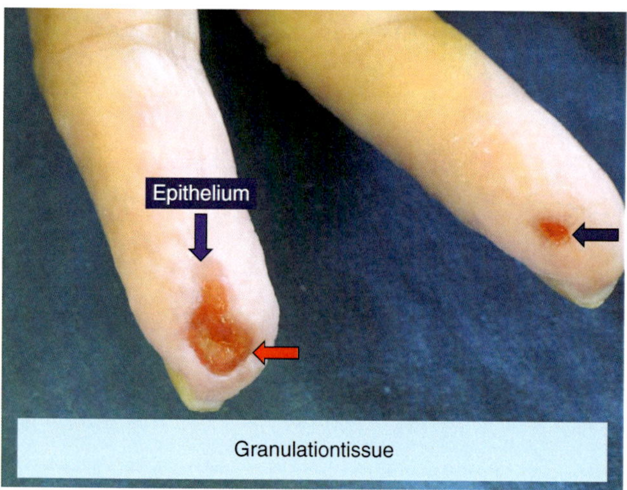

Granulationtissue

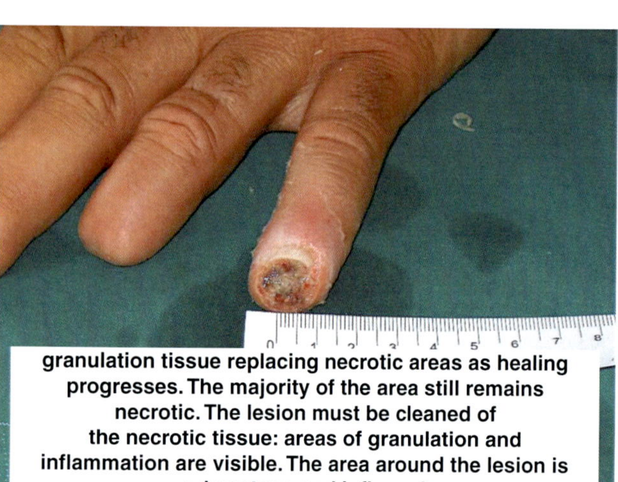

granulation tissue replacing necrotic areas as healing progresses. The majority of the area still remains necrotic. The lesion must be cleaned of the necrotic tissue: areas of granulation and inflammation are visible. The area around the lesion is edematous and inflamed

Fibrin

An elastic filamentous protein derived from fibrinogen by the action of thrombin.

It is a component of the inflammatory exudates and usually covers the bottom of the ulcer.

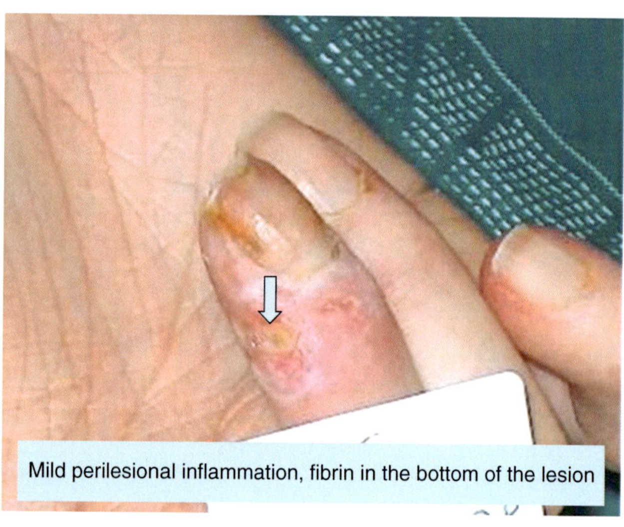

Mild perilesional inflammation, fibrin in the bottom of the lesion

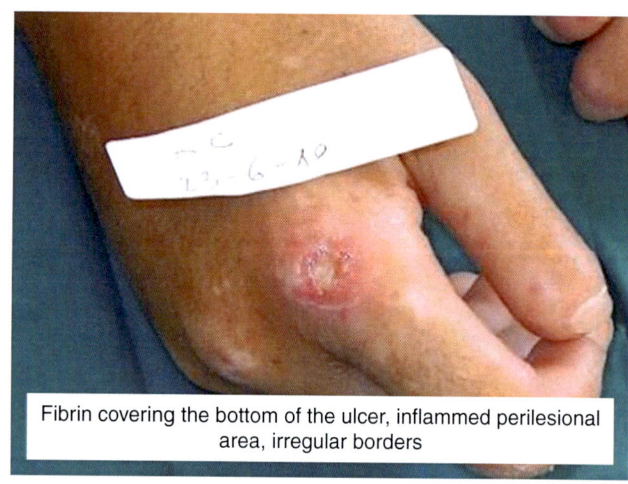

Fibrin covering the bottom of the ulcer, inflammed perilesional area, irregular borders

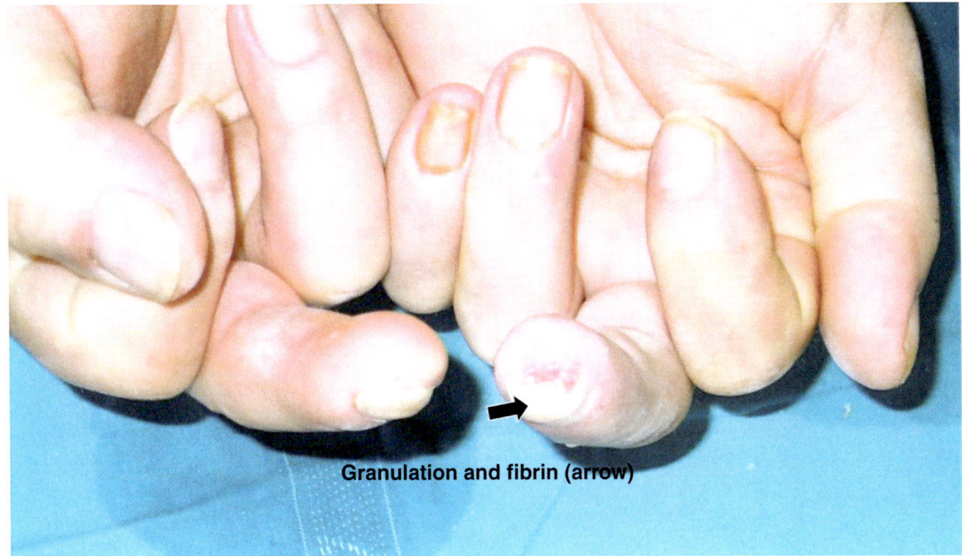

Granulation and fibrin (arrow)

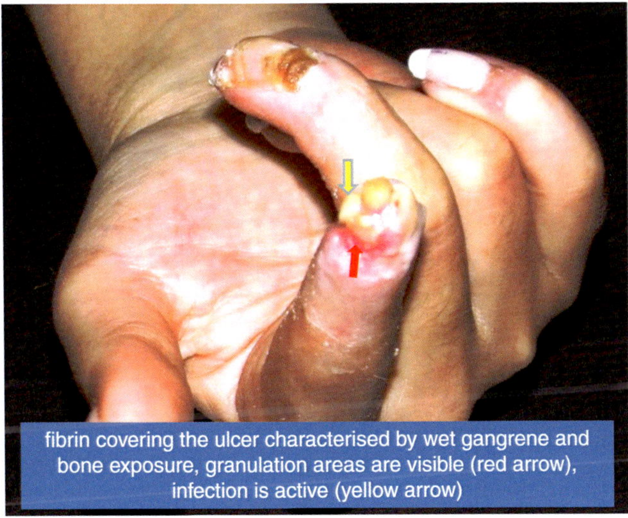

fibrin covering the ulcer characterised by wet gangrene and bone exposure, granulation areas are visible (red arrow), infection is active (yellow arrow)

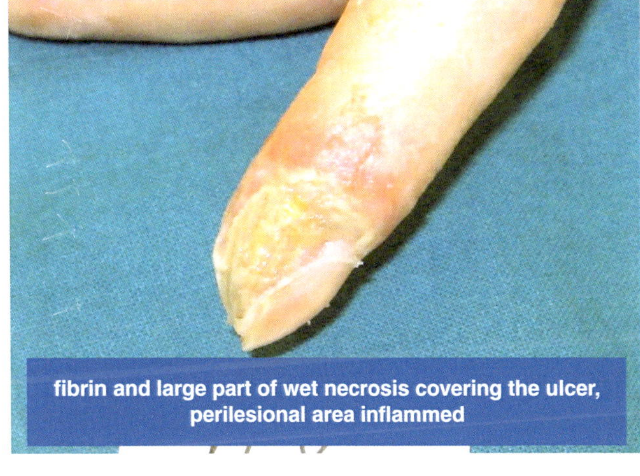

fibrin and large part of wet necrosis covering the ulcer, perilesional area inflammed

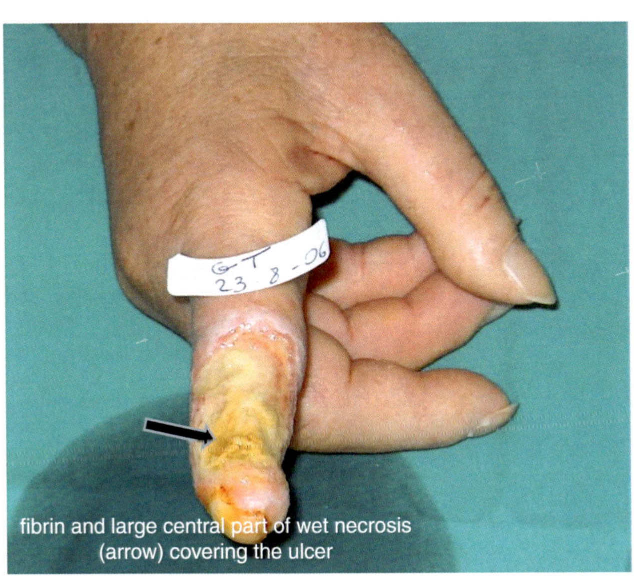

fibrin and large central part of wet necrosis (arrow) covering the ulcer

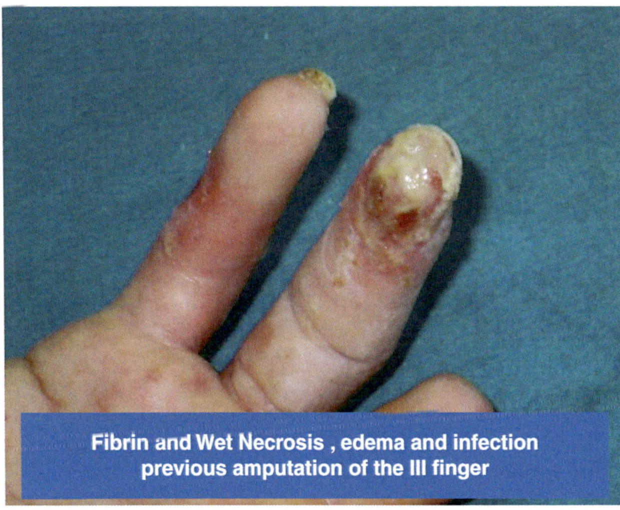

Fibrin and Wet Necrosis , edema and infection previous amputation of the III finger

Index

© Springer Nature Switzerland AG 2019
M. Matucci-Cerinic, C. P. Denton (eds.), *Atlas of Ulcers in Systemic Sclerosis*, https://doi.org/10.1007/978-3-319-98477-3